REVERSING

MULTIPLE

SCLEROSIS

REVERSING

MULTIPLE SCLEROSIS

9

EFFECTIVE STEPS
TO RECOVER YOUR HEALTH

CELESTE PEPE, D.C., N.D.
AND LISA HAMMOND

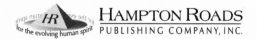

HAMPTON ROADS
PUBLISHING COMPANY, INC.

for the evolving human spirit

Cover design by Susan Shapiro
Cover art by Photo Researchers, Inc. and PhotoDisc
For information write:

Hampton Roads Publishing Company, Inc.
1125 Stoney Ridge Road
Charlottesville, VA 22902

Or call: 804-296-2772
Fax: 804-296-5096
e-mail: hrpc@hrpub.com
www.hrpub.com

If you are unable to order this book from your local
bookseller, you may order directly from the publisher.
Call 1-800-766-8009, toll-free.
Library of Congress Catalog Card Number: 00-111725
ISBN 1-57174-226-3
10 9 8 7 6 5 4 3 2
Printed on acid-free paper in the United States

Dedicated to my companion,

Jerry Kessler

Without his love,
support, and encouragement
this book would not have been possible.

With Love,
Celeste Pepe

Table of Contents

Section III: Controlling Your Destiny—Beating MS

Acknowledgments

By Celeste Pepe, D.C., N.D.

There comes a point in each person's life when a crossroads is reached, and a decision must be made that will change the course of life as they have known it until that moment. My moment came shortly after I was diagnosed with multiple sclerosis. I had a choice: to accept the prognosis of conventional medicine and resign myself to a steadily declining quality of life, or to fight, to refuse to accept what I had been given as fact and find a way to alter what was considered to be inevitable. I chose the latter, and began a five-year journey into the world of alternative healing, searching for what I knew had to be out there somewhere: a means to rid myself of this unwanted disease, a way to cure MS.

Through perseverance, diligence, and an almost obsessive refusal to quit and resign myself to my fate, I was ultimately successful. Some of the damage left by the disease remains: an occasional weakness in my leg and other minor traces. But even these continue to fade with the passage of time. I believe that they will one day vanish completely. I believe myself to be well, having achieved health through the scientific application of natural substances and cleansing therapies. During the course of my journey, several people were essential to my success and overall well-being. I would like to take this opportunity to thank them for all that they have done.

First and foremost, I would like to extend my love and appreciation to my beautiful daughter, Sara. From the first moment in Hawaii when my illness became apparent, to the long hours spent composing this book, Sara has always been there for me. In my darkest, most frustrating times of searching, her bright smile, warm hugs, and a wisdom and compassion far beyond her years have kept me going. Although others may have had their moments of doubt, Sara never wavered. Her faith in me was safe harbor in the midst of my medical storms. I love you, honey. You have always kept Mommy's heart singing.

Love and thanks also to my companion, Jerry Kessler, to whom this book is dedicated. Jerry has enhanced and completed my life. His warmth, intelligence, and inner strength gave me an emotional pillar to lean on. He has kept me grounded with his insightful opinions and solid common sense, made me laugh when no one else could have, listened to me vent, and comforted my fears. Though he sometimes questioned the options that I chose, he always believed in me. For all that he has done for me, and for all he continues to do, I thank him from the bottom of my heart. Without him, my healing and this book that I have written to help others, would not have been possible. I love you, Jerry. You are a gift to my life, and I thank God for you.

I'd also like to thank my mom, Ramona Pepe, for the love and support she has shown throughout my illness. Mom often brought me articles and information that she could find on MS and its treatments. It was she who first brought me the research on MS as a virus, a piece of knowledge that proved instrumental in my final victory, and many other clues that ultimately led to my success. There is a bond of love between us, as mother and daughter, which has given me strength and comfort always. Thanks, Mom. I'm so glad I have you in my life.

My sincerest appreciation also to my friends, Leanore Izen and Christa Peterson, for all of their assistance and support. Leanore helped me to use spiritual principles to view my MS as a challenge rather than a blow, as a mission rather than a sentence of doom. In the earliest days of my illness, she helped me find the courage to begin my search for healing. If she had not been there to counsel and encourage me, I might never have made the decision to try and find a cure. Christa is also a wonderful friend. I am so fortunate to have such an experienced nurse as a close personal friend. She was so vital to my successful experiences with bee venom treatment, assisting with the therapy while helping me deal with the emotional battles that are so often a presenting symptom of this disease. Thank you both, my good friends.

Thanks to Dr. Jonathan Wright and Dr. Mitch Cantor, good friends who are learned men in their respective fields. Jonathan introduced me to Dr. Bradford Weeks, who became instrumental in my final success. He also recommended the fatty acid testing that became one of the first steps toward restoring the imbalances in my body. An accomplished medical professional and noted alternative healer, Jonathan provided me with much insight and valuable suggestions during my search. Dr. Mitch Cantor's commitment to keep abreast with the latest developments in human dentistry was the reason I became familiar with the work and practices of Dr. Hal Huggins, and later, Dr. Steven O'Dell. He initially recommended the mercury filling removal and the DMPS chelation therapy that became vital protocols in removing the excess mercury and other heavy metal toxins in my body. Both of these men contributed significantly to my awareness and choice of therapies that led to my healing. I thank them both for their friendship, insight, advice, and knowledge. I will always be grateful to them.

I'd also like to thank my Zaca Lake family, Rose Farrington, and Melody Pierson Foster for their endless hours of transcription and compilation of the materials that would become the basis for this book. They worked hard without complaining and gave me invaluable assistance. Thank you, ladies. I appreciate all that you have done to help make this book possible.

Two of the people most instrumental to my success are clinical nutritionists, Robert Santoro and Albert Weyhreter, founders of BioCybernetics Inc. and developers of the BCI analysis system. Bob and Al taught me the BCI system long before I had MS. My familiarity with it led to my reasoning that if perfect elemental balance were achieved, then by definition, no illness or imbalance condition could exist in that system. They also provided me with the beef concentrates that ensured I received the proper amounts of essential amino acids while I was experiencing dietary restrictions, and the Sphyngolin Myelin Beef Protein so crucial to diverting the virus away from the myelin it was previously attacking and destroying in my system. I have always valued their friendship, and have benefited immensely from their knowledge and skills in the field of nutrition.

My endless appreciation is also extended to the learned medical men who treated me during my search to find a cure for my MS. Dr. Hal A. Huggins and Dr. Thomas E. Levy, for their work on my mercury fillings and their education on excess metals trapped in the body and their effects. I thank them also for their introducing me to DMPS chelation, so necessary to the removal of excesses in my system. My thanks to Dr. Steven O'Dell for taking up where they left off, completing my chelation and working with me through my fatty acid testing and ozone therapy. He gave me many valuable insights that would prove excellent clues to my proper course of action. I was fortunate to have the expertise of so learned a trio at my disposal.

Much gratitude to Dr. William Crawford and Dr. David Watts for their treatment of my MS as a virus, one of the final keys to unlocking the hold the disease had on my system, for their work with EBV, and their research into its relation to multiple sclerosis. They have contributed so much to my healing process. Dr. Crawford's experience with the Nieper protocols and calcium orotates helped to bring the virus under submission, to begin to push it from my body, and to restore the elemental imbalances in my system. Dr. Watts's superior analytical skills and his extensive knowledge of nutrient therapies were key to restoring my body harmony and optimum function. Their continued work with me has been instrumental in the restoration of my overall balance and health.

Special thanks are due to Dr. Bradford S. Weeks, for his work with vitamin and nutritional therapies, and his vast knowledge of apitherapy and bee venom treatment. His recommendation of BVT therapy led to the restoration of mobility and feeling in my leg, numb for nearly four years at that time. He also prescribed my vitamin and hormonal replacement therapies that halted the progress of the disease and were also instrumental in restoring my body's nutrient balance. Thanks also to him for taking the time to read this book while still a manuscript, and for his comments and compliments. I am privileged to have him for a doctor and a friend.

Recognition and appreciation are also due to Dr. Matthew Van Benshoten and Dr. Joseph McSweyne, accomplished acupuncturists and masters of the ancient arts of Chinese herbal medicine. Their treatments kept my body mobile and my system clean of impurities, and they introduced me to the Zero Dairy, Zero Sugar protocol that was to become such a large part of my nutritional plan during much of my healing process. Their combination of the old and new ways of medicine has greatly benefited me and others who suffer from a broad base of autoimmune dysfunctions.

Dr. Wayne Miller and his father, Dr. Robert Miller, continue to help me strengthen my body and return it to its former flexibility through the latest in chiropractic medicine. Working with non-force treatments and an exacting awareness of the relationship between the skeletal and neurological system, they have been responsible for the mobility I enjoy today and for the restoration of my athletic abilities. I continue to work with them regularly, and hold an intense amount of respect for their combined skills in a field I know very well. I am grateful for their medical advice and professional camaraderie.

I must express my appreciation to Dr. Theodore Cherbuilez for all the help he has given me in the completion of this project. His gracious interview, input, and suggestions on BVT were invaluable and crucial to the completion of that portion of the book. Thanks also to all of the learned doctors and scientists who contributed so significantly to my final nutritional plan that I follow to this day. Dr. Roy L. Swank, Dr. Barry Sears, and Dr. Peter J. D'Adamo are a credit to their respective fields and some of the most brilliant minds in medical science. Their knowledge of nutrition, elemental food substances, and blood and cellular composition were the final keys to my success. Applying the principles of these internationally recognized experts was the final step in my journey. I appreciate their years of research and thank them sincerely for choosing to share their knowledge with the world through their books.

The final two people that I would like to recognize provided crucial assistance to my ultimate victory and the writing of this book. First, my very warmest thanks to Mrs. Pat Wagner. Pat made it possible for me to find the courage to try BVT and to continue the therapy until my leg was restored to full feeling. She taught me the practice of BVT, answered my many questions, and provided comfort and emotional support. I thank her also for her generous contributions to this book. Despite the demands on her as a BVT practitioner, lecturer, and grandmother, Pat made the extra time to complete her informative interview and aid in the compilation of the chapter on BVT and apitherapy. Thank you, Pat, for your help and your friendship.

Last, but certainly not least, I would like to extend my very special thanks to my writer, Lisa Hammond. I have felt throughout this chapter in my life that I have been divinely led through many circumstances and decisions. Seemingly out of the blue, as these things usually are, I found my way to Lisa. I don't think that I could have made a better choice in a writer. From the first day that I spoke with her, as she listened so intently to my story and the vision I had for this project, she has been an irreplaceable asset. Her exceptional writing skills and expert research abilities enabled me to present my personal story and the scientific data in this book in a way that the reader can understand and enjoy. Throughout the long hours we spent together, I have valued her keen intelligence, cynical New York humor, and innate ability to see clearly what I wanted to present and make it happen. I would welcome the opportunity to work with her again in the future and am glad to have been her client. Thanks, Lisa. You have made this book a victory to be proud of.

Celeste Pepe, D.C., N.D.
Solvang, California

Acknowledgments

By Lisa Hammond

The first contact I had with Dr. Celeste Pepe was via the telephone on a cold and crisp morning in March of 1999. Despite the mountain of work upon my desk, I was to spend the next three hours listening to this pleasant and cheerful Californian voice tell me a most amazing story. I must admit, my first reaction to this complete stranger who announced that she had found a cure for MS was a silent, *Yeah, right!* My second reaction was far more visceral, as I continued to listen, waiting with typical New York skepticism for the flaw, the catch, the payoff pitch. There was none. No one could doubt the sincerity in that voice. I agreed to take a look at the project.

An extraordinary aspect of operating in the capacity of ghostwriter is the diversity of projects to which one is exposed. I may compose a political speech this month and edit a murder mystery the next. The caveat to the job is that one must choose carefully, as only one project at a time can be written. I have a writer's penchant for immersing myself in the work at hand, much as an actor in a film or play. During the time of the undertaking, I become a temporary expert on the subject at hand, especially on a project such as this one.

After my initial review of Dr. Pepe's materials, I decided to accept the assignment: to write the personal story of one woman's courageous journey from incurable illness to optimum health, against all odds and the prognostications of futility and doom from the medical community. I began to see the importance of the message behind the story: that multiple sclerosis, a disease that cripples over 300,000 Americans, and countless others worldwide, can indeed be *cured*. That in itself is incredible.

Far more sobering was the thought of the benefit that could be derived by others afflicted in a similar way. Not only would they have the possibility of success, they would be able to accomplish their own victories in far less time than the five-year period of Celeste's own healing, because they would have readily at hand the treatments that she spent the time and energy to search for and embrace. The impact of the book would be twofold. It was to be Dr. Pepe's uplifting and inspirational story of victory, certainly. However, ever the consummate teacher, Celeste decided to add additional chapters that would effectively serve as instructional materials for the reader. It was her desire to share her story with others afflicted with MS, and to educate as well, to show the readers in clearly understandable steps how they could accomplish the same triumph for themselves.

This was my challenge: to develop Dr. Pepe's notes and audio lectures into a cohesive work that would potentially benefit thousands of persons afflicted with this debilitating disease. From it stems my short, but important, list of those to whom I am most grateful.

First and foremost, I would like to thank those whom I love most: my family. My teenagers: son, Thomas, and daughter, Casey, who carried on bravely while their mother remained sequestered with mountains of research, crumpled wastebaskets of paper, and the ever-present tape recorder, frequently unable to tear myself away from the project. Casey plans to become a chef. At fourteen and a half, she is, admittedly, a far more proficient cook than I shall ever be. Little girl, you do make the best coffee on Earth, so help me. Thomas, considering a career in law enforcement or the military, maintained order in our home with an efficiency that belied his nearly seventeen years while still finding the time to pursue hockey, honing his already considerable skills in that difficult and physically demanding sport. He also unfailingly cared for my considerably overweight and aging Norwegian Forest cat.

Tom, Indy is undoubtedly alive and fat today because of you. Thank you, with all of my heart. I am so proud of you both. You are, and will always remain, my very best works.

My eternal gratitude to accomplished musician and writer Jim Siegrist, my companion and confidant for so many years. He was always there to listen, encourage, and support me, and temper my bouts of self-pity while I was trying to understand unbelievably difficult medical terminology, at times overwhelmed by the task of explaining the concepts in lay terms the average reader could understand. Possessing a brilliantly creative mind in his own right, Jim well understands those periods all writers endure, when one stares at the ceiling and cannot compose a grocery list, juxtaposed by others where the gift flows and the sound of the keyboard echoes until the rosy fingers of dawn appear on the horizon. Thank you, 'P.' I love you dearly and will always be your number one fan.

I'd like to thank my staff at URI, my own firm, particularly Bob Kirkswieller and Lily Fanning, who untiringly manned the office, took my messages, and reminded me constantly when I was supposed to be elsewhere.

Special thanks to Claire Newcomb, Ed and Cindy Triggs, Lloyd Crain, Crystal Joyce, and John Muuss for their unfailing moral support. Thank you, my friends. You have been my buffer between sanity and the world of the budding psychotic.

My sincere gratitude to Dr. Theodore Cherbuilez and Mrs. Pat Wagner for their efforts generously donated to this project, for their forthright and detailed interviews so essential to the chapter on bee venom treatment (BVT). I shall always appreciate the charm and Old World courtesy of Dr. Cherbuilez throughout our several conversations, and the time expended by this learned and internationally respected member of the medical community in answering my questions and assisting with my overall presentation of this important chapter. Mrs. Wagner's warmth and cheerful demeanor were a most welcome experience as she constantly made herself available to me despite the demands on her time as a grandmother and full-time practitioner of BVT.

My appreciation and thanks are also extended to Robert Santoro, C.N., head of BioCybernetics, Inc., for his patient and detailed explanation of the BCI analyses and their significance to the healthy person and the MS patient. His input and guidance were essential to my successful explanation of the BCI procedures in clearly understandable terms.

I would also like to sincerely acknowledge the assistance of the following: Michelle Ferris of Ferris Apiaries for her expertise in beekeeping and the wonderfully useful materials she graciously provided; The Linus Pauling Institute and Oregon State University for access to their materials on the life and works of the late Dr. Linus Pauling; The A. Keith Brewer Science Library and the German MS Society for access to their materials on the life and works of the recently departed Dr. Hans A. Nieper; MedLine; BioMedNet; the University of California and the USDA for access to the medical information, studies, reports, and articles so essential to establishing the credibility and scientific feasibility of Dr. Pepe's treatment choices.

Thanks also to the many scientists, researchers, and medical professionals who have devoted their lives to the eradication of disease and the betterment of the human condition. Their constant exploration of the uncharted regions of science and medicine has allowed Dr. Pepe and others to achieve that which was once thought to be impossible.

And finally, I'd like to thank Dr. Celeste Pepe for allowing me the opportunity to work with her on this project. She has truly been a delight, witty and irrepressibly cheerful. I found her to be a beautiful, classy, and absolutely sincere individual. We are quite opposite in style and personality, but I think that the balance of her California sunshine and my New York night have combined to create a book that the reader will learn from and enjoy. Thanks, Celeste. I am proud to have been a part of it all.

Lisa Hammond
Southampton, New York

Prologue:
What Constitutes
"Controversial"?

What constitutes "controversial"? Is it that radio personality poking irreverent fun at society's luminaries? Is it the rock star whose choreographed sadomasochism gyrates across the stage to platinum dance tunes? Is it that new wonder drug that miraculously reduces our larger friends to knife-hipped fashion statements? Is it an automobile that runs on solar power, gay parents, neo-Nazis, abortion?

The answer, quite obviously, is *yes*. All of these can be described as controversial. The list of persons, activities, and topics that create controversy is as endless, and as diverse, as human nature itself. That is as it should be. For, defined at its lowest common denominator, controversy is *change*.

Change. A departure from the mainstream, the accepted, the familiar. A new thought, action, or creation that redefines an existing condition. Change is as ancient as Socrates, as current as Scientology. Change is seldom initially popular, and not all changes are good, decent, or beneficial. And, throughout the vast expanse of human history, change has brought with it controversy.

Controversy is a healthy extension of the process of change, the interaction of human minds, cultures, and morals.

History teaches that often the greatest changes in the human condition were brought about only with immense controversy, often violent and deadly: the Crusades, the French Revolution, the Second World War.

Not always violent, controversy has also paved the way for some of the most beneficial changes mankind has effected in the most fundamental areas of culture and society. Socrates taught in the peristyles of the Greek aristocracy, Columbus sailed at high tide, Edison worked late in an attic. And, one morning, on a beach outside of a little town called Kitty Hawk . . . All of these events created great controversy, but each resulted ultimately in the positive progression of human existence.

Perhaps the most current controversy has been created in the field of medicine, the treatment of the human biological condition. Explore the history of medicine and you will find nothing but controversy in every instance where great change was effected. When Florence Nightingale walked into a battle tent and knelt beside a wounded soldier, society was horrified. Today, the nurse is one of the most vital components of successful medical practice, indispensable to both the doctor and the patient. Colleagues laughed at Alexander Fleming and his moldy bits of bread. Now, millions of people owe their lives to the wonder of penicillin.

The list of pioneers who dared to brave the voices of controversy and pursue their ideas is long and proud. Against sometimes seemingly impossible odds and opposition, these courageous individuals persevered, and the quality of human life was improved tremendously.

Medicine today is a particularly volatile field. Debates rage over a variety of treatments, procedures, and medications, from birth control options to the use of experimental drugs in the war upon chronic illness. Utilizing the lightning advances of modern technology, medicine has adapted in the pursuit of its ultimate goal, the eradication of ailment and disease.

Modern medicine faces several challenges in the search for cures to the most serious of illnesses prevalent in society today. Although the killers of the previous two centuries, such as polio and measles, have been rendered ineffective and all but eliminated or neutralized, the world today is faced with a fresh set of horrors. This list is long as well, but far more deadly: AIDS, cancer, multiple sclerosis, muscular dystrophy, ebola, herpes, Parkinson's.

Millions of global citizens suffer and die from a host of diseases presently labeled "incurable." Billions of dollars have been spent in the search for the keys that will unlock the secrets to the causes of serious afflictions. Although advances in the treatment, or more accurately, management, of these afflictions are made, no "cures" are found.

Why? Perhaps that is the most controversial question of all. Why aren't these diseases already eliminated? With all of the funding, and all of the state-of-the-art facilities, hasn't anyone been able to find even *one* cure?

Perhaps the cynically sinister explanation could be that modern affliction is big business, a tremendous source of revenue for a myriad of corporations across a broad expanse of industries. Keeping people alive, allowing them to cling to their existence, even in the most limited form, is an extremely lucrative enterprise. The pharmaceutical industry is a powerful government lobby, as are the medical equipment manufacturers, the health care insurance industry, and the elder care field. A "cure" for a major disease would eliminate the need for the drugs that "manage" it, the specialists who "treat" it, the equipment necessary to "live" with it, and the billions paid to insurance plans that "cover" it. Perhaps the influence of those interests has shifted the emphasis to "management" under the misnomer of "treatment," and away from elimination, or cure.

Until as recently as the twentieth century, the field of medicine has not been financially lucrative. Driven not by currency but by compassion, the pioneers of medicine labored under sometimes appallingly impoverished conditions to complete their experiments, their research. With very little fanfare and even less monetary gain, tremendous achievements were realized. Today, the inverse seems to hold true. Billions are spent, but few breakthroughs are seen. Is big business the obstacle to progress? Or, is the true obstacle simply viewpoint?

Perhaps the reason that this trend prevails is not so cynical a one after all. The mainstream of researchers may indeed be oblivious to the influence of these factors. These medical detectives are truly committed to the elimination of modern-day illness. *They may simply be looking in the wrong places for clues.*

Around the globe, brilliant minds are beginning to seek elsewhere for the answers, probing other courses of action, looking simultaneously forward and backward in history. There is a growing movement toward the past, a return to, literally, our roots. And to plants, vitamins, proteins, and minerals, the most basic building blocks of the human body.

This book serves a dual purpose: It will present the story of one woman's courageous battle and ultimate victory over one of the most dreaded afflictions in society today. It is also an instruction manual, a step-by-step procedural, a prescription for victory.

Are the diseases we face today truly "modern"? Or, are these diseases out of control because of modern medicine? Does the answer to the elimination of these killers lie in our future, in some as yet undiscovered wonder drug that, like penicillin, will cure these ailments? Or, does it lie in our past in arcane natural remedies older than recorded humankind?

This growing school of thought and practices is painted with a broad and often scathing brush labeled "alternative medicine." The term implies questionable credibility, an image of flaming torches and old women, of carnival barkers on the back of wagons, of communes full of barefoot people who grow their own wheat germ and keep chickens in pyramid-shaped coops. Although over 48 percent of Americans have tried some form of these healing methods, alternative medicine, in the eyes of the mainstream medical community, is often understood to mean *caveat emptor.*

It is an image as absolutely incorrect as it is undeserved. Today's pioneers of alternative medicine are Nobel Prize winners, eminent scientists, physicists, physicians, and nutritionists. More than just advocates for a "return to nature," these individuals have begun to back their claims with something that the mainstream medical community has had in short supply: results.

The fact of the matter is that alternative medicine *works.* People are being cured of diseases presently considered incurable. Persons once too debilitated to exist without constant medical care are returning to normal, active lives, often healthier than they were prior to the onset of their illnesses. Could it be that these modern-day practitioners are performing feats of herbal magic, creating the illusion of health? Not likely.

Quite the reverse. These respected professionals are blowing the dust from the volumes of history, reaching into our natural past. They have not discovered a new miracle drug or therapy. They have instead changed their viewpoint. When faced with scaling the sheer face of the mountain that is modern medicine's route to a cure, they have simply chosen to walk around to the other side of the mountain, and choose a path that, although overgrown and ancient, is still the surest route to the pinnacle: a cure for the condition they are fighting.

As expected, their methods are a source of controversy. Whether from financial interest or accepted school of general thought, the bulk of the medical community is either uneducated or dismissive of many of these methods of treatment and eradication of disease. Some may react with indifference, some with resentment or even hostility. Why? Because alternative medicine is change, the catalyst of controversy.

This book serves a dual purpose: It will present the story of one woman's courageous battle and ultimate victory over one of the most dreaded afflictions in society today. It is also an instruction manual, a step-by-step procedural, a prescription for victory. It is controversial on two fronts.

First, this book will give you a glimpse into my personal life over a five-year period: from the time I was first diagnosed with MS to my present-day state of health. It will also take you through significant incidents that occurred earlier in my life, prior to the onset of the illness, as I strive to discover the root cause of the disease. On the face of it, this doesn't appear to be all that controversial. After all, I have never been an international spy or a member of a royal family in exile. I am a doctor, in two fields. And therein lies what some may consider controversy.

In an effort to help those suffering now as I was then, I let the reader get to know Celeste Pepe, the person. Many of my medical colleagues will disapprove of this approach, arguing that allowing the reader access to my thoughts, fears, and emotional conflicts compromises my credibility. They believe that in order to achieve the proper relationship with patients, a certain distance must be maintained. I disagree. Although I pride myself on my professionalism, I felt that it would be far more helpful for the MS patient reading this book to know that, even though I am a medical professional, I experienced many of the same fears, doubts, and frustrations that they are feeling. Many times, I felt unsure, confused, or alone. I battled with the mood swings and emotionalism that is often so much a part of MS and any serious illness. I struggled with willpower when giving up some of the things I enjoyed during various therapies.

I have told my personal story here as if speaking to a good friend, holding nothing back. I want those who have MS to know that I did not attain my healing through some special strength or superior ability to handle a crisis because I am a doctor. I achieved this victory because I was willing to make a commitment, to fight for what I wanted, and to never, ever give up. I want them to know that they can realize their own success and improved health by following the steps that I have taken, and that they, too, need to persevere. By revealing the highs and lows, the triumphs and setbacks, the joys and despair that I have experienced, other MS patients will know that they are not alone. Maybe, knowing that someone else has gone through what they are dealing with and has emerged victorious on the other side could give them the courage to pursue these healing protocols for themselves. If I can convince just one MS patient to try these healing techniques, then the efforts and expense incurred in the writing of this book will have been well worth it.

In the second section of this book, I will show you, through actual analyses, test results, and verbatim interviews with eminent physicians and others successfully treated with these alternative healing methods, that MS can be reversed, and cured. It is my desire to open a door of hope to millions of MS patients and those with other life-threatening diseases who search desperately for a cure in a world that presently offers them *no other option* than resigned acceptance of their fate. Using the chapters in the second section will allow MS patients to duplicate the steps that I have taken and achieve their own optimum results using the alternative healing methods that I have learned.

My purpose is not to fly in the face of mainstream medicine, or to point a finger of accusation at the medical industry, government, or practicing physicians. Regardless, undoubtedly some of those entities will indeed take exception to the contents and term them controversial. Even some of the members of my own field of naturopathic medicine may take exception to some of the substances that I review and recommend, or the choices that I made in certain situations. I never began this search considering what other members of the medical community or people in general may think of my decisions.

No, after my own diagnosis, I refused to accept the pronouncements of conventional medicine that insisted that my return to health was an impossible hill to climb. I simply walked around to the other side of the mountain. I sought for, and found, the answer on another road. My five-year journey began as I set out to find the cure on an alternative path. A journey the MS patient today can also choose to undertake. A journey to wellness, to victory. A journey to a cure.

Section I:
My Personal Road to Recovery over MS

If you are ever diagnosed with a life-threatening disease, you must pursue, with all of your might, every doctor, of all varieties, with every healing modality known to them, and never give up, until you find the ones that heal you.

–Celeste Pepe

1

Why Me, Lord? A Life Turned Upside Down

It wasn't raining, but it should have been. The gray California sky hung leaden, threatening, the tired clouds heavy with their unreleased burden. I should have taken it as an omen, but of course I didn't.

The day had begun innocently enough on our beautiful, sprawling ranch in California's canyon country. Recently back from a trip to Hawaii, I had started the morning in my usual way, with meditation and exercise. I felt good, actually better than I had in days. Much better than I had in Hawaii, where I had suffered the mysterious and frightening episode that sent me to several doctors for a battery of tests upon my return.

The trip to Hawaii was supposed to be special. More than just a much needed vacation from the busy schedule I kept as a practicing chiropractor, this was to be an adventure with the person dearest in the world to me, my ten-year-old daughter, Sara. Her father and I had divorced some time before, and she made her home with him in New York City. Being on opposite coasts did not allow us to spend a lot of time together. We had planned to spend every day doing something new and exciting.

One of the events we had planned was a day-long hike up the mountains of Kauai. Sara had never been hiking before and was excited by the prospect of this new adventure. We had begun on a beautiful crystal clear morning, the kind that Hawaii seems to have the exclusive patent on. The mountain was not overly challenging, but the climb was long and somewhat strenuous, especially as we began to reach the higher altitudes along the face. Victory lay at the top, of course, and all of the exertion was worth it as I shared the wonder in my daughter's face as she stood surveying the wonder of God's Earth that is that stunning ring of volcanic islands.

It was during our descent that the nightmare began. My legs began to feel numb, the muscles sluggish, unwilling to respond with their normal strength and agility. I put it down to exhaustion and pushed on, believing that some well-earned time in a hot bath and a good night's sleep would soon cure what ailed me. It soon became apparent that my problem was far worse.

Something was terribly wrong. My legs grew heavier, the muscles wooden, almost rigid. Silently, I began to be afraid. We were far from any portion of the resort where help could be easily obtained. The hiking trail, though well marked, had no handrail or walkway to assist the hiker, the assumption being made, naturally, that anyone who came this far would, by definition, be physically fit enough to make the return journey unassisted. Worse by far than my physical difficulty was watching the growing look of concern in my daughter's taut face, the increasing note of panic in her voice as she asked me what was wrong. Although I kept reassuring her that I was just "getting old and tired," it was painfully apparent even to her young eyes that I was, to put it politely, lying through my clenched teeth.

Halfway down a mountain that I swore had doubled in height since our ascent, it happened. My legs refused to work at all. I fell to the ground, Sara's frightened scream echoing in my ringing ears. I could see that I had scraped some skin off of my knees and calves, but I couldn't feel it! I was effectively paralyzed. With Sara in tears and with an effort born of sheer desperation I made it down the rest of the way on my backside, propelling myself with my hands, tearing the skin off my palms and breaking my nails to the quick as I fought to control this sudden dead weight that was the lower half of myself.

By the time I made it down the mountainside, a great deal of the feeling had returned to my lower limbs, and I put it down to possible lumbar strain, brought on by overexertion and lack of oxygen to my muscles from the demands of the climb. Sara was overjoyed, and, although I had my doubts, I said nothing, relieved that her confidence and sense of security had been restored by my pronouncement of plain old back strain.

I wasn't so sure, however, and resolved to be examined in California as soon as I returned there. Unbeknownst to Sara, this wasn't the first time that my muscular lack of response had concerned me. I had been having some difficulty with the step aerobic portion of my routine for a couple of months. I kept falling off the step equipment near the end of my workout. My ankles seemed to invert, to turn on their sides as if I were ice skating for the first time. I had thought it was simply encroaching age. After all, I was 42, and my standard 45-minute step routine was strenuous.

At the local hospital facility in Santa Barbara, I was examined by Dr. Willis, the neurologist in residence. She suspected lumbar, or spinal, problems and took several tests, including an MRI of my lower spinal area to determine the problem. I underwent all of the tests she recommended, determined to get to the root cause of this creeping malaise. Dr. Willis's demeanor was clinically detached, virtually emotionless as I explained my concerns. I don't know if it was her personality, or the fact that I was a chiropractor that engendered this cold response.

Unjust as it most certainly is, a large portion of the medical community views chiropractic professionals as pseudo-scientists, a group of fringe shamans, either consummate grifters playing at being "real doctors," or medical school failures who couldn't make it "all the way." The truth is that chiropractic, in the hands of a dedicated professional, is as legitimate and exacting a medical science as heart surgery, or any other specialty field.

I underwent the procedures and returned home to the ranch to await the results. And so, the scene was set, the players perfectly positioned the morning destiny grabbed my life in an irrevocable grip, changing my world forever.

I was standing in our southwestern-style kitchen on this particular morning, the flagstone floor cool under my feet, the clouds obscuring the normally caressing sun, absently staring out of the sliding glass doors toward the corrals, watching the horses enjoy the freedom from a night in the stall.

Even on this overcast and gloomy day, the ranch was still breathtaking. I never failed to see the wild beauty of the landscape or realize the pure insignificance of man beside it. All of our lives in all of their moments mean less than nothing to mountains as old as time. They were here before us, and would stand, mute guardians of the oldest secrets, long after the memory of humankind was a whisper in the lone trees far above the timberline. And so, lost in thought, I didn't hear our cook, Kurt, join me at first. He called my name, and something in his tone made me turn and stare hard at him.

"This came for you this morning. I was across in the office at the time, and they asked me to bring it over here for you." He held out a sheet of paper toward me, his face too carefully expressionless, his body too still.

I took it from him, automatically scanning the header. It was a fax from Dr. Willis's office at the clinic in Santa Barbara regarding the results of the tests that had been performed. My heart beating faster, I read the message, the cold, impersonal tone biting with an antiseptic sting.

FINDINGS: Multiple focal and confluent areas of increased signal on long TR and inversion recovery sequences are seen in the deep and periventricular white matter, predominately around the lateral ventricles but also around the fourth ventricle. The lesions are very extensive and patterned. . . .
Frontal, parietal and temporal lobe involvement is shown.

CONCLUSION: Findings strongly suggestive of multiple sclerosis.

I stood frozen as waves of immeasurable fear swept around me while each word burned before my eyes, piercing my heart like grotesque and deadly darts. As a doctor, those chilling words held more terror for me than perhaps for another with less knowledge of the human condition as a whole. I reeled from the pronouncement that gripped me with icy hands, a verdict of misery and doom that I could not accept.

Multiple sclerosis. Dear God. Time really does freeze during your most horrible moments as the chasm of fear yawns before you. I remember gripping the edge of the counter for support as the room shifted and somehow became unstable. Dimly, I could hear Kurt's voice, as from a distance, telling me not to panic as I suddenly understood his uncharacteristic behavior. I lifted my locked stare from the page and stared blindly through him as my mind raced, desperately seeking escape from a reality too awful to contemplate.

His tone strong and infinitely calming, Kurt continued to talk to me, the words beginning to penetrate as the roaring in my ears lessened.

"Don't freak out too much, really, Dr. Celeste. This isn't so bad. I have a cousin who's had MS for years, and it's really amazing how much of it can be treated with diet and nutrition."

"What?" I focused on his honest, kind face, suddenly listening. He noticed the change in my response and smiled reassuringly.

"Sure," he repeated. "A lot of this thing can be managed with diet. My cousin isn't cured, but he's living a nearly normal life. You're a nutritionist. This should be easy for you!"

Easy? I know he meant it encouragingly, but I almost laughed. Yes, I was a nutritionist. In addition to holding a chiropractic degree, I was also a fully accredited Doctor of Naturopathic

Medicine. For years I had successfully counseled my patients on the benefits of a healthy lifestyle, of the value of nutritious eating. But this was entirely different. This was me!

I managed to smile weakly as he continued, seemingly unaware of the gauntlet of emotions rushing furiously through my heart. "I'll be happy to get a copy of his diet from him, and you can check it out, ok? I'll call him this afternoon and see if he can fax it over here. Don't worry!"

"Would you do that, thanks? I would like to see it." I had to get out of the kitchen, away from his well-meaning advice and attempts to comfort me. I needed to be alone. I needed to think. I shifted, pushing off the counter. "Thanks for the advice. I need to take a couple of moments, okay? I need to sort this out."

He smiled understandingly as I turned to leave. "Sure, no problem. It's a big blow. Although I can't know exactly what you're feeling, I'm sure right about now it's plenty rough. I'm here if you need me, and I'll get that diet info for you right away."

I nodded my gratitude and then I was out of the kitchen and down the hall, heading blindly toward my room, the fax tightly gripped in my icy, nerveless fingers. I spent the next several hours alone in my room, my mind seeking desperately to recall every scrap of information I ever knew about this incurable and often fatal disease.

On the one hand, my life had already been touched by this mysterious crippler. My dad, Sam Pepe, had been diagnosed at the age of 31 as having MS by the U.S. Navy. He had continued to live with the disease for years. Although he did have his medical problems, he was never debilitated, except at the very end of his life, at which point he had contracted a number of concurrent problems in addition to the multiple sclerosis.

On the other hand, my questing mind leapt unbidden to the images of celebrities afflicted with this scourge, people like Richard Pryor and Annette Funicello, visualizing the obvious ruin their lives had become, the daily agonies and indignities they suffered. I didn't think that I would be able to bear that, and wondered if I would have the courage to end it all if it ever got that bad.

I also spent the prerequisite amount of time feeling sorry for myself. Although we all may be noble publicly, in private, at least for a few moments, it's usually an entirely different matter. Someone once asked the late Gene Roddenberry, the talented creator of *Star Trek*, if his success was attributable to the old adage, "Face each day like a lion instead of a mouse." Gene replied, "It's more like: 'Face each day like a lion and shake in bed each night like a mouse.'" Well, I certainly felt at least that small, and sat there for moments uncounted too terrified even to think at all.

The afternoon wore on as I began a pattern of thought that would become almost routine in the months to follow. I began to review my life, trying to recall what, if anything, I might have done that made me a candidate for this disease.

It was early evening when Jerry returned from his meeting in Los Angeles. Although I often accompanied him, enjoying the drive and my various activities while he engaged in his busy schedule as owner of a large international corporation, this time he had gone down alone while I had slept in, still not one hundred percent recovered from my Hawaii experience.

I stood facing the window as he entered our room, his voice full of tired warmth and affection as he greeted me. We had been together for over three years, but a complete stranger could have seen the naked desolation in my face as I turned toward him.

"What's wrong?" In an instant he had crossed the room and stood beside me. Mutely, I gestured to the wrinkled fax lying on my vanity table. His face questioning but concerned, he read its contents. I watched him closely, and saw him blanch as the import of the words sank into his consciousness. He stood silently for a long moment, and then spoke, his voice gruff and businesslike.

"This is a mistake." He walked toward me again, the language of his body aggressively defensive. "This can't be what is wrong with you. There's got to be an error somewhere."

"There's no error, Jerry. It has to be true," I answered, my own voice low and strained, barely audible.

"Why? Because of that crap in Hawaii? I thought you said it was back strain." He shook his head defiantly. "No way, Celeste. You can't be this sick. It has to be a mistake. We'll get the test redone, by a *good* doctor."

"This *was* a good doctor, Jerry. And a good hospital." I stepped forward and took the fax from him, replacing it on the vanity and smoothing it reflexively. "And a good test."

"Bullshit, Celeste!" The words exploded from him, as if by the sheer forcefulness of them he could alter the circumstances, make it right. "This *cannot* be what is wrong with you! I won't accept this!"

He crossed the room and grabbed me, almost too hard, enveloping me in his great bear hug that I had always found so reassuring, so safe. Now I stiffened, feeling trapped instead of comforted. He continued, his voice calmer, the man of reason, one large hand stroking my hair. He pushed me back slightly, looking down intently into my face.

"Look. It can't be true. Look at yourself," he said, turning us both to face the full-length mirror on the opposite wall. "You're *healthy*, Celeste. You're trim, fit, beautiful. This thing puts people in wheelchairs, for God's sake! You'd look . . . well, sicker if you really had this thing the damn test claims you have."

"I don't know, Jerry," I said slowly, fighting a hope that I knew to be false. I rested my head on his broad chest, surveying our reflected image. I *was* healthy, in appearance at least. My physical body was in excellent shape, and looked far younger than my forty-plus years. My hair was full and shone with the vitality of good care and a great cut, my smile cosmetically perfect, my face relatively unlined.

He was right. This was not the image of a sickly waif or some frail creature subject to fainting spells at every turn. I ran, I swam, I rode horses, I exercised for hours. My exercise regimen was twice what most people would even attempt to perform on a regular basis. Jerry was right. I didn't look sick. Maybe . . .

My uncertainty must have shown in my face, for he brightened visibly. "Sure, it must be a mistake. We'll just have you do the test over again. And besides," he added, releasing me to walk to the dresser again, staring accusingly at the paper that had torn a hole in his well-ordered world, "even if you *do* have it, you probably only have a minor case of it. I'm sure it can't be all that bad."

I stared at his back with growing frustration. This was so like him, I thought with mounting resentment. Jerry never accepted anything that didn't fit in with his plans. That quality had made him an excellent businessman. It also made him, at times like these, a difficult partner. He also tended to minimize the afflictions of others, which could make him both a difficult boss and mate. It was almost as if my illness was inconvenient for him, so therefore, it was either a mistaken diagnosis or nowhere near as serious as I made it out to be.

I stood there silently, feeling almost cheated, and very alone. I don't know what reaction I expected, or was hoping for, but this definitely wasn't even close. Knowing that any further contradictory response on my part would only instigate an argument I couldn't handle right then, I sighed silently, feeling defeated.

"Okay, Jerry. Maybe you're right. I'll take the test again."

"There you go, babe," he encouraged happily. Feeling in control of the situation again, he stepped behind me, squeezing my shoulders for emphasis. "It'll be fine, you'll see. We'll get you the finest medical diagnosis money can buy. You'll be past this thing in no time."

Turning toward the walk-in closet, he shed his jacket, casually dropping it over a chair. "I'm going to grab a quick shower before dinner. Find out what we're having, would you? I'm starving."

He disappeared through the adjoining bathroom door, not looking back, confident that he had handled yet another crisis. I stared after him, desolate and empty.

There was really nothing more to say anyhow. Jerry would have his way. He usually did. I would take the tests again, with doctors *he* chose, in a situation where he could remain firmly in control. I knew the results would have to be the same. I also knew that Jerry would never accept them unless he was certain that there had been no error, no possible mistake. And maybe, not even then.

Sleep that night was far from blessed relief. My dreams were vivid, disturbing, full of frantic surrealism. I was lost in a thick and swirling mist, knowing that somewhere beyond it was God. I searched for Him, certain that He had the answers, answers I desperately needed to keep from losing my sanity and my will to survive.

Why had this happened to me? Why was I chosen? Was this a payment for sins, known and unknown? Was it a genetic failure, a distortion of my DNA that made it more susceptible to damage? Was it some childhood sickness, returned in a more virulent and deadly form to attack me once again? I'd already had my share of difficult episodes in my life, and I really didn't think I deserved this. The questions of my conscious mind became the dreams of my unconscious as I strove desperately for the understanding that I needed to handle the devastating reality my life was about to become.

I awoke from the dreams with no new answers. No epiphany had been mine. The room was dark, and I was sweating. Jerry snored peacefully beside me, oblivious to my waking start. Absurdly, I wanted to shove him, to wake him from his unconscious bliss to feel just a little of the uncertainty and fear I was feeling.

In frustration, I almost leapt from the bed, grabbing my notebook from the night table. Stalking to the overstuffed chair by the balcony window, I flung myself into it and flicked on the small light on the occasional table beside it. I began to write, the words coming furiously from the pen, almost of their own volition. I had questions. God was *supposed* to be omnipotent. I wanted, needed, *demanded* answers. I wrote:

Dear God,

I am afraid. The shock I felt has gone, only to be replaced by fear and the wild desperation of a rabbit in a snare. Why did this happen? Why is my life to be shattered by MS?

Is MS really just a virus I didn't handle when I was young, as some doctors believed? Is it the result of the mononucleosis I contracted at seventeen, after moving from Camarillo to L.A.? Or, does the MS stem from the cause of the virus: the desolate heartbreak of losing the boy I loved and the deep, fierce resentment of my parents that I felt, blaming them as I did for the loss?

Dear Billy, the boy who was so unsuitable for me in their eyes that they uprooted my world and moved the family to the airport area of Los Angeles, to a neighborhood I hated, leaving my high school friends behind? You know that my resentment of the situation was so strong that it was palpable. It colored everything I did, as did my loneliness, until finally I fell ill with mononucleosis. Is MS the virus returned, or are they totally unrelated?

I need answers, God. My logical mind craves a reason. Everything I've ever been taught screams to me that there has to be an explanation. My career, my world, is built on cause and effect. This can't be different. I need to know why!

And beyond the why, the what. Or more accurately, the what now? I'm a doctor! I'm supposed to be healing the world. And now, it is I who desperately seek healing.

Is this why I was chosen, selected to bear a burden this great, knowing that I must begin a race against time upon which my very survival depends? You promised me in your Word that you would never give me more than I could stand. Are You saying that I can stand this?

I certainly don't feel like I can. I want to run, screaming, until I outdistance this terrible twist of fate. I want to wake from this nightmare and find I am safe in the arms of the man You have given me to love, and find that none of this awful reality ever existed. Or is this where faith comes in? Is this where I let You carry me, the place in my life where only one set of footprints lines the sand?

How do I treat, even cure, this crippling disease? Kurt, our cook, has told me that one of his family members, similarly diagnosed, was combating the effects with a regimen of herbal medications, nutritional supplements, and alternative medicines. Is this where I come in? Am I to seek a cure for this silent destroyer of lives?

And, finally God, where? Where do I start? Not with the hospitals, and not with the doctors. Not with the institutions in which my world was based, in whom I had put my trust for so long. Not with these same individuals who now were telling me with great sympathy and greater finality that there was basically no other option. There was no cure. The best that they could offer was to help me adapt to my deteriorating existence.

That's not good enough!

There are so many threads that I can follow, like so many clues to a heinous crime. Which ones? Is the answer in the herbs, Your first medicine, given to man when the world was new? Or does it lie with nutrition, the subject so dear to my heart, and of which I have acquired so great a knowledge? I've heard reports of even more dramatic treatments like bee venom, treatments far outside the realm of conventional medicine. Is there a message in this for me? Or, am *I* the message?

Is this why You put it upon my heart to study medicine? As I pray to You, I see the path before me now as a challenge, a mission given to me. I will, I *must* find a way to beat this thing.

I need Your Strength, Lord. The strength to carry this burden without allowing it to crush the spirit and the life from my body. The strength to never acknowledge defeat, no matter how arduous and unfruitful the path that lies before me now may seem.

I also need Your Healing. I am happier now, at 42, than I can remember being except for brief moments in my already eventful life. That inner happiness will allow Your Healing

Power to flow through every fiber of my being, through every organ, every vessel, every cell. Bless me with Your Healing and Your Strength, Lord, so that I may begin the journey that You have set before me.

Thank You for my answer, God. A few hours ago, I was terrified. Now, I feel a growing resolution, almost an exhilaration, an anxiousness to begin my quest. Although I may never know *why* I've gotten MS, I thank You for helping me come to the realization that I can, and will, accept the challenge before me. And, with Your Guidance, I will emerge victorious in the most important fight of my life. Amen.

I leaned back against the big chair, physically and emotionally spent. I might not have had all of the answers that I needed, but I did have direction. I would do this. I would beat this thing. I returned to bed, knowing that the alarm would soon ring in a new day. It really would be the first day of the rest of my life. I curled around Jerry's comforting bulk as he mumbled in sleep, unaware that I had passed the last few hours in the chair by the window. Yes, my existence had been dramatically changed. I would have to redefine my life. Not as an MS sufferer. No, I would begin the search for a cure, emerging on the other side of this trial as an MS survivor.

One crimson ray from the emerging sun shot a long finger of benediction over the bed to splatter in splashed brilliance against the bedroom door as if in cosmic agreement with my resolution. I smiled, sighed deeply, and finally slept.

2
From Despair to Determination —Accepting the Challenge

The test results were the same the second time around. Jerry had sent me to the best facility he could find, the Samsun Clinic in Santa Barbara, California. My first visit was about two weeks after I returned from vacation. There, I was introduced to Dr. Curatalo, one of the leading doctors at the facility. He ordered that all of the tests I had undergone previously be reconducted, with the addition of a complete MRI series.

An MRI takes a series of detailed pictures of various parts of your body: spine, bones, and brain. This information would be more conclusive and more complete than the initial tests, and, in theory, give a more definitive answer as to the root cause of my physical problems.

Dr. Curatalo's demeanor and "bedside" manner were far different from the cold and sterile actions of the individuals at the first clinic. Dr. Curatalo was a very competent, thorough, and dedicated doctor who saw beyond the illnesses of his patients and took into consideration their emotional state when delivering his diagnoses. Shortly after I had gone to his offices for the testing, I received a very pleasant call from his nursing staff, requesting that I return for a new appointment to discuss the results at my earliest convenience.

In the early summer of 1994, I found myself sitting in Dr. Curatalo's large and well-appointed office while he delivered the diagnosis that I already knew would come. He broke the news to me as gently as he could, attempting to reassure me without sugar coating what was an extremely serious finding. I appreciated his concerned manner, and naturally, I quizzed him hard as to what my options were from this point on.

Leaning forward in the comfortable leather chair, strain evident in both my face and voice, I asked him, point blank, "So, how long does it take to cure this MS?"

I heard the great sympathy in his voice as he replied gently, "Celeste, perhaps you have misunderstood me. There is no cure for multiple sclerosis. All we can hope to do is manage the disease, allowing you to experience the fullest life possible under the circumstances."

The rebellious nature of my youth flared inside of me, refusing to accept this pat answer to the destruction of my world. "What do you mean, there's *no cure*?" My voice was hard and brittle. "Surely some people must get better!"

"Although some people do manage to live with the disease," he answered, still patient, "I will not lie to you and give you false hope. There is no statistical evidence that shows anyone has ever been cured of MS. There are medications, however, that will help you cope with it, both physically and emotionally."

I sat completely still, the import of this thorough and accomplished medical man's words settling into my soul. After a minute, I spoke again. This time, my voice was flat, devoid of all emotion as I posed, for the first time, the question that had whispered at the edges of my mind since the moment I had first read the fax in my kitchen.

"Are you telling me that I am going to die?"

Dr. Curatalo's face relaxed. "We all die, Celeste. No one is immortal, as much as we may wish it so. If you are asking me if MS is going to kill you, well, I am not sure that I know the answer to that. My most educated guess would be no, or at least, not for a long period of time. It appears that you are in an early stage of the disease, when the drugs I am prescribing have proven to be the most effective. They will allow you to live a nearly normal life and slow the progression of the disease."

Multiple sclerosis, then, is the appearance of multiple scars, or lesions, along the protective casing that surrounds the human nervous system. MS interrupts the flow of impulses from the brain to the different sections of the nervous system, reducing sensation, motor control, and eventually most voluntary motions, especially the use of the body's extremities, the arms and legs.

I still wanted to know more. My life was too full, too rich, to be taken away from me with one cruel stroke. How much of a change would this be? The questions tumbled out of me almost without volition as I sought to gain a complete picture of my impending future, or lack of one.

"Am I going to be crippled? Is my leg ever going to get any better? Will I have to stop doing all of the things that I love to do, that I *have* to do? Will I still be able to be a doctor, to see patients? Or, do I have to give it all up and sit in a wheelchair waiting to die?"

Dr. Curatalo smiled, seeking to calm my mounting fears. "I don't think that you need to go shopping for a wheelchair tomorrow, Celeste. And, I see no reason, at least at present, why you cannot remain in your own practice. In fact, work is the best therapy for a lot of people, especially professionals like ourselves. As I said before, modern medical science has developed several drugs that will help you to fight the progress of the disease."

I exhaled hard, frustrated. "Will these drugs fix my leg? I can't stand this limp, this weakness! I feel . . . helpless! And, quite frankly, it's pissing me off!"

He never took his eyes from my face as he answered, still in the same calm, reassuring tone. "I don't know if they can.

These medications are meant to slow the progress of the disease so that you can manage your condition. They are not known to repair already existing damage. You may have to face the fact that your leg will never again be what it once was. Again, I want to be completely honest with you. There is no cure for MS, Celeste. You will have to learn to accept that, eventually, and to work with what you still have available, using the drugs I recommend to maintain your present level of physical health. There really is no other option."

No other option. The words echoed inside my head, crashing against the walls of my reason. I stared upward at some indeterminate point on the ceiling while the conflict raged within me. My emotions were almost out of control. Later, I was to learn that extreme mood swings were experienced by many MS patients as a result of the chemical and hormonal imbalances that accompanied the disease. Dr. Curatalo sat silently while my brain took the time to register this information.

Several minutes passed before I finally dropped my gaze again to meet his. This time, the words came slowly, dull with defeat. "What drugs do I have to take for this?"

Sensing that I was now ready to move along with the discussion, Dr. Curatalo responded in the brisk tone of a confident medical man. He reached across his desk toward me, holding out a small booklet. As I took it from him, he began to explain its contents.

"This is a drug called Betaseron. It is a beta blocker, which means that it interferes with the antibodies in your system that attack your nerve endings and cause the damage." Noting the uncomprehending look on my face, he continued. "Look. Read the booklet, and also read," he reached for several sheets of photocopied information and passed it to me, "these articles I had my staff gather for you on multiple sclerosis. They explain the disease, and how it affects your nervous system, and your body as a whole."

Most people are unaware of the specific type of damage done to the nervous system of the MS-afflicted patient.

Sclerosis is the medical term for scarring. Multiple sclerosis, then, is the appearance of multiple scars, or lesions, along the protective casing that surrounds the human nervous system. I will explain in the second portion of this book exactly how this scarring occurs and progresses. Suffice it to say here that MS interrupts the flow of impulses from the brain to the different sections of the nervous system, reducing sensation, motor control, and eventually most voluntary motions, especially the use of the body's extremities, the arms and legs.

I took the group of papers, grateful for some printed information that would answer my ever-growing list of questions. Dr. Curatalo advised me to begin the Betaseron treatment right away. "My nurse can teach you the self-injection procedure, if you are not already versed in it. I also want to prescribe something for depression and sleeplessness, either Zoloft or Valium. You will need to begin to take these daily as well. I will send you home today with some beginning dosages, and you can have the prescriptions filled at your local pharmacy. These should help you to deal with your depression, anger, and mood swings."

My eyes already scanning the information he had given me, I nodded, only half listening. I focused again as I realized that he was continuing, preparing to send me to yet another diagnostic facility.

"I also want to refer you to the University of California at Los Angeles medical research facility. Dr. Meyers, the head of that facility, is one of the foremost experts on MS in America. I think that you will be more readily able to accept this diagnosis if you have a second opinion from such a highly regarded institution."

The notion that I would now be relying on daily dosages of tranquilizers bothered me intensely. Once again, I put the question to him. "Are you *sure* that there is no other way to treat this condition?"

Dr. Curatalo was understanding in his reply. "I see here that you are a naturopath, and so I understand that the idea of drugs to maintain your balance is foreign to you. I respect your beliefs. However, in all seriousness, I really do recommend that you begin to take these. Depending upon your progress, we may discontinue some, or substitute others as time goes on. There really is no other option here if you want to maintain a nearly normal existence."

No other option. Those words again, words that denied all hope of life as I had known it ever being possible again. Dr. Curatalo was correct in his assessment of my reservations. A naturopathic doctor differs from a conventional M.D. on several significant points. Foremost is the naturopath's firm belief that illness can be cured and deficient conditions corrected through the use of naturally occurring substances as opposed to conventional medical treatments utilizing manufactured drugs. We treat our patients through the use of vitamin and mineral therapy, physical rehabilitation exercises, and nutritional education.

He shook his head, seeing that I was still having difficulty coming to terms with the diagnosis. "Let me call my nurse. She will set you up with some sample dosages of these medications so that you can begin your regimen today."

He reached for his interoffice phone, but I stopped him. "Wait," I said, my voice determined. "I'm not sure I want to take this stuff just yet. It says here that in some cases, the side effects can be pretty severe."

He sighed, but replaced the receiver. "Well, those are rare cases. Most patients can take Betaseron with very little or no difficulty." I continued to shake my head in the negative. Dr. Curatalo offered a compromise.

"All right. Although I do not agree with you, I do respect your decision. Let me make a call to UCLA and have you go there for a referral and re-examination. After we receive the results, perhaps then you can begin the recommended protocol with less resistance. I will have my staff call you at home as soon as I have obtained an appointment for you. Until then, try not to worry, and do avoid any strenuous activity until we can get you started on the Betaseron."

I rose from the chair and thanked him for his thorough diagnostics and caring concern. He insisted that I take some sample packets of Naprosyn, a pain medication compound that contains an anti-inflammatory agent that might help to reduce the swelling and numbness in my leg. He also gave me Zoloft and Valium packets, instructing me on their use and suggesting that I use only one at a time, to see which I preferred as a counter to depression and mood swings.

As a courtesy, I took the pills, knowing that never in my life would I swallow any of them, except possibly the Naprosyn. Naprosyn is essentially the prescription strength equivalent of the over-the-counter medication Aleve. It can be effective in many circumstances, and used sparingly would probably cause no ill effects. He grasped my hand warmly as we shook on departure, again reassuring me that this was not the end of the world. I smiled thinly in response and left his office.

Jerry, as I expected, still refused to accept the diagnosis, even though this doctor was of his choosing. He continued to minimize my condition, anticipating my trip to Los Angeles, certain that the MS experts there would be sure to confirm that I had only a mild case that would probably go away sooner or later, or at least not get any worse.

I was beginning to resent his attitude. He was so unable to deal with anyone else's affliction or suffering. I had watched him take exactly the same attitude with members of his own family, his mother and his daughter. I swear, sometimes I was convinced that if my arm were pulled completely off, Jerry would insist that it was only a flesh wound. However, if he got so much as a scratch, it was time to call in a full-time, live-in nurse. It was so unfair, yet so typical of him.

My difficulties with Jerry, especially in the beginning of my illness, were typical of common reactions exhibited by the family members of many newly diagnosed MS patients. Spouses, children, and family members are used to the role the patient has always fulfilled in the home and family unit. A serious illness such as MS threatens to permanently alter that role. Initially, many of those close to the patient find the idea frighteningly unacceptable. Instead of lending support just at the time we patients so desperately need it, often our thoroughly human loved ones respond with negative emotions that range from anger to complete denial.

Sadly, the fact is that some of those close to you may never be able to come to terms with the fact that one so dear to them has developed a life-threatening condition. With some it is the fear of, or unwillingness to accept, the increased demands inevitable when dealing with a loved one's illness or chronically debilitating condition. Providing care and shouldering responsibilities that were formerly the province of the afflicted person may be more than they think that they can handle. With others it may simply be the inability to face the very real fear of the unknown and the possibility of loss: their loved one may die. Unfortunately for those of us who are afflicted, understanding why those close to us react in these ways does not make any of the negative reactions easier to bear. We want them to be there for us. We need them to support, comfort, and reassure us. It can be hard and very lonely when they don't, or can't.

Dr. Curatalo's office called the next day. The appointment with UCLA was scheduled for June 27, 1994. This created a new series of complications. California is huge. Los Angeles was over a three-hour drive away from where we live outside of Solvang. We would have to leave very early on the morning of the appointment, drive there, have the tests, and endure another drive home in the evening. Jerry, of course, insisted on coming with me, perhaps feeling that his presence would cause the doctors to realize that this was not at all serious after all.

The drive to Los Angeles was largely spent in silence on that bright June morning. Normally, I find the sunrise along the Pacific Coast Highway breathtaking. That day, I hardly noticed it, lost in my disjointed thoughts. I have always been a person who plotted her course, who thought things out in advance. This time I had no plans. I was caught in limbo, with no clear course of action pending the results of these new tests. Jerry had attempted to make the trip lighthearted, but I saw it only as a further attempt to minimize my condition. After several surly responses and half answers from me, he gave up and stared out of the opposite window, or spent the time on the telephone, doing business. Our driver wisely sensed the mood in the car and said nothing either, concentrating on the road.

The medical research facility at UCLA was state of the art and bustling with activity. The waiting rooms were decorated with cheerful paintings and bright colors; the students and staff were immaculate in their white lab coats and nursing uniforms. I laughed to myself as I thought how much the scene resembled those doctor shows of the 1970's, where no one got bloody, tired, or emotional, and everyone went home cured.

Dr. Meyers was brisk and businesslike when we met. He spoke very highly of Dr. Curatalo, and told me that he would perform the same tests, including a second MRI series and a spinal tap. Jerry sought confirmation from Dr. Meyers that someone as healthy as myself could not possibly have a serious case of the disease, but Dr. Meyers refused to be drawn into the conversation, stating only that we would have to await the results of the testing before any further determination was made. This did not please Jerry, as he was accustomed to immediate answers from his employees. Dr. Meyers, however, was not to be pressured into a position, and so Jerry was left to his own devices for the next few hours while I underwent the barrage of testing.

It was late in the afternoon when all of the tests were complete, and I was exhausted. My leg was stiff and aching, my back was sore from the spinal tap, I was hungry and developing an uncharacteristically fierce headache. Dr. Meyers rejoined us both briefly in the waiting room, to inform us that he would discuss the results of the tests with me the following morning. He recommended we spend the night in Los Angeles and return to the medical center the following morning for a meeting in his office.

Dinner that evening was a bleak affair. I was not in the mood for conversation, and made no attempts. Although we were checked into the Beverly Wilshire, a beautiful five-star hotel, it could have been a tent for all the difference it made to me. I slept fitfully, uninterested in my surroundings or Jerry's romantic advances.

The meeting the next morning with Dr. Meyers shed no new light upon the issue. We met in an examination room. The minute I saw him, I knew the results were the same. He placed my MRI photos on the lighted x-ray board and pointed out the lesions that were clearly noted in the pictures. He explained that these lesions were the damage already done by the disease, and how their number would probably increase as the disease progressed. Although his demeanor was nowhere nearly as cold as Dr. Willis's had been, his manner was still far more detached than the warm style of Dr. Curatalo.

He confirmed Dr. Curatalo's initial diagnosis, explaining, as I had already known, that there was no mistake. He also went on to explain that, contrary to what Jerry believed, my case of MS was not "slight" or "mild." As these were the first tests that I had undergone, there was also no way to determine the rate of the disease's progression through my system. Only the passage of time and repeated testing would be able to determine that fact accurately.

Our meeting was brief, lasting less than ten minutes, and ending with his recommendation that I return to Dr. Curatalo for continuing care. When I posed the question of options to him, much as I had done to Dr. Curatalo, his answers were identical: he recommended that I begin the Betaseron injection protocol and take a prescribed series of antidepressants to control my emotions. I knew that he would offer no additional or alternative solutions, so I thanked him for his time and left the examination room. On the way out of the medical center, the nurse on duty at the desk gave me a pamphlet from the Multiple Sclerosis Society of America, suggesting that I contact them regarding an MS support group in my area.

Jerry was waiting for me. As soon as he saw my face, he could tell that the news was not good. Not wanting to create a scene in the medical center, I walked outside to where our driver was parked. He could plainly see that my test results were not encouraging. Although too much of a professional to intrude with questions, he did place his hand gently on my elbow as he opened the back door of our limo. The touch was unusual, but strangely comforting. He drove us regularly, but always kept our contact to one of polite distance. Though he said nothing, all of the sympathy he felt was in that gentle touch. The comfort of it brought the sting of tears to my eyes, and I turned and smiled thinly at him, silently acknowledging his support.

Once inside the car, Jerry was not at all as supportive or comforting. In fact, he seemed almost angry with me, as if my contracting MS had been done deliberately to inconvenience him. I resented his attitude and his failure to give me the comfort I felt that I deserved and should be able to expect from someone who supposedly loved me. Before we had gone too many miles, his irritated tone of voice and my sullen, sarcastic answers had developed into a full-blown argument.

Our driver concentrated on the highway, pretending to be deaf and dumb as unkind words were hurled around him. The argument eventually degenerated into resentful silence on both sides. The rest of the trip was spent in stony silence on my part, while Jerry made endless business calls, acting, to my mind, deliberately jovial with the persons he was speaking with, as if to put a spiteful emphasis on our falling out, somehow attempting to convey the fact that all of this was my fault.

I stared out of the blackened privacy glass of the window, hot tears of resentment and self-pity streaking my face. The harder I tried not to let him see that he had hurt me, the more difficult it became not to cry. I bit my lip hard, forcing myself to concentrate on the pain and not the tears as he chatted and guffawed away on the telephone. Finally, I managed to get myself under control, and sighing deeply, closed my eyes and settled back against the comfortable seating, wishing the ride were already over so that I could get away from him and be by myself.

I had almost lapsed into unconsciousness when I heard the voice. *Celeste.* I started visibly and sat upright in the seat, causing Jerry, who was still on the phone, to look at me curiously. I shook my head to clear the cobwebs, glancing at our driver. He was intent on the road ahead and had obviously not called to me. I settled back against the seat, and the voice came again, low and clear. *Celeste.*

Suddenly, I was listening, hard. I knew this Voice, having heard it once before, long ago. I knew that it was the Voice of God. *Yes, God,* I answered silently. *I am listening.* A long moment passed, and it was almost as if I were alone in the car. Then, as clearly as I could hear Jerry, I heard it again. *My child. Do not fear. I have a purpose for you.* Almost fearing to breathe, I waited for the Voice to continue. It did, in that strong clear tone, strange, yet familiar, awesome, yet beloved. All of the power and wisdom of all of the ages was in that Voice, and my heart leapt to it like a flame to a rush of life-giving air.

You must understand. This is your karma, your destiny. I have brought you out upon this path, and I have been beside you. Before you were, you were with Me, and I with you. You knew this was why you had come. You chose this walk, to return at this time, in this body. It is your destiny to heal My people, to give hope where there was none, to ease their suffering and so to glorify My Name. You are here to find the cure for this affliction that besets and destroys My innocent, without favor or cause. You will walk this path, and I will light your way. Only obey, and trust. I will show you what is to be done. Do not fear, for this is what I have planned for you. Trust always, for I will never fail you . . .

I sat stunned, unmoving, as waves of infinite peace washed over me. I felt lifted, my tormented mind clear for the first time in weeks. *Amen, Father,* I whispered silently, *thank you.* This was what I had prayed for, sought God for, that first awful night in my room. I knew that the Voice was indeed the Almighty, the Giver of all Life, the Ruler of the universe and all that lay beyond.

I sat, almost transfixed, and reflected on the other time that I had heard this Voice. It had been almost seven years earlier, while I was still married to Paul Kerr and had a full and successful chiropractic practice in New York City. I was heavily into a spiritual practice known as Eckankar, which involved chanting the Name of God during times of meditation. As this practice involved other vocal singing, chanting, and verbal expression during the ritual, I normally conducted my daily sessions in our garage, on an old mattress I had laid out on the floor.

On this particular day, I had been into my meditation for fifteen to twenty minutes, and had entered a deep spiritual level. I was chanting, using the Name of God. In the tenth level of Eckankar, He is called Sugmad. I was seeking the wisdom of God in treating my patients. My practice involved more than chiropractic techniques. I treated using aromatherapy, sound, and color therapies to restore the inner balance of the whole person. Adjusting the bones was only part of the solution. I believed then, and still believe, that in order to cure the patient, one had to treat the root cause of the ailment, to restore the body's spiritual and emotional harmony.

Suddenly, I heard the Voice. It sounded as if it were coming from the roof of my garage, yet it filled all of the space, reverberating both inside and outside of my head. It said, *Celeste. Put your hand upon your patient, and ask in the Name of Sugmad, 'Let His Will be done.' You will be My instrument, and I will show you how to heal the afflicted one.*

On that day, I sat straight up in the middle of the meditation, snapping instantly to full consciousness, and said out loud, "What did you say?" The Voice, with infinite patience, repeated what I had heard again, word for word. I was thunderstruck. Then, suddenly, I began to laugh. How foolish of me! Of course God would know what the patient needed. God knew everything. He would absolutely know just what each patient needed for perfect health and harmony to be restored. All I needed to do was obey Him, and the answers would come. And they did. From that point forward, I have always been able to tell just what patients who place themselves in my care need most, which therapies to use, which remedies to apply, simply by placing my hands upon the patient and seeking the Wisdom of God in each situation.

Remembering that day, which I shall always call "God in my garage," caused me to laugh out loud again now, suddenly relaxed and happy for the first time in weeks. My ebullience was short-lived, however, because my outburst caused Jerry to turn from his endless conversation and ask me what was the matter. When I shrugged and said nothing, for some reason unwilling to share my moment, he shot me a look that implied that I was disturbing him while he was conducting important business, and he wished I would desist. I rolled my eyes in aggravation and flounced back against the seat cushions again to stare out at the rolling highway in silence, savoring my moment silently, alone with my thoughts.

Once we reached the ranch, I immediately got out of the car, refusing our driver's assistance, even though my left leg was aching and I was half afraid I would fall in the driveway. It's very hard to stalk up the walkway when your leg is killing you, but I managed, going straight up to my bedroom and closing the door with a decided "leave me alone!" slam.

I sat on the edge of the bed for several long minutes, thinking of and staring at nothing. Then, my female instincts took over, and I wanted to talk to someone. Not Jerry, as he was not being at all supportive, and the harsh words between us in the car still rankled. But, now that the diagnosis was definite, confirmed three times in fact, I wanted, needed to reach out and contact those people whom I considered to be close to me.

My mom, Ramona, and I hadn't been close over the previous years. The rift that was created between us during my high school years had never fully healed. Even so, it is a truism that in times of crisis, everybody needs their mom, and I was no exception. I reached for the phone and dialed, surprised that my hands were shaking. Mom answered almost immediately, and suddenly, I was no longer a successful professional and well-traveled woman. I was ten years old again, and I burst into tears as I choked out the news of my disaster.

Mom was great. All of the distance that had existed for so long between us melted away. She was shocked and fearful for me, but also loving and reassuring. The stubbornness and strong self-will of mine that she had so often criticized me for she now explained patiently would help me to pull through. Mom is one of those people who always wants all of the information available on any given subject, and she queried me in depth about MS, the doctors that I had seen, and the tests that I had been through.

As each detail was gathered from me, she seemed to find just the right thing to say that was both reassuring and supportive. I began to feel much better as I gave her the full story, marveling that the bond between us still existed, deeper than conscious thought, even after all of these years and so much bad water under the bridge. I told Mom that I didn't think that the doctors had any solution for me other than a series of drugs that would help to prolong my existence. I felt that perhaps this was my calling, my mission, to find a cure for this awful disease. Surprisingly, Mom agreed with me, revealing for the first time that the drugs that had been given to my dad never helped him fight MS. She said that she always knew that I would take a different path, and that my training in nutrition and exposure to alternative medicine would probably prove to be very useful in my search for a cure. We talked for almost an hour, and I was much calmer after I hung up the phone.

For the first time, I began to see beyond the awful diagnosis. There *had* to be other options. I just needed to find out what they were. I walked into my bathroom, splashed cold water on my face, and combed my hair, the feeling of desolation subsiding. I heard our cook calling me to dinner from the bottom of the stairs. I really didn't feel like going down to dinner with Jerry. I wasn't up to any more bickering, and I still resented his lack of support when I needed him the most. I went to the door of my bedroom and called down to Kurt, asking him to please bring me a tray, I wanted to eat in my room.

The next few hours after dinner were largely spent on the phone with the other important people in my life, including my daughter, Sara, my close friend from my college days, Leanore, and even my ex-husband, Dr. Paul Kerr. The conversation with Paul was not a good one, and it left me feeling empty, even though our relationship had been over for almost five years. He was cold and stiff, offering no sympathy, comfort, or reassurance. Paul had always been wrapped up in Paul, and he certainly hadn't changed. I quickly realized that I would get nothing positive from him, and I asked to speak to our daughter, Sara, who was living with him at the time.

Sara was scared, although I tried to reassure her. I have always tried to be honest with my daughter, but it was very difficult to explain a disease that I didn't fully understand myself. I so wanted to be with her, to hold and reassure her, to give her a comfort that I myself did not entirely feel. But she was in New York with her father and I was in California, so I contented myself with telling her not to worry, that I was fine, and that the doctors would be able to help me, even though in my heart that was certainly the last thing that I believed. Even though at that point I was not sure that it was the truth, I needed to convince the person that I loved the most that her Mom was not going to die. Sara has always been a delight in my life, a bright, loving, naturally compassionate child. It touched my heart as I heard her trying so hard to be brave, trying to offer me comfort when I knew that inside, she must have been absolutely terrified. I finally hung up the phone, after promising to spend time together with her very soon.

Clearly, the most supportive of all of the people that I contacted besides Mom was Leanore, my friend from my college days at UCLA. We had become close when we were both in a photo workshop class in 1973, and the bond between us had remained strong throughout the years. Her first reaction was intense dismay. She expressed so clearly the injustice that I was feeling, that I was a good person and did not deserve this cruel twist of fate.

That night, true to form, Leanore became a positive force once again. After sympathizing deeply and expressing all of the love and concern that I value her for so highly, she began to pump me up, to lift my thoughts to a higher purpose. She agreed with me that the thought of there being no other option had to be wrong. There had to be other options. They were just, as yet, undiscovered. I told her about hearing the Voice, just as I had told her the first time that I had heard it in my garage, all of those years ago.

Leanore believed me, of course, just as she had the first time. She has always been one of the most spiritually enlightened persons that I have ever known, in touch with herself, her God, and her world. Excitedly, she said that my hearing the Voice only confirmed what she already believed, that if there was anyone on Earth that could find a cure for MS, it would be me. She told me to look back at my life, and all of my experience and exposure to nutrition and alternative medicines. She reminded me that I had been a chiropractor and naturopath for several years, and had exposure to methods and avenues not open to many other people, much less others suffering from multiple sclerosis. If the answers were not to be found within conventional medicine, then they had to be out there in the alternative practices. She agreed with me that this was to be my challenge, a path that only I was destined to take, to find this cure, and to bring it to the world, acting as living proof that it worked.

Even though I had heard the Voice, her conversation that night was just what I needed to build my courage, to turn my focus from myself to the problem, to start on my search to defeat this affliction. At the end of our conversation, I knew that I was ready, that I could do this. MS would *not* defeat me. I would find the cure, saving not only myself but those who would come after me, overcoming this silent killer that had ruined the lives of so many.

It was well after midnight on the Pacific coast when I finally finished speaking with Leanore. Jerry had come into our bedroom somewhere during the conversation, and I had changed phones to the one that we had in our bathroom. Although most of the time I felt Jerry's insistence on having a dozen phones in the house was overkill, that night I was grateful. I finished my call to Leanore from the luxury of a nice, hot bathtub while Jerry went to sleep. I was almost cheerful when I returned to our darkened room, falling quickly into a deep and mercifully dreamless sleep less than five minutes after my head hit the pillow.

I came down to breakfast to find Jerry at the table. He was normally a hearty eater, but his plate was still largely full and growing cold. He appeared to have been pushing the food around distractedly without eating much of it. He glanced at me, saying nothing as the cook served my favorite breakfast of bacon, fluffy scrambled eggs, toast, and freshly brewed coffee. I also did not wish to fight anymore, and so kept silent, devoting my attention to devouring the delicious items on my plate. I soon became aware, however, that he was fidgeting in his chair, obviously wanting to say something to me, but feeling very awkward about beginning.

Jerry is a complex and difficult person to know, and harder sometimes to understand. An astute businessman and owner of an international vitamin firm that he built from the ground up to become one of the foremost manufacturers and distributors of vitamin and nutritional products worldwide, Jerry has always been more comfortable with his business relationships than his personal ones. Accustomed to power and knowing absolutely how to wield that power when necessary, Jerry hated to be in situations that he could not control, could not bend to his own considerable will. His first marriage had failed largely due to his fanatical devotion to his business and his inability to express his personal feelings and show his appreciation for those close to him in personal life.

Jerry is a large and handsome man, with well-defined features, a broad face, intelligent eyes, and an infectious laugh. He is almost a decade older than I, and we had already been together for several years before this major event occurred in our lives. We had met one another in the spring of 1991, on Long Island, in New York. Jerry owned a holistic healing center called Body, Mind and Soul, located on Long Island in the town of Huntington. I had become aware of the establishment through a patient of mine, who informed me that the center was seeking a nutritional counselor.

My own practice was in the Soho section of New York City at the time, although I, too, was living on Long Island. I was becoming entirely sick of the daily commute. Those of you who live on Long Island will know instantly what I mean, but for those of you who have never been to New York City or the 128-mile island that is attached to it, let me explain. Long Island has a population of over 2 million people, New York City over 8 million. These two bodies of land are connected by three bridges and one tunnel. Need I say more?

Therefore, I was most interested in investigating an opportunity to practice nutritional counseling, my first love, in a town that was only a 15- or 20-minute drive from my home. I met with the people who ran the center and was soon in practice there as a nutritional counselor, scaling back my practice in the city to one or two days a week.

After a short period of time had passed, the suggestion was made that I might want to bring my chiropractic practice there as well. The vice president of Natural Organics, the company Jerry owns, arranged a meeting between Jerry and myself so that I could sign a non-liability waiver, releasing the center and Natural Organics from any consequences should any legal difficulties arise from my practice while on the premises. We met and hit it off immediately. Unlike my relationship with Paul Kerr, who considered nutrition an unimportant hobby,

Jerry and I had much common ground as both of us were involved in vitamins and nutrition. Our marriages were virtually over, and the immediate chemistry between us soon developed into something more intimate. A native Californian, I had always wanted to return home to live. After Jerry purchased the ranch in the Canyon country, north of Santa Barbara, it didn't take much convincing on his part to get me to move back there with him.

Our relationship, like everybody's, had highs and lows, but it was basically solid, which is one of the reasons that I was so hurt when he failed to show support for me after I received this devastating diagnosis. So, that particular morning, I concentrated on the breakfast in front of me, loath to have any more negativity between us. I was about two thirds of the way through the meal when I could feel him staring at me. I continued to look at my plate, deliberately eating each mouthful, knowing that something was coming, but not at all certain what it would be. Jerry cleared his throat several times, shuffled his chair back and forth, and finally spoke. When he did, what he had to say was shocking.

"Celeste," he began, uncharacteristically hesitantly. I didn't look up, so he repeated my name, more urgently. "Celeste. Look, I . . ."

He stopped for a moment, as if deciding just what he wanted to say. This got my attention, and I finally looked up at him, because Jerry usually has plenty to say. As soon as I met his gaze, he drew breath, and launched into the conversation, like a swimmer who suddenly decides to dive into cold water.

"Look, Celeste," he repeated. I was surprised to see the earnestness in his face, to hear the tension in his voice. "I'm . . . I'm *sorry* about yesterday. I was pretty rotten to you, and I really didn't mean to be."

I just sat there, amazed. Jerry was definitely not one for apologies. When we had fought before, he'd never apologize. He'd just wait until enough time had passed so that he thought I would forget about it, and then acted as if nothing had ever happened between us. He wasn't finished, though. It was as if, once he'd made the decision to get through that part, the rest of it was easy. The words almost tumbled over one another as he continued.

"I really am sorry. I don't know why I acted like that. I think that I was just afraid. Afraid that you were really sick, and that I couldn't do anything about it. Afraid that . . . that I would lose you, that you were going to die. I couldn't handle that."

If a puff of wind had blown on me in that moment, I'm sure that I would have fallen off of my chair. Jerry, no doubt noting my look of stunned amazement, rose from his chair to move and take the one beside me. Grasping my hand in his, he continued earnestly, his eyes never leaving mine.

"Celeste, I really want you to understand that I *mean* this. I want you to have the finest care available, so that you can fight this thing. You can go back to Dr. Curatalo, and he'll start you on the treatment right away, before this gets any worse."

I looked at him, this man that I loved, touched to the heart that I did mean a great deal to him, after all. But, especially after the conversation that I'd had with Leanore the night before, I didn't want to pursue that route. I had to tell him, and I wasn't sure how he'd react. Withdrawing my hand, I placed it gently on the side of his face. My own voice was warm, but determined, as I answered him.

"Jerry, dear," I began, looking into his face and searching his eyes, "I've made my own decision about this. I don't want to go back to Dr. Curatalo. I don't think that he can help me."

"What do you mean, you don't want to go back? I thought he said that if you began treatment right away, you could keep this thing from getting any worse. You just can't ignore it!"

"I don't plan to ignore it, Jerry. But, I don't think that Dr. Curatalo has the answer. In fact, I *know* that he doesn't. I don't want to 'manage' my MS, living my life with Betaseron injections for the rest of my existence, because I certainly wouldn't call it a 'life.' I'm a nutritionist, Jerry! I don't want to start my day with Valium, and end it with Zoloft. I *don't*, Jerry. I would rather die than do that."

My voice shook from the passionate conviction I felt. As I said the words, I realized how much I meant them. I, who had devoted the majority of my adult life to the pursuit of nutrition and the harmony of the inner being, was not going to live tied to needles and pills. I needed Jerry to understand and accept this. I grabbed his hands, my voice and face fiercely intense as I explained what I was going to do.

"Conventional doctors don't know what to do! The only thing that they can offer me is a road that I won't travel. They said that there is nothing that they can do to change the fact that I have MS, and I'm sure that they were telling the truth. But, that's not good enough. It's nowhere *near* good enough. I can't just *live* with this, Jerry. If these doctors don't have an answer for me, then I'm going to find someone who does. There has *got* to be an answer out there, somewhere, and I'm going to use every last bit of my energy to find out what it is. I am not going to live my life with multiple sclerosis. I'm going to find a way to cure it. I believe that this is my destiny, my challenge. I believe that I was brought here, now, at this time, for this purpose. I'm either going to find a cure, or die trying."

> *"There has got to be an answer out there, somewhere, and I'm going to use every last bit of my energy to find out what it is. I am not going to live my life with multiple sclerosis. I'm going to find a way to cure it."*

He drew back from me, his face dark, his brow furrowed. His eyes flashed, and I waited for the explosion that I was sure would come. But, regardless, I was adamant. I would not follow these conventional protocols. I'd seen the end result for people, famous people, who had, and their lives were irrevocably ruined. I would not walk this path, and all the Jerrys in the world could not force me. I had chosen my course, and, even if it meant leaving him, I would not deviate from it now that I had made up my mind.

All of my thoughts in that moment must have shown in my face, for the explosion of anger that I expected did not come. His face lost its dark aspect, and he sat for a long moment in silence. When he did speak, his words surprised me, coming slowly, as if from a man who, waking from a dream, discovers he's found himself in an even greater nightmare. "All right, Celeste. I'm *trying* to understand. If you don't want to go back to Dr. Curatalo, then you don't have to. But, what are you going to do? You have to do something!"

"I *am* going to do something. I am going to learn all that I can about this disease. What causes it, how it starts, what damage it does. Then, I'm going to find out how to reverse that damage, to rid my body of this thing, and restore it to health. I'm not exactly sure where that will lead me, but I think that if conventional medicine does not hold an answer, then perhaps alternative medicine may. I'm going to start exploring that avenue. In the more than ten years since I graduated from chiropractic college, I've met many wonderful healers who operate outside the realms of what the medical community deems conventional treatment. I'm going to start with them, and see where that leads me."

He looked at me, hesitant, and more than a bit confused. "You mean holistic medicine? Herbs and stuff like that?"

"Possibly. You know that we had wonderful success with Body, Mind and Soul. We cured a lot of people while we were there, using only natural remedies. I think the answer may lie in that direction. I plan on finding out."

"I agree with you there, but only to a point. Celeste, those people had bad backs, headaches, allergies, and skin rashes. They didn't have something that was going to *kill* them, for God's sake!"

"That's true," I admitted, "but, if it worked on their ailments, who says that the same methods would not work on something more serious? Jerry, you know that the medical community never wants to accept something that they haven't thought of themselves. Remember laetrile? Nobody wanted to believe that apricot pits could fight cancer, so it never got approved. There have got to be other treatments like that out there, outside the realm of what the American Medical Association says is acceptable. Treatments the big drug manufacturers hope never get approved, because the money's in the illness, not the cure."

He drew back, looking a little offended. "I don't want people to stay sick, Celeste, and I'm a big manufacturer."

I laughed, but gently. "Yes, dear, but you manufacture wellness drugs, vitamins, and nutritional products made from natural substances that help people to restore their bodies and stay healthy. You don't make endless pills and potions that prolong the suffering, and other pills and potions that make them too numb to feel the disease that's eating away at their bodies and their lives."

He also laughed now, his face brightening. "That's true. I insist that our products are made from only natural things. The only stuff that's ever in them that may be the least bit artificial is the bonding agents we use to keep the pills in a form people can take. Do you think we make things that you can use to cure MS?"

"Possibly. I'm sure that maintaining a proper nutritional balance has got to be important. In fact, I *know* that it *has* to be. But that's what I'm going to do. I'm going to find out the answers. I want to know what the body lacks, or has too much of that invites MS, and then try to stop the progress and reverse the process. I don't know where that will lead me.

"Perhaps the answer is not even in this country. The drug people wield an awful lot of power over the government and the AMA. You know how hard it is to get approval for something new, whether it's treatment or medicine. Sometimes it takes years, even decades. How many people died of AIDS before the government let them take AZT? I don't have years, Jerry. I want to, I need to find a cure now. I'm treating the most important patient I've ever had, *me*, and I'm not going to fail her."

Jerry leaned forward and enveloped me in his big arms, pressing my head to his chest. I could feel all of his love flowing into me, giving me strength. Jerry was not normally comfortable with showing his deepest emotions and his voice shook slightly as he spoke to the top of my head, "You're also treating the most important patient I've ever known, Doctor. You're healing the woman I love. You better not fail her."

I raised my face and kissed him, long and tenderly. "I won't. She is, after all, all of the world to me."

He drew back from me then, looking long and earnestly into my eyes. When he spoke, his voice was deep with conviction, and his words made me know that I had his full support at last.

"Look. You do whatever you have to do. Go wherever you feel that you need to, see whoever you think will help you find the answers you need. No matter where this leads, no matter what it costs, I'm there for you. I'll use everything that I have at my disposal to help you. All of whatever influence I may have, every dollar I've ever made. All that matters is that you get well, that you *beat* this thing. Nothing else is important. Whatever it takes, you do it. I'll be there, doing whatever I can to help you. I love you, Celeste. And, even though I admit that this scares the hell out of me, I believe in you. I *know* how good you are. I hired you, after all, didn't I?"

"Yes, but I think you had ulterior motives at the time!" We both laughed, the tension broken, hugging one another close. I knew that he spoke honestly. It was often difficult to get Jerry to see your point of view, especially if it differed from his, but once he made up his mind he stood resolute. It was a quality that made him a formidable businessman, and sometimes such a difficult partner. Now that he'd decided that my course of action was valid, he'd support me all of the way, from the first to the last.

And he has. Throughout what would become a five-year journey to healing, toward finding a cure, Jerry has always been there. He has never said anything that I wanted to do was too radical, too costly, and some of the things that I was to try were to prove horribly expensive. No, Jerry was firmly on my side from that day forward, and there he would stay, and has stayed, to this day. I love and appreciate him for it, and always will. I will never forget that his support and his considerable resources helped me to save my life, and, with the writing of this book, possibly the lives of countless others as well.

Breakfast ended that morning on a happy note, our disagreements and the MS for the moment forgotten. We laughed and joked together as if none of this had ever happened. I felt wonderful for the first time in weeks. I was upbeat, positive, and lighthearted. I felt like I could change the world, that I could conquer this mountain. Little did I know just how high the mountain was.

3

In My Beginning—Removing the Poisons, Searching My Life for Clues

My first steps on the road to a cure over the next few days were largely spent on the telephone. I did return to Dr. Curatalo's office one more time, to explain that I had decided not to begin the Betaseron protocol. Although obviously concerned for my health and disappointed that I would not accept the standard treatment he had offered me, he respected my decision as one medical professional to another, even though he disagreed and doubted that I would be successful in my attempts to find an alternative treatment and cure.

The first two weeks after my visit to UCLA, I spent several hours each day on the telephone in addition to my normal daily routine. My left leg was still stiff and unresponsive, but I was determined not to let it impede my progress, so I continued to exercise in our training room each morning. My normal exercise routine lasts about forty-five minutes to an hour, but with my leg in this condition, I had to reduce my workout to twenty to thirty minutes.

It's been said that Californians are obsessed with looks and vanity, and that we are the mecca for plastic surgeons. I can't confirm or deny that perception, but I will say that we probably are confirmed exercise addicts. Nearly everybody in California works out, or at least has a plethora of training equipment somewhere in their homes. Maybe it's due to the fact that we have so much film media in the state, with Hollywood and Burbank and all of the other places where movies and television are produced. Or, maybe it's because we are such a physical recreation state. We ski in the north, ranch in the canyons, and swim and surf our 840 miles of coastline. It's hard to hide unwanted fat in tight ski pants or skimpy bathing suits.

I have always been more concerned with health than my waistline or dress size. A healthy body is naturally trim, although not necessarily rail thin. I think that my exercise routine, and living the natural lifestyle that I had practiced for so many years prior to the onset of the MS, worked dramatically to my advantage. It is much harder to repair a body that is barely functioning than one that is already healthy and in good shape when injury or illness occurs.

My belief in this theory was confirmed by one of the earliest telephone calls I made in my search for an alternative treatment for my MS. I have always loved the Olympic Games, watching as much of them as I can every time they take place. I love the excitement, the competition, the sportsmanship, the human interest side of so many of the athletes' stories. One of the stories I remembered clearly was of Jimmie Huega, a member of the 1976 U.S. Olympic ski team. Jimmie was a champion skier long before the 1976 games, but those were special. I'd like to take a moment to tell you about him here.

Jimmie Huega was a competition skier from a very early age, having gathered an impressive list of medals and trophies before he ever entered Olympic competition. Judged to be one of the best and the brightest stars of U.S. competitive skiing, Jimmie was diagnosed with multiple sclerosis in 1970, at the pinnacle of his career. The news was devastating to himself, his family, and his teammates. It seemed that his dreams of Olympic competition and a normal life were over. He dropped out of the athletic scene for the next six years, following his conventional doctors' orders and leading a non-strenuous, sedentary life until he couldn't take it any more. He came to a decision that he was not willing to let MS run, and ruin, his life.

Jimmie began to exercise and train, rebuilding his body, his strength, and his mental outlook on life. He began to ski again, and in 1975, rejoined the U.S. Olympic hopefuls. Not only did he make the team that year, he went on to earn a bronze medal in the 1976 Olympic Games. He has gone on to be a champion in a far broader sense, proving that one does not necessarily need to lie down and wait to die when one has contracted multiple sclerosis.

Always active in his home community of Avon, Colorado, in 1984 Jimmie successfully opened a scientific research facility, the Jimmie Huega Center (JHC), with the full support of his family, friends, and neighbors in that beautiful and historic Eagle County town. The JHC is supported by private donations and community fund-raisers, including the annual Jimmie Huega Marathon in the Squaw Valley and Lake Tahoe areas of Nevada, and the Mountain Bike Express series of fund-raisers, held in various parts of Colorado and throughout the northwestern states.

Pursuing the Center's mission to "Re-Animate the Physically Challenged," Jimmie and his expert staff specialize in working with the multiple sclerosis patients and their families. Their emphasis is on nutrition, general health, physical fitness, and the psychological well-being of not only the patient, but the families of the afflicted, helping all to live fuller, more rewarding lives of independent self-sufficiency.

I contacted the JHC in the midsummer of 1994, shortly after my return from UCLA. Although I regret that I never had the opportunity to speak with Jimmie personally, I had a wonderful conversation with a member of his staff. Upbeat, cheerful, and positive, she reassured me that MS was certainly not the end of the world, and confirmed that my commitment to a continued exercise program was absolutely the right thing to do. She told me that Jimmie firmly believes that God created all of us a certain way, with bodies that were designed to function properly, in fitness and health. Jimmie believes and teaches those who come to his clinic that if you do not use your muscles, you will most certainly lose their function. She encouraged me to continue to exercise daily, pushing my body to the limit, especially my damaged leg, in order to maintain the mobility that I still possessed and to rebuild that which I had lost.

Although I was warmly invited to visit the Center at any time, I have never had the opportunity, as yet, to actually go there and experience it for myself. I felt that my path lay along other, more immediate avenues, because I was already exercising daily, a routine I started years before my diagnosis. I do, however, recommend his clinic highly for those MS patients who live in the Colorado area, or who are seeking a highly regarded treatment facility that not only specializes in this affliction, but is also headed by a man who knows exactly how you feel and what you are going through. I also urge those of you who are financially able to support the JHC and its continuing efforts to help MS patients and their families obtain both physical and spiritual wellness. MS is not only a physical crippler. It can damage the patient emotionally as well, and any facility that recognizes that fact and works to fight against it is certainly a most excellent cause worthy of support.

In those early days, I proceeded to go through my entire address book of associates, friends, and colleagues, past and present, in an effort to obtain leads and ideas pertinent to alternative treatments for MS. I called everyone that I knew, doctors, nutritionists, and people not in the medical field at all. I asked each of them if they had ever had any experience, clinical practice, or exposure to alternative medical treatments for multiple sclerosis. Most of the answers I received, I'm sorry to say, were in the negative. I was seeking concrete alternative forms of healing, methods that had been tried with positive results by others.

Those I contacted who answered in the affirmative, or who gave me the names of others who could help me I questioned extensively on their methods, experiences, and results. I took notes of every positive conversation and obtained solid leads that were to prove to be very useful later in my search.

One of the most important calls I made proved not to be to an alternative medicine practitioner at all, but to a friend of Jerry's and mine, a wonderful dentist from Long Island, Dr. Mitch Cantor. Our friendship with Mitch dated back to the days when we were all living on the Island, and we saw him socially whenever we were in New York, which was several times a year. He, like all of our friends, was shocked and dismayed at my news. But, in addition, Mitch also had what proved to be a very valuable suggestion to offer.

Mitch is the kind of dentist who is never content to practice simply with the knowledge he has already gained. He is constantly seeking to improve his skills and broaden his horizons, to expand his knowledge of dentistry to improve the quality of care he gives to patients. Because of the way that he views and approaches his profession, I also benefited. Mitch had attended a seminar not long before I spoke to him. There he was introduced to the work of a prominent dentist and well-known author with an alternative point of view, Hal A. Huggins, D.D.S.

Dr. Huggins's Colorado-based practice provides dentistry of a different sort to his patients. Dr. Huggins is the author of over fifty articles and three widely read books. His brand new work, *Uninformed Consent* (Huggins and Levy 1999), expands upon his previous book, *It's All In Your Head: The Link Between Mercury Amalgams and Illness* (Huggins 1993), and deals with the primary focus of his practice, which is dental toxicity. Dr. Huggins believes that many of the autoimmune diseases prevalent in society today, including but probably not limited to multiple sclerosis, Alzheimer's, Parkinson's, Lou Gehrig's, lupus, and breast cancer, are caused, or at least exacerbated, by toxic mercury amalgam fillings placed into the teeth of the patient over the course of a lifetime of dental treatments.

Mercury fillings are the most common form of cavity treatment used by the majority of American dentists today, as they have been for nearly 150 years. These fillings, technically referred to as amalgams, are comprised of a compound of materials, including silver, cadmium, copper, zinc, beryllium, nickel, and other substances. In the second section of this book, you will see how an over-accumulation of these metals in your system can give rise to toxic levels, causing multiple complications. Not only found in fillings, these materials are routinely included in many other dental replacement or cosmetic correction materials, including crowns, caps, braces, and bridgework.

In defense of your dentist or orthodontist, who may be a caring and dedicated professional, he or she may not even be aware of the growing number of studies that show that these materials often turn toxic in the system, especially if the patient treated may have an inborn sensitivity or hidden allergy to them.

Most of the states in this country do not require dentists to inform their patients as to the possible complications that may arise from the placement of these fillings into the mouth, or to inform or offer their patients alternative materials. Because revealing these facts is not required, this may also be the reason your dentist does not have this information. California recently passed a law that requires dentists practicing here to distribute a printed fact sheet to their patients prior to dental care, advising them as to the possible dangers arising from the use of this type of filling or orthodontic device, and alerting them as to what alternative materials may be available as a less hazardous choice.

The California State Legislature is currently considering an additional bill that would require not only that dentists alert their existing or prospective patients as to the toxic potential of these materials prior to the placement of them into the patient's mouth, but also that the patient sign a release form agreeing to their use after being apprised of the possible risks. This bill may indeed have been passed into law by the time this book is published.

Mitch not only alerted me to this new information and to Dr. Huggins's book but he additionally suggested that I go to see Dr. Huggins to have my own fillings removed and replaced with nontoxic materials. At the time he made the suggestion, in 1994, my mouth was replete with mercury fillings, some of which had been placed there in early childhood.

I found all of this fascinating and said as much to Mitch. I thought that I would consider it as something I might want to try. Then, he told me something that convinced me that I had to check this out, and at least speak personally to this most unusual dentist. Mitch told me that Hal Huggins also had MS!

I was intrigued and eager to learn what Dr. Huggins believed about mercury toxicity, and about his experiences with multiple sclerosis. Perhaps there were treatment options that he had explored that I was not aware of, and that perhaps I could also try, or at least consider. The very next day, I obtained a copy of *It's All In Your Head: The Link Between Mercury Amalgams and Illness*. I found it to be fascinating and frightening. I read with growing horror how the fillings, crowns, caps, and orthodontic braces we have all received from early childhood from our kindly dentists could be slowly poisoning us every day of our lives.

I am not going to go into a detailed history of the use of mercury or silver amalgam fillings here. Suffice it to say that, as is so often the story in so many areas of life, these fillings came to be widely used simply because they were cheaper than previous substances such as gold, and easier to compose in the dentist's office than porcelain. Cheaper and easier allowed the dentist to treat a greater number of patients and reduce the overall cost of dental repair. It also allowed for a wider profit margin. Even today, many members of the American Dental Association (ADA) consider these fillings or orthodontic devices to be "safe" when in the mouth, even though these substances would be considered highly toxic if ingested in other forms. This makes no sense.

For instance, in recent years, consider the growing concern for toxic mercury levels in fish due to pollutants found in the waters where the fish are harvested. Toxic levels of mercury and other substances found in these fish and shellfish have been proven to cause brain damage, certain types of cancer, and a number of other illnesses and complications. How can it be advisable to avoid eating contaminated fish or shellfish, yet allow many times the concentration of mercury found in an average serving of these food items to be placed in our mouths as a permanent repair of tooth decay?

After I finished reading this excellent, well-researched, and enlightening book, I became convinced that even if excessive mercury had nothing to do with MS, it would be advisable to have these fillings removed from my mouth and replaced with other, safer substances without further delay. Especially now, when my body needed to fight this illness, I could not see how it could possibly be beneficial to ask it to deal with the effects of mercury poisoning at the same time. Several days later, I contacted Dr. Huggins's office and conversed with him briefly. I flew to Colorado, where Dr. Huggins would examine me and discuss the feasibility of removing the mercury fillings from my mouth.

The treatment was to last more than two weeks. I stayed at a lovely hotel not far from Dr. Huggins's office in Colorado Springs. During that time, I went to his office each day, where he began to remove the mercury fillings from my mouth. He would remove one to three each day, beginning with the oldest first, and replace them with nontoxic alternative fillings made of porcelain. Naturally, while I was undergoing treatment, I had the opportunity to learn more about Dr. Huggins himself and about his own case history with multiple sclerosis.

At the time, Dr. Huggins had already been suffering with multiple sclerosis for several years. He had been initially diagnosed with MS in 1968. As the technology of the time did not include the ability to do an MRI, Dr. Huggins has never had an MRI, even now. Maybe just as well, because researchers are beginning to learn that repeated MRIs can exacerbate the MS patient's condition. Now sixty-four years old, Dr. Huggins's own left leg is failing him, and he walks with a cane to support his weakened limb. He believes that his MS is a result of his thirty-six-year exposure to the mercury compounds he worked with in his dental practice. In his own case, Dr. Huggins is now highly sensitive to many substances—particularly fresh seafood—that never bothered him before contracting these symptoms. His reaction is so severe that he cannot go to a restaurant that serves fresh seafood due to the adverse reaction he will experience if he even smells the fish served there.

One of the interesting methods that Dr. Huggins uses during his dental treatments is to place magnets on the face of the patient to control the pain that is normally felt during the filling removal and replacement, instead of employing the standard numbing agent, novocaine. Although somewhat skeptical at first, after experiencing this for myself, I was most impressed by how effective these magnets were in pain management. Another portion of the treatment involved the daily use of a low-heated sauna. Not only relaxing and soothing, the sauna, set at about 102 degrees Fahrenheit, allows the body to remove the excess mercury through perspiration, further reducing the levels in the patient's system.

I now firmly believe that the removal of mercury fillings is essential to the health of many patients, and a good health choice for others who may not be experiencing any adverse reactions to the compounds. However, before you elect to undergo this treatment, I strongly caution you to investigate the dentist who will conduct the removal. Mercury removal if done incorrectly can be dangerous to your health. Mercury released improperly or unchecked in the body can cause a multitude of immediate or long-term adverse effects. If you make the decision to replace your old fillings, I urge you to be certain that the dentist you choose is familiar with the hazards and has experience with the procedure.

While I was undergoing the treatment, I also had non-dental tests that were extremely important. Dr. Huggins shared his practice with another wonderful, enlightened medical man, Thomas Levy, M.D., the co-author of Dr. Huggins's latest book, *Uninformed Consent*. Working in concert with Dr. Huggins, Dr. Levy handles the non-dental procedures for all the patients at the facility, including scheduling various testing procedures and nutritional counseling. As a naturopath and nutritional counselor myself, I appreciate the depth of knowledge and range of expertise exhibited by Dr. Levy. A warm and caring professional, Dr. Levy is always accessible to the patients and performs a vital function in this excellent practice.

Dr. Levy had asked that I bring with me my most recent MRI to examine my brain for mercury. Dr. Huggins placed the MRI on a lighted examination board and indicated the areas where there appeared to be indistinct regions. Referring to these areas as "brain fog," Dr. Levy showed how these indicated the mercury that was leaving the system. It remains trapped between the brain and the skull walls as a gaseous substance unless flushed from the system with procedures like chelation. (I explain more about chelation in the next chapter.) Dr. Levy believes that this mercury is in fact leaving the system of both the autoimmune and typically "healthy" patient every time chewing occurs and that it accumulates in this area of the body. It is essential that this excess mercury be released from the system, thereby reducing and eventually eliminating toxicity.

Dr. Levy also ordered a blood analysis to measure the level of mercury present in my body. The test results were disconcerting. An acceptable range for mercury in a healthy individual should be less than 3 units. My numbers came in at greater than 12 units! That is over four times the acceptable level and indicated severe toxicity.

Because of this finding, Dr. Huggins and Dr. Levy recommended that I undergo chelation to expedite the removal of the remainder of this substance upon my return to California, thereby bringing my levels into the acceptable ranges once more. They advised that I undergo about twenty-five chelation sessions after the filling removal and replacement was completed. They would provide me with a referral to a facility that could complete this necessary step in removing the toxins from my overloaded system.

The test for excessive mercury made me begin to think that perhaps other substances had also reached toxic levels in my system, throwing it out of balance and thereby creating susceptibility to any number of complications. I determined to have a complete system substance analysis upon my return to California. I would undergo a series of tests known as BioCybernetics Analysis, which I will explain in more detail later.

During my stay in Colorado, I found myself with quite a bit of time on my hands while not at Dr. Huggins's. I began to research multiple sclerosis, learning as much as I could about the scientific nature of the disease and the possible causes of its origin. I read dozens of articles from eminent scientists and researchers throughout the world regarding the physical nature of MS, its symptoms, the damage it causes to specific areas of the body, and the prognosis if unchecked or treated conventionally.

One of the theories that I found to be most fascinating was that MS is not genetically, racially, or geographically determined, as was thought until recently. Scientists are beginning to theorize that MS is instead a virus, either introduced into the body when a certain set of elemental conditions is present, or perhaps as the current expression of the mutation of an older illness that had never been completely eradicated from the system, even though all outward symptoms had ceased and the patient appeared to have "gotten well." This mutation could be the result of an illness experienced as long ago as childhood, lying dormant for years until re-manifesting itself as MS.

With this intriguing possibility in mind, and with time on my hands, I began to examine my own personal history, searching for the clues that might lead me to the answers I needed to drive this illness permanently from my body.

I'm a California girl, born and bred. The daughter of Samuel Pepe, an Italian-American and lifetime Navy man, and Ramona, his Norwegian-American wife, I made my appearance into this world in 1950, in San Diego. The second of five children, I had three brothers, Sam Jr., born in 1948, Max, born in 1952, and Jim, two years later, in 1954, and one sister, Rose, born much later in 1961. My dad was away at sea far more than he was at home, and my mom raised the five of us largely alone, as did so many career servicemen's wives.

My dad came home from the sea for good in 1964, at the age of 44. Although having been diagnosed with multiple sclerosis himself by Navy doctors at the age of 30, he had remained in the service for another fourteen years. Dad was initially a pilot, serving aboard an aircraft carrier. When he was diagnosed, the Navy grounded him from flying, and he spent the rest of his career serving in other capacities. No tests like we have today were ever performed upon Dad. I wonder in retrospect if what he had contracted was instead what is today known as the Epstein-Barr Virus (EBV), as he was able to continue his Navy service for more than a decade after he was afflicted.

One of the theories that I found to be most fascinating was that MS is not genetically, racially, or geographically determined, as was thought until recently. Scientists are beginning to theorize that MS is instead a virus, either introduced into the body when a certain set of elemental conditions is present, or perhaps as the current expression of the mutation of an older illness that had never been completely eradicated from the system.

None of the medicines ever prescribed for my father did anything to change or improve his condition. Although he was confined to a wheelchair at the end of his life, I don't think that his MS, or EBV, was responsible for that. He had contracted cancer and had undergone quadruple bypass heart surgery. Dad left us in 1987, at 67. I didn't see much of him while I was growing up, something that I will always regret. He was a wonderful man and a good father when he was at home, although we did get into a major conflict during my high school years.

My mom, Ramona, is in her seventies now. She maintains not only her beauty, but an energy level far greater than that of many women twenty years younger than she. A major incident occurred during my teenage years that was to cause a wide rift between us. This split lasted until I was diagnosed with MS, almost a quarter century later.

Since my diagnosis we have grown closer, not only as mother and daughter on terms of mutual respect, but as two women who have faced major challenges in their lives. Today, Mom is interested in nutrition and health and is always on the lookout for new information about MS. Mom often sends me articles and newspaper clippings about MS and has been one of my strongest supporters, even though it seemed sometimes that I was taking far too many risks on far too little evidence. Although I admit that I will never be able to reconcile some of the incidents, those things are in the past for both of us. Instead, we build upon the foundation we have created together over the last five years, and I think that I value her more now than I have at any other time in my life.

Samuel "Skip" Pepe, Jr., my brother, was two years older than I. I always looked up to him, and we were very close. He served in the Army in 1966 and was sent to fight in the Vietnam War. Although he survived his tour of duty, in 1977 he was tragically killed in a fire at the age of twenty-nine. The remainder of my siblings are living today. They have experienced their own medical problems throughout the years, but none have been diagnosed with MS or any other serious or life-threatening illnesses.

Looking back in an attempt to find the cause of my own MS, I remember the first serious illness we experienced was the measles. All of us children contracted it except Rose, who was not yet born. The disease raged through our home in the middle 1950's, ricocheting from one child to another. I was the last to contract it. My case was the worst of the four of us. My brothers all recovered within one to two weeks, but my illness lingered, lasting a month or more. I continued to be weak for quite some time afterward, but was assumed to be cured as time went on and I returned to a normal childhood.

I don't recall any other serious illnesses until I reached age 16. I slipped and fell down a flight of stairs during a teenage argument with a young man named Bobby. Although I didn't realize it, a visit to our family doctor a few days later revealed that I had broken my coccyx, what's commonly known as the tailbone. It had deviated to the left, and even to this day has never fully healed.

After seemingly recovering from this injury, I entered into a serious relationship that was to cause an almost irreparable rift in our family. It was 1967, and I was in my junior year at Camarillo High School, an honor student and junior co-captain of our cheerleading team. Life was full of California sun and fun, and I fell in love with a boy named Billy Medina. I thought he was the best person I had ever known. We went everywhere together, inseparable as only teenage couples can be. He was handsome, kind, caring, and funny. I loved him dearly, and thought of him in terms of forever.

In the eyes of my parents, Billy was the farthest thing from an ideal choice of a date, much less a long-term mate. My father hated him. Dad tried everything he could to separate us. He restricted my movements, eavesdropped on my telephone calls, and grilled my friends in an effort to be certain that I had nothing to do with Billy. Our home became a battleground. The fights were constant, hurtful, and spiteful on both sides.

I could not understand my father's objections. Dad didn't hate Billy for his academic ability: he was an excellent student. He didn't hate him for the way his daughter was treated: Billy always treated me like a princess. No, Dad hated Billy for a far less noble reason, one that really surprised me, seeing how many years he had spent in the military, where all kinds of people were found. In a word, Dad hated the first real love of my life because Billy Medina was Mexican.

My father was one of the most racially prejudiced people I have ever known. In his eyes, there was no way that his nice Italian daughter was going to be touched by someone "not of *our* kind." It was out of the question, too horrible to even be contemplated. I began to feel that I hated my Dad, and was angry at my mother as well, feeling that she should have understood and supported me. She didn't. I made up my mind that regardless of how they felt, there was no way that I was going to stop seeing Billy. I loved him and had no intention of giving him up. There was no way that they could make me.

I was wrong. I had no idea how far my father would go to end our relationship. My parents sold our home and moved the entire family. The public reason given was that my father, employed by Hughes Aircraft, was being transferred, but he let me know in no uncertain terms that the only reason he accepted that transfer in the first place was to do this to me. We moved to an affluent, almost exclusively white suburb of Los Angeles known as Playa Del Ray, located near the Los Angeles International Airport. I was miserable. I lost weight, becoming almost skeletally thin, and experienced a deep and growing depression.

I never saw Billy again, at least, not for years afterward. We did run into each other one more time, in 1974. We were both students at Long Beach State University. The meeting was brief and bittersweet. Although I finally did get the chance to explain to him what had happened, our worlds had grown so far apart that there was no possibility of our old relationship ever resuming. I have never seen or heard from Billy Medina again since that day I saw him on campus.

I entered Westchester High School in Westchester, California in the fall of 1967, my senior year. There was a great deal of stress at home between myself and my parents. We barely spoke, and arguments were commonplace. I became more withdrawn as the depression worsened, growing weaker as I ate less and less. One morning, I didn't come down from my room. I was too weak to move. Until that time, my parents had considered the change in their daughter to be childish sulking over the move and the end of my relationship. They assumed that I would eventually "get over it."

I was extremely ill. Depleted by months of emotional trauma and lack of proper nutrition, I had wasted away to almost nothing. Only semiconscious, I was rushed to the hospital. The diagnosis was mononucleosis and acute depression. I asked my mother about this period recently, and she told me that the doctors never did pinpoint the cause. They prescribed no medications but recommended complete bed rest and fruit juices. I remained bedridden for the next six weeks before eventually returning to school. Slowly, I emerged from my self-imposed exile. I have always been naturally outgoing and friendly, and soon I was enjoying school again. After all, it was my senior year.

The rest of 1967 was not to pass without further injury. A group of us had gone to Big Bear Mountain, a ski resort, looking forward to a day of fun in the snow. The day started out beautifully. We spent several hours on the slopes. Early in the afternoon, some of us decided to go tobogganing. Four of us got a sled and climbed in at the top of the toboggan run. The sun had been shining brightly all morning, and a thin and almost invisible sheet of ice had formed. Unaware, we ran along the top of the course, each of us jumping aboard the sled as it began to pick up speed and began to descend the slope.

The thin ice coating was an ideal surface for a flying sled. We shot into the first turn, screaming with delight. Snow flew from the runners as we leveled out, the toboggan slowing somewhat as we reached the first flat plateau. The scenery whizzed by us, people and trees blending into blurred dark spots against the gleaming white landscape. It was an exhilarating ride. My long hair whipped across my face, the cold air bit at my lungs.

We had gone about two thirds of the way down the slope when it happened. A small branch lay in the path. We struck it, and it caught under the rear left runner. I was seated as the third of four. The rider behind me was a tall young man. He grabbed the end of the branch and pulled sharply, attempting to dislodge it. The sudden shift in his weight caused the rear of the toboggan to fishtail sharply. We shot up over the small embankment of plowed snow and down the other side. The sled hit a broken pine log about ten feet long but only about four inches in diameter. Not enough to shatter the sled, but enough to flip it and send all of us flying into the air.

I was still very thin and flew about ten feet from the crash. I landed with my lower back across another downed limb about the size of a baseball bat. I heard a small sound and felt a sharp pain in the lowest part of my spine, just above my previously broken tailbone. The back of my head hit the snow, and I lost consciousness.

At the hospital, x-rays revealed that I had broken my sacrum, the spinal bone located just above the coccyx. The pain was excruciating. I spent Christmas and the New Year on the living room couch, able only with the aid of crutches to reach the bathroom on the ground floor. My friends stopped by often, bringing other new friends with them. By the time I was mobile and had returned to school again, my circle of new friends had grown to be almost what it once was in Camarillo.

The rest of the school year passed uneventfully except for a car accident I had while driving alone through the L.A. suburb of Inglewood. Hit in the rear, I did sustain a whiplash injury. I wore a soft cervical collar for about two weeks. I graduated from Westchester High School with honors in 1968.

I met Tim Milse shortly before graduation. He became my first serious relationship since I had moved to the area. Tim and I had been intimate for several months when I became pregnant. My parents favored immediate marriage, but Tim's parents objected to our union. I was happy about the pregnancy and looking forward to the child, even without a marriage to the father. It appeared that I was about to become a single mother.

The situation changed radically when Tim was ordered to report for the draft that summer. Tim did not want to become a soldier and sought a way out of the legal obligation. He discovered that fathers were exempt from service provided they were legally married. Tim Milse and I were married in the San Fernando Valley in 1969. Oddly enough, we honeymooned in Solvang, the town just outside of the ranch I live on today.

We returned to live in the Los Angeles area and our beautiful daughter was born late in 1969. I fell in love with her instantly and couldn't wait to take her home. However, tragically, we were never to leave the hospital together. The baby developed respiratory difficulty. Despite all of the best efforts of the doctors and their staff, our daughter died of bilateral pneumonia two days after she was born.

The death of the baby drove me, I think, even closer to the edge of insanity than the loss of Billy Medina. I was angry. Angry at my parents, my in-laws, angry at Tim. Perhaps most of all, I was furious with God. How could He let this happen? Bitter, enraged, and disgusted with the injustice of it all, I felt that since God had certainly turned His back on me, I would turn my back on Him. I was not to enter a church for another ten years.

Less than a year after the baby's death, I had emergency gall bladder surgery. Doctors never determined what exactly caused the organ to malfunction. I still have significant scarring from the operation. After my recovery, I attended West Los Angeles Junior College and obtained an Associate of Arts degree. My marriage was never solid, having been more of a convenience than a commitment. It ended in divorce in 1972.

In 1975, I worked as a TWA stewardess. At this time, I began to become interested in vitamins and nutrition. I was dating a young man named Steve Remphis, a weight lifter who introduced me to the vitamins and supplements he was taking regularly. I began to explore the subject of nutrition myself.

I decided to study nutrition at California's Long Beach State University. I would study during the flights, and attend classes when not flying. On one of those flights, I had a conversation with one of the passengers, a chiropractor. He asked me if I had ever considered becoming a chiropractor. I had not. He explained that chiropractic would be a wonderful way to combine my desire to help people with my growing knowledge of nutrition. Although the idea was intriguing, I put it to the back of my mind, my classes and full-time job already consuming most of my time.

I was also taking elective courses at UCLA, including Kirlian photography, the Russian technique of photographing auras. It was there that I met Leanore, forming a friendship that is still strong. I obtained my bachelor of science in 1975. I continued working for TWA and decided to continue my education in nutrition and began to attend the University of Bridgeport to obtain my master's degree. It was while I was at UBC, I met a man named Buddy Pasero, a chiropractor and lecturer. Buddy was a handsome man of Italian descent. I found him to be intelligent, energetic, charismatic, and a lot of fun. We began dating, and, although neither of us realized it at the time, he was also to be instrumental in determining my life's direction.

One winter evening in late 1975, we were enjoying drinks in my apartment when the conversation turned to my studies in nutrition. Buddy was the second person to ask me if I had ever considered chiropractic work. He echoed the sentiments of the doctor I had spoken with on the plane: that I was smart enough to gain the skills, that I had a naturally compassionate desire to help people, and that chiropractic would be an ideal way to help those in pain while counseling them on the proper nutrition to keep them healthy.

I explained that I didn't have the time. I loved my nutritional studies, and with my flight job, I didn't see how I could take on additional classes. He suggested that I change my focus. I could suspend or reduce the studies for my master's and start to study chiropractic care. I hadn't considered taking the classes at all, much less putting my hard-earned education in my chosen field on hold. I said as much to him.

I'll never know if his next remark was in jest, or half serious. I only know that for me, it was the gauntlet, thrown at my feet with an arrogant flair. Looking at me over the rim of his glass, he said, "Celeste, I guess I was wrong about you. I guess you're just *too stupid* to go to chiropractic school after all. You'd probably never be able to understand it anyway."

Well. Celeste Pepe, honor student, who had paid her own way through school as a waitress on the ground and in the air was not about to let that just fly by. In the silent moment between us, I could hear the gauntlet land. Eyes flashing, I snatched it up, responding with a determined salvo of my own.

"Oh, really?! The hell I couldn't! I could take all of those classes, ace the test, and become the kind of doctor you could only *hope* to be!"

Buddy laughed in that way that men have when they are humoring "the little woman." I wanted to choke him. He spread his hands wide and grinned, insisting that he was only teasing me. I didn't care. That idiot remark rankled. I was determined to show him just who was stupid. I would go to chiropractic school.

Buddy and I still remain friends today. Years later, after my daughter Sara was born, I called him. Buddy had become a fine doctor with an excellent reputation and a large, well-established practice. Even though our practices follow different methodologies, I respect his abilities, and I thank him heartily for challenging me to excel that night. Throughout the years, my patients have benefited from my acceptance of that challenge.

I did indeed begin to study chiropractic medicine. In 1980, I began to attend classes at the Los Angeles College of Chiropractic (L.A.C.C.), located just outside of Los Angeles in Whittier, California. I was also beginning to discover a new spirituality through the practice of Eckankar meditation. Shortly after enrolling at L.A.C.C., I again sustained a significant injury.

Driving a Volkswagen Beetle, I was involved in an auto accident. A speeding pickup truck ran a stop sign and my "Bug" slammed into the side of it, flew into the air and landed two hundred feet away. I was knocked unconscious and sustained a compound fracture of my right ankle, my third broken bone in less than ten years. The only positive was that the injury gave me the opportunity to concentrate on my studies. A flight attendant on crutches was a flight attendant on the ground.

The classes at L.A.C.C. were difficult and detailed. The study of the skeletal and nervous system of the human body is an exacting science. Errors in treatment could hurt the patients more severely than their original injuries. We began to make rounds with experienced chiropractors, observing their diagnoses, treatments, and the manner in which they interacted with their patients.

During this time I met Paul Kerr, the man who was to become my second husband. Not an outstandingly handsome man, he was dark haired, of average build, and over six feet tall; he was one of the most intelligent men of my age I have ever met. Paul was a chiropractic lecturer at the school. We began to study together. We had so much in common. We had the same Catholic upbringing and similar tastes in music, recreation, and entertainment. Our outlook on life was also in harmony. We fell in love.

Paul and I were married in February of 1981. I finally made my peace with God. My marriage was the first time that I had returned to church in over ten years. Our beautiful daughter, Sara, the joy of my life, made her appearance in 1981. Sara was big and beautiful, requiring a Cesarean section. The birth was difficult, and the doctors informed Paul and me that further pregnancies could carry a greater risk. I underwent a tubal ligation in 1982. I have never had any other children.

I received my Doctor of Chiropractic (D.C.) in 1983 and

was eager to begin my new life in practice, although I still wanted to pursue my degree in nutrition. Paul and I had dreamed of going into practice together, perhaps opening the Kerr Chiropractic Center. We could rotate shifts, and I would be able to spend time at home with Sara. After graduation, however, I was shocked to learn that Paul had formed his own plans.

Far from content with his own degree, Paul decided that a D.C. was not an adequate theater for what he considered his own exceptional medical talents. There didn't seem to be the potential for enough prestige in chiropractic medicine to suit Paul, who always craved recognition. Instead of entering into practice, Paul wanted to continue school, becoming an M.D., perhaps a surgeon. I initially supported his decision, even when he wanted to continue his studies in New York. Looking back now, I think that this was my first indication that Paul Kerr was interested most of all in Paul Kerr. He was not about to modify his own plans to make room for mine.

I was adamant about obtaining my nutritional accreditation. In 1984 I earned my second degree, becoming a Doctor of Naturopathic Medicine (N.D). After a short stint in Minnesota, where I got my first taste of real practice with a wonderful doctor, Russell Desmares, we were off to New York City.

Shortly after we arrived in 1986, I was accepted at the Manhattan practice of Dr. Randolph Meltzer. Paul began four years of surgery fellowship. I worked while Paul attended classes, sharpening my skills on the wide variety of patients in Dr. Meltzer's office. The exposure and experience that I gained there has been invaluable throughout the rest of my professional life.

Years later, as I researched multiple sclerosis, I recalled how a complaint could take many different forms and degrees of severity with differences in the gender and racial history of the patients. Undoubtedly, this same diversity has been the biggest impediment to science's discovery of the definite cause of this disease with conventional research. Although many detailed, long-term studies have been conducted over the years, I don't think that any study has included people from such a diversity of origin. It would be interesting to see the results.

After a year with Dr. Meltzer, I felt that I had gained the experience I would need to operate my own practice. In 1987 I opened an office in the Soho section of New York City. Luxuriating in the time I could spend with each of my new patients, I began to find my practice was placing increasingly more emphasis on nutritional counseling.

It was during this time that I developed the "Heart Songs" technique that I am best known for and still use in my private practice today. This healing module not only treats the bone or joint injury of my patient but also addresses the total person, physically and spiritually. Combining sound, music, colors, aromatherapy, Bach flowers, nutrition, vitamins, and chiropractic adjustment, Heart Songs restores the body's inner and outer balance. A body and soul in harmony can release healing energy to repair damage and restore optimum health. I have taught the complete technique to other progressive chiropractors and portions of it to licensed massage therapists and nutritional counselors. All have reported success with their patients, enjoying the satisfaction of seeing a patient who had come to them in pain and stress leave refreshed and restored.

Paul had nearly completed his fellowship. I thought he would soon be taking the exam for his M.D. and begin his own practice. Paul had come to another decision, one that would make his career but irrevocably damage our marriage. He had decided to become a cardiac surgeon. Before I begin to sound equally self-absorbed, I need to mention that Paul's original decision to further his education was already a strain. I spent very little time with our daughter, and almost never saw him, our schedules were so diverse. All of our expenses were my responsibility, requiring long hours at Dr. Meltzer's and later at my own office. Still, I believed in the partnership of marriage. I wanted my husband to be a success, of course. I knew that when he finished school, our financial stress would ease.

It was a strain, however. Not only was I exhausted, I was missing my daughter's early development years. I had handled the overwhelming situation because I thought it was for a finite time period. Paul assumed that he could pursue his goals and I would deal with the prolonged demands on my time and our finances. I resented his attitude and told him as much. Paul was unrelenting. He apologized, explaining that I was such a good wife to him that he never thought that I would mind carrying the burden a little while longer.

I *did* mind, though, very much. I felt I had already made too many sacrifices for Paul's career. My practice was beginning to thrive, however, and for Sara's sake I agreed to continue to support the family while he studied cardiac medicine, on one condition. I owned land just outside Sedona, Arizona. When Paul graduated, I wanted to move west. He could complete his fellowship in either Arizona or Southern California. He readily agreed, and before long, life returned to its status quo.

Almost two more years passed. Paul would soon receive his accreditation and we could leave the New York area. I went briefly to Arizona in the fall of 1989 to obtain my license to practice chiropractic in the state. I returned home just before Thanksgiving to find that the rug had been pulled out from under my unsuspecting feet once again.

Paul was now a cardiac surgeon, a title that would give him the prestige he craved. I was to find out on my return that the deserts of Arizona were not even considered on his list of fellowship choices. His desire was to remain in New York, where he could realize his ambitions. He had no intentions of going anywhere. Furious, I felt that he had lied to me for two years. He would have agreed to anything that would further his plans. We had terrible fights over the next several weeks. I began to realize that more was wrong with my marriage than a conflict in career plans.

Christmas was approaching, and we had an eight-year-old to consider. I focused on preparing for the holiday. Paul was hardly there, so the illusion of holiday happiness continued. I'm glad now that I spent so much time with Sara that holiday season. It was the last time we would be together as a family. Christmas Day brought joy and laughter to my young daughter, as it should have done. Paul and I pretended to be a loving couple. Sara went to bed that night happily exhausted.

Paul and I remained awake after she had gone to bed. We hadn't spoken much lately. Like a lot of spouses in this situation, there had been other things that I had failed to notice. I had been so busy working and spending my free time with my beautiful child that I didn't see the other little clues telling me something else was terribly wrong in my marriage. Perhaps I never would have noticed anything if Paul had at least listed a facility in Arizona as one of his choices for fellowship. But he didn't. He had lied to me. I felt used, hurt, and increasingly angry. Inevitably, there's one little incident, the final puzzle piece that completes the picture. Usually it's something quite innocuous.

During my holiday shopping I had quizzed my daughter on her heart's desires with that age-old question, "So, what do you want Santa to bring you this year?" There was a gift that she really wanted but could not describe to me. She kept telling me that Daddy knew. One morning I decided to call Paul at the hospital and see if he could give me a better description of this much wanted item. I reached the nurses' station on Paul's floor. The nurse who answered thought she recognized my voice. Cheerfully, she said, "Sure, Julie, I'll get him for you. I just saw him in the hall. Hold on . . . "

Julie? All of the doctors Paul worked with were men. Paul got on the line, but I didn't say anything about this odd incident. In fact, I asked him quite pleasantly if he knew about the toy that Sara wanted. Thankfully he did, and I got off of the phone as quickly as possible. I felt sick. The refusal to consider my wishes was bad enough, and now *this* . . .

I said nothing in all the days leading up until Christmas. I never called to find out if he was really at work. I didn't need the additional pain. Christmas night, however, I felt suddenly tired. Tired of the lies, tired of the extra workload, tired of pretending that we had the perfect family. In short, I was tired of Paul. I was seated in the parlor, sipping some heated wine. Over the rim of my mug, I asked him quietly, "Who's Julie?"

He jumped as if he'd been shot, then recovered, but not quickly enough. In that instant, I no longer had suspicions. I *knew*. And the knowing made me furious. I firmly believe that nobody fights like Italians. From the clouds on my face, this storm was shaping up to be a whopper. Paul could have done any number of things in that next moment that would have diffused the situation. He could have acted surprised, wounded, amused. Every wife wants to doubt herself when she gets to this point. It takes a lot for a woman to want to break up her home, especially if children are involved. But, no, Paul didn't do any of these things. He became condescending as if speaking to a retarded child.

"What the *hell* are you talking about, Celeste? What are you implying now? Is this some new tack of yours? Gonna hold some bullshit you've cooked up in your head over mine? You think this'll make me say, 'Okay, honey, screw New York! Let's move to Boy Howdy, Arifuckingzona' so I can spend the rest of my life as kindly Dr. Paul, with his dog and his pickup truck? Well, it won't. There is no way that I'm moving to some backwater, Neanderthal state that doesn't even have daylight savings time! I didn't go through all of this for that!"

Arrogant prick! I exploded. "*You've* gone through?! What did *you* go through? You went to school, playing doctor in some hospital while I worked my friggin' butt off to pay for everything that this family needed! I'm here trying to figure out how to spend more time with my kid and still pay for our lives while you're out there trying to figure out how to spend more time with *Julie* and who knows who else without fucking up your meal ticket! You *bastard!*"

The battle raged on. When it's ending, you drag out the heavy artillery that you've stored for ages, the really hurtful stuff that doesn't get used unless you no longer care if the marriage is destroyed. I told him that'd I'd had an offer of a job in Sedona and would leave without him if he didn't honor our agreement. I also wasn't paying one more bill. The responsibility for the house and our family were all on his head now. I had taken my turn, and now it was his. Of course, he could always get *Julie* to help him pay for it.

He countered with the threat that I'd never see Sara again if I left. That stopped me, but only for a moment. It would be hard for Sara if I took her with me at that time. She was on winter recess from the school, teacher, and classmates she loved. She wouldn't even get the chance to say good-bye. My father had done that to me. I'd be damned if I would do it to her. I couldn't take her with me and I didn't want to leave her. I loved Sara more than anything in the world. The thought of life without her was horrifying. I hesitated, and Paul saw it. It didn't suit his purposes that I leave just now. Smiling at me, he offered what he thought was the perfect reason to stop this nonsense.

"C'mon, Celeste. You know you're not leaving. Look, it's not as if we can't work this out. I'll get my appointment to a hospital right here in New York where everything is happening. We'll get a bigger house, Sara can go to private school. We'll get you a nice office in Great Neck. You'll get better patients and make a lot more money. Besides, it's not like you can't do what you do anywhere, is it? It's *only* chiropractic, for Crissakes! That nutrition thing is a nice extra you can always add to the bill. It's not as if you were doing heart surgery."

I stood for a long moment letting his thoughtless words sink in. He was so self-absorbed. Not only didn't he care about my feelings, he didn't think that what I did was at all important. It was a nice hobby that the missus could play at while he was doing medical miracles. Never mind the fact that he had once been a teaching chiropractor. No, Paul had gone on to be a *real* doctor. I knew that I could no longer live with this man, not another day. In a voice as hard and as quiet as stone, I spoke only one sentence to him.

"Go straight to hell, you selfish, rotten *bastard*." I went to our bedroom and slammed the door behind me. I flung myself across our bed, too emotionally drained to cry. I lay there for a long time, finally falling asleep.

As it happened, a very dear friend was getting married in Kansas City in two days. We were invited to attend the wedding. I decided to go alone. I needed to get away, to think things out, and this was the perfect opportunity. Sara would have to understand. If not now, then someday. I explained to her that I was going to the wedding. Daddy couldn't go, but I had to or my good friend would feel very sad. I didn't tell her anything else. Always sensitive to the feelings of others, Sara agreed that I should go to make my friend happy. And so, on December 26, 1989, I found myself on a plane to the Midwest. I knew that my marriage was over. I just hoped that my relationship with my daughter would not be.

After the wedding, instead of returning to New York I flew on to Tucson, having decided to accept the position that had been offered to me earlier that year. They understood that I couldn't start right away. I had my practice in New York to conclude, and now I would have a divorce to deal with as well. I remained in Arizona for about a week before returning to New York. I stayed in a downtown hotel and saw Sara as much as possible, but our times together were difficult. She didn't understand why I had left. Her father had tried to convince her that Mommy didn't care about her. Although she fought buying into it completely, I knew how relentless Paul could be. I'd thrown a wrench into his plans, and this was his revenge. He was trying to turn my daughter against me.

Many times after our visits together I found myself in tears. As much as I'd tried to prevent it, my kid was suffering. Paul was using her as leverage between us. To this day, I regret that Sara ever had to go through that. It was so unfair to her. Finally, I had enough of Paul's deceptions. When summer came again, I returned to New York and took my nine-year-old back to Arizona with me.

Sara loved Arizona. I spent lots of time with her, exploring, riding horses, hiking, visiting the local Indians. I repaired all of the damage that Paul had done. In my turn, I did nothing to injure her belief that he also loved her.

Paul sued for custody in his divorce papers, as did I. The court recommended I remain in visiting distance during the proceedings. After that wonderful summer in Arizona, I resigned my position and returned with Sara to New York. She was so happy to see her father that I questioned the wisdom of pursuing the divorce. Paul had his fellowship now, self-supporting once again. We could reopen the proceedings when Sara was older, better able to handle the breakup.

After speaking with close mutual friends, I realized that such thoughts were unrealistic. Paul was openly involved with other women. I gave up. My thoughts were for Sara, but she couldn't possibly benefit from watching her parents live a charade. No, it was over. Neither of us considered our marriage to be worth saving.

The divorce was a nasty four-year battle. When it was over, I didn't want to stay in New York any longer. Jerry and I had become involved by that time, and when he invited me to live with him on the ranch, I accepted. Sara chose to remain in New York with her father. I think she felt sorry for him, afraid he would be lonely.

Today, Sara attends a fine Northeastern college and lives with friends. She splits her holidays between us. After he remarried, Paul became much more agreeable to Sara's visits during the remainder of her school years. We speak now on matters related to our daughter, and he consults me when decisions need to be made. We've moved on with our lives. I don't think that there are regrets on either side. There are none on mine, anyway.

Five years later, in 1996, I opened my own healing facility. Located in Solvang, California, the Healing Valley Wellness Center (HVWC) combines all of my chiropractic and naturopathic practice techniques. I have also added sauna, spa and water therapy, professional muscle massage, ozone therapy, and other alternative healing techniques. HVWC was a full-time job, and I thrived on it. I never failed to put in at least some time there each week while I sought a cure for my own affliction.

I still own the Center, although I temporarily suspended operations in order to be able to devote my time to this book. I plan on reopening the facility when this project is completed. I will focus on MS patients and their families, offering lectures and healing and teaching sessions that will educate the patients and help expedite their own healing.

I was to learn through further research into emotional and physical traumas and their effects on MS that the major incidents in my life may have indeed played a part in the condition of my immune system and overall physiology. All of us have emotional highs and lows in our lives. It is part of the human experience. However, it is my belief that extreme emotional episodes, including prolonged stress, may have adverse long-term effects, enhancing the likelihood of contracting severe or debilitating illness. I will discuss specifically how these episodes and injuries may have been contributing factors to my MS in later chapters.

I was to learn through further research into emotional and physical traumas and their effects on MS that the major incidents in my life may have indeed played a part in the condition of my immune system and overall physiology. It is my belief that extreme emotional episodes, including prolonged stress, may have adverse long-term effects, enhancing the likelihood of contracting severe or debilitating illness.

I finished the sessions with Dr. Huggins and Dr. Levy in less than a month. Before I left, another blood test was ordered to check my mercury levels. They had dropped, but remained at about ten units, three times the recommended safe amount. Dr. Huggins recommended I undergo chelation therapy, a series of injections that would remove the remaining excess mercury from my system. I decided to undergo the therapy, but I couldn't remain in Colorado Springs for the sessions. Dr. Huggins referred me to a California progressive dentist, Dr. Stephen O'Dell. I would contact him upon my return.

I returned home in time for the holidays in 1994, eager to begin the chelation therapy. But first, I wanted to talk to an old friend, a clinical nutritionist by the name of Bob Santoro. Bob had developed a phenomenal testing method for determining not only the level of heavy metals and other possibly toxic substances in the system, but virtually every substance found in the blood, tissues, and other components of the body.

After the tests that specifically measured only mercury, I began to wonder what other essential elements of my internal composition were presently in excess, or even lacking. Could these imbalances have contributed to my contraction of MS? And could their continued misalignment enable the disease to grow stronger, to progress through my system? I was determined to find out as I began the next stage of my journey.

4
Looking Inside—BioCybernetics, Chelation, Ozone Therapy

I was glad to be home in California. I was glad to see Jerry. I had missed the ranch and our staff. I was also eager to continue my search to be rid of MS, and in California I had all of the contacts of my professional and social life at my disposal.

Jerry was delighted to see me. The restful period that I had spent in Colorado had certainly helped, as had the daily saunas. My leg was still slightly unpredictable, but so much better than it had been when I left. I wasn't using a cane, and I felt full of energy, even after the flight and lengthy drive back to the ranch. I had returned just before Jerry's birthday, and plans had been made to celebrate at one of our favorite places in Santa Barbara, a continental restaurant with a bar and a dance floor.

I have always loved to dance. I was a cheerleader at Camarillo High, I knew formal dancing, and, yes, I loved those disco nights. I was always one of the first out on the floor and the last to leave. I could dance for hours, still going strong long after my companions were collapsed in their chairs. I hadn't gone dancing since before I'd gone to Hawaii, before this whole thing started. I was delighted by the idea. As soon as we reached the ranch, I hurried inside to shower and change for the evening.

I spent a lot of time getting ready. I have always loved beautiful clothes and a wide variety of styles. I found just the perfect dress to wear to the place we were going, a tight black sheath covered with a very fine crystalline web, nearly invisible in normal light, but that would glint like sparks under the mirrored lights of the dance floor. My hair, my face, my nails, soon everything was perfect. I almost ran down the steps to join Jerry, waiting by our bar for me. With a woman's secret satisfaction, I noted the look of pleasure on his face as he took in my appearance. We shared a quick drink together, and then we were off to the long white car patiently waiting outside.

Even though I had been with Jerry for several years, times like these always made me feel like a princess, or maybe a famous movie star. He never spared expense for anything he wanted to do, or anyone who was with him. When you were out with Jerry, it was first class all the way. We chatted happily during the drive, Jerry interested in my adventures in Colorado, listening intently to all that I said, occasionally interjecting a question or comment. After a short drive, we'd arrived at the restaurant. Once inside, I found that our good friends were waiting for us. And so, three other couples joined us at a large, well-placed semicircular booth near the dance floor. We could watch the dancers while we ate.

These were very good friends of ours, people whom we enjoyed, and who likewise enjoyed us. Most of them had not seen me since my diagnosis. They, too, were interested in my story as I brought them up to speed through our meal. Flatteringly, the remark was made several times that I looked so fabulous, they were sure that I must be almost well. Perhaps they were right. Perhaps the root cause of this disease was indeed mercury poisoning, as Dr. Huggins firmly believed. Maybe after I had finished with chelation therapy, I would be cured.

A warm and cheerful glow surrounded our circle of friends as we finished our meals and leaned back, relaxing against the leather seats. We chatted pleasantly while, on the dance floor, the partners twirled and gyrated, moving to the infectious beat of a popular dance tune. I began to feel the music inside of me, and soon, when someone suggested we join the moving figures, I was one of the first to slide from my seat, my body already enveloped in rhythm almost before my feet touched the polished, gleaming floor.

We had been dancing for a short time, perhaps ten minutes, when I began to feel something was wrong. I began to feel a twinge in the muscle of my left thigh. Out of practice, I thought ruefully. I danced on, whirling around Jerry to spin away and then back again. Prancing backward, I brushed up against another dancer, knocking us both slightly off balance. He laughed from above me, and I, too, smiled an apology, words impossible over the volume. My mind was seized by a sudden, disturbing realization. I spun again towards Jerry, and he saw the cloud pass across my face.

"What's wrong?" he asked, shouting to be heard above the din.

"Nothing!" I answered, and smiled up at him, continuing to move to the music. I came in close to him and we danced together, my face too close to his chest for him to see my expression of growing concern. There was, however, something definitely wrong.

I didn't feel the man who had danced into my leg. In an effort to make it seem part of my dance moves, I slid both of my hands down the sides of my thighs, twisting seductively in front of a very appreciative Jerry. I reached my knees, the panic beginning to rise within me concealed from my partner as I kept my head slightly lowered, my long hair hiding my face. I slid my hands upward, curving the tips of my fingers slightly so that the nails were in contact with my stockinged limbs. My right leg felt the pressure of my long nails, the skin instinctively shuddering against it. My left leg felt nothing.

A dead numbness stretched across my thigh, beginning just above my knee and traveling to my hip. I dug my index nail into my leg, noting with clinical detachment that it had been hard enough to break the skin. Nothing. No twinge, no pain, not even the sensation of pressure. The only concrete evidence I had that even suggested that I had scratched myself was the welling line of red that grew on my skin.

Suddenly, I was seized with the fear I would fall. I had to sit down, get off of the dance floor before I couldn't feel anything at all. The tune that was blasting was coming to an end, and I finished the dance. As people clapped and laughed, engaging in hurried conversations before the beat began again, I wove my way through the other dancers and returned to our booth.

Those last few feet were terrifying. I kept imagining that my leg would give out at any moment. I think the idea of public acknowledgment of my weakness, and the embarrassment of losing my feet in front of all of these strangers was far more loathsome than fear of the actual fall. I collapsed into our booth, my heart pounding. My companions were still out there, and so I sat massaging my leg muscles while I attempted to gather my thoughts.

"There you are!" Jerry's hearty voice boomed into my reverie. I started and looked up at him. My face showed immediately that something was wrong, and an instant later he had slid into the booth beside me, his voice full of concern. "What is it, honey?"

I saw no reason to bluff him. The numbness had grown since I had been sitting there, reappearing below my left knee and extending down my calf. I was beginning to lose feeling in my toes. As the feeling in my leg receded, my fear grew. With growing dread, I realized what was happening. I had felt this way before. My leg had acted just like this on that mountainside in Hawaii.

"I can't feel my leg, Jerry," I answered him, my voice low but obviously shaken.

I saw fear reflected in his eyes, but, typical Jerry, he needed confirmation. "What do you mean, Celeste? What's wrong with you?"

I had no patience for this right now. Exasperated, I burst out, "I mean, I can't feel my fucking leg! No thigh, no calf, no friggin' foot! I can barely make it move, and I don't think that I can stand on it, let alone walk. Tell me . . . what part of that statement is obscure?"

His face lost all of its color as he realized I was deadly serious. "Oh, God. Do you want to call the paramedics?"

I almost struck him. "No, I don't want the parafuckingmedics! I want to get out of here. *Now!* Go find our driver and get him to bring the car up to the door. I'll lean on you. I'll make it. I just want out of here before it gets any worse, and I end up looking like an idiot."

"What should I say to our friends? We can't just *leave*. They're our guests."

He was right. Of course it would be rude to our friends to leave them flat, without so much as a goodnight. At that moment, though, the teachings of Emily Post were not foremost in my mind. Distractedly, I replied, "I don't *care* what the hell you tell them. Tell them I'm sick, tell them I'm drunk. Tell them I'm tired from my trip. Look, tell them I've been abducted by space aliens for all I care right now. Tell them whatever you like, but get me out of here!" He rose to do as I asked, but I grabbed his arm, stopping him as he headed back out onto the dance floor to find our companions. "First, find our driver and get the car."

In the end, I was left to explain it myself to our friends. While Jerry was locating our driver and the car, one of the women that we were with returned to the table. Laughing and out of breath, she flopped into the booth beside me. "Well, this is a switch! You're usually still dancing long after we've given up, gasping for oxygen." She leaned forward, smiling. "You okay, honey?"

"Absolutely," I lied. "Just perfect." My years of experience as a flight attendant, skilled in the delivery of soothing political answers to passengers stood me in good stead as I smoothly provided the perfect answer. "I'm just a little tired. I only got back into town earlier today, after all. I really am falling asleep. I think we'll be leaving. Jerry's already gone for the car."

My companion detected no subterfuge in my reply. A fine hostess in her own right, she responded beautifully, just as I'd hoped she would. "You sit here, Celeste. I'll go get the others so that we can all say goodnight. Come to think of it, we've got a babysitter that has school in the morning. I'm sure her mother won't appreciate it if we stay out too much longer. And," she laughed, putting her hand gently on my arm, "you know how hard it is to get a good sitter nowadays!"

I could have kissed her. Still laughing, she floated off into the dancing crowd to find her husband and our other friends while I sat in the booth, waiting for them and Jerry, trying to look cool and unconcerned. While I had the chance, I maneuvered my largely dead limb with my hands under the table, moving it into a position that would allow me to rise from the table gracefully on the support of Jerry's arm. I hated to lie, especially to such valued friends as these, but I didn't see the need to ruin everybody's evening with the truth. There was nothing they could have done about the situation, anyway.

Jerry returned to find me seated with all of our friends, sharing one last drink for the road. If my conversation seemed a little too scripted, my eyes a little too bright, no one noticed but Jerry, and he covered for me beautifully. We were able to leave the club without anyone we knew well noticing my distress. Outside, Jerry practically lifted me into the car. Our driver, concerned but discreet as always, gave me a look that spoke volumes but offered no other comment. Once inside the car, Jerry gathered me into his arms. I went willingly, and spent the rest of the ride home curled in his embrace, gripping his hand hard, staring at and saying nothing. At the ranch, he looked down at my leg and then at my face, questioningly. Woodenly, I shook my head. He exited the car, scooped me up in his arms, and carried me to our bedroom.

Balanced on the edge of the bed, I undressed, throwing my clothes carelessly onto the floor. I pulled a night shirt over my head and slid between the covers, my left leg totally unresponsive now, like it was encased in a heavy plaster cast. I lay there for some minutes before I realized that I was crying. I didn't bother to check the tears, which began to flow faster down my makeup-streaked cheeks. I felt Jerry come into the bed beside me, settling down himself. I made no effort to disguise my emotions. With a wordless sound, suddenly he gathered me to him, stroking my hair and uttering those soft sounds of comfort that pass between mates at times like these.

I thought I was doing so well. My leg had been almost normal for the last couple of weeks. I had energy, I felt great. Dr. Huggins firmly believed that mercury poisoning was the cause of MS, and he had removed it from my teeth. Then I had the saunas, and Dr. Levy's new test showed that my mercury levels had dropped. Why, then, did this happen? If I was getting better, why was my leg doing this to me? Did this mean I was getting *worse*, or I was too far gone for the filling removal to help? This was so damned unfair! After bottling it all up for so long, I finally broke down. I cried as I hadn't since the day my infant daughter was buried. Jerry held me close, saying nothing but offering all of the comfort in the world by his silent, encompassing arms. I sobbed for a long time, finally falling asleep out of emotional exhaustion.

I couldn't walk for a week. During that time, Jerry showered me with presents: flowers, new perfume, Bavarian chocolates, candied fruit. I finally begged him laughingly to stop bringing me things to eat every time he came through the door, or I would soon be too fat to ever get out of the bed, no matter how good my leg felt. The next day, he suggested I return to Dr. Curatalo, perhaps to get a shot. I was adamant about not taking the Betaseron, even after this incident, and he subsided without pressing me further.

While I was bedridden, I continued to search for a cure to this condition, driven now more than ever by the notion that I was racing against time. I didn't want anything else on my body to go numb before I figured it out. My leg was not bouncing back, by any means, and I heard the small voice of a growing concern that whispered that it might never return to normal. I also knew I had to look beyond mercury poisoning as the cause for my MS. There had to be other factors that either contributed to or influenced the disease. I needed to determine what these were and discover how to correct or eliminate them.

One of the practices that I had followed for several years prior to my diagnosis with MS was directly related to the nutritional counseling I gave patients while at Body, Mind and Soul. As do many other doctors, I received numerous magazines, publications, and articles related to my field. Sometime during the fall of 1990, I read one such article on alternative approaches to nutrition entitled "Space Age Nutrition Through BioCybernetics." It was written by a Dr. Diamante. It discussed a new theory on nutrition being researched and developed by a New York team of clinical nutritionists, Robert Santoro and Alfred Weyhreter.

Santoro and Weyhreter had developed a new type of computer-based data analysis that would record and interpret data gained from hair, blood, and urine analyses. This program would not only record the data on almost every element present in the human body and measure each concentration, but also analyze that data and make the nutritional recommendations for each patient on an individual basis. Naturally, I found this exciting, because such a procedure, if viable, would eliminate a lot of the guesswork that went along with nutritional counseling. Some excesses or deficiencies of nutrients were not symptomatic unless the condition was chronic or severe, and several symptoms cross correlated to a number of different nutritional imbalances.

I called Bob Santoro shortly after I read the article. I wanted more information about their procedure. Perhaps it was something that I could either directly utilize in my own practice, or steer my patients toward as testing they should consider having performed for themselves. Bob is a wonderful, dedicated professional. A bit shorter than average, slightly built, with dark hair, he is a definite contrast to his counterpart,

Al Weyhreter, who is a tall, robust man. Both, however, have passionate conviction about nutrition and their program. At our initial meeting, I instantly liked Bob and was most impressed by the depth and detail of the research he had done. We discussed our relative viewpoints on nutrition as the cornerstone of health, and I was pleased to discover that our views were similar. Bob had been involved in the field of nutritional research and study for nearly ten years when I first met him.

He explained the process of BioCybernetics, and the theory behind its development. As he opened up this new line of thought to me, I realized that not only was he a dedicated scientist, he was a wonderful teacher as well. A member of the International American Internal Association of Clinical Nutritionists, he is the author of several articles and published studies in the nutritional field.

He left me with one such study for my review, written with his colleague, Al Weyhreter. Published in the *Journal of Applied Nutrition* (Santoro and Weyhreter 1993, 45:48-60), it explained how the level of elements necessary for optimal organ function could be affected by the ingestion of nutritional supplements distilled from corresponding animal organs. For instance, when attempting to restore function or repair damage to the human pancreas, Santoro and Weyhreter used nutrients originating from a pig's pancreatic organs. These organs are specially processed to remove not only the fats, but any chemicals, pesticides, or other contaminants that may also be present.

When the process is complete, only the proteins and enzymes that comprise the essence of these organ tissues remain. These remaining substances are then molded into pill form, which the patient takes orally. These nutrient substances, when released through digestion into the bloodstream, find the corresponding organs in the human body and become part of their substance, restoring functionality and beginning to repair the damaged human organ by regenerating the organ cells.

These two scientists confirmed their theory by applied clinical research. The procedure was tested on two human organs—the liver and the pancreas—and one gland, the thyroid. The tests were conducted on diverse groups of patients of varying sizes, results measured by their own beginning data and control or placebo groups. In the case of the thyroid trial, Santoro and Weyhreter were able to show that the T-4, or thyroxin level inside of the gland, can be changed by the ingestion of these nutrients. Low T-4 readings could be increased after the raw organ concentrate was taken by the patient for a measured period of time. This is especially significant to those suffering from thyroid imbalance, as, even presently, conventional medicine routinely prescribes the artificial supplement Synthroid for the condition. These clinical tests proved that the same results could be achieved through the use of natural nutrient supplements instead, with none of the side effects possible with the artificial substance.

As is common with most new studies published that contradict established knowledge or prescription procedure, Santoro and Weyhreter's work was challenged later by a physician in Texas who disputed their findings. In response, the team sought out and obtained the services of an independent biostatistical analyst to confirm or refute their findings. They selected the globally known and widely respected Susan Shott, eminent professor at Chicago's St. Luke's Hospital, to perform the reanalysis. Without predisposing her to awareness of their desired conclusion, the researchers submitted the raw data to Professor Shott. Her conclusions confirmed their findings on all points, and Santoro and Weyhreter published a follow-up article shortly afterward that illustrated her confirmation of the accuracy of their testing procedures and the data generated from them.

I was so impressed by their technique that I immediately made plans to attend their next lecture series. Taught by both men, these classes explained the three types of tests required to gather the data on each patient, the BioCybernetics procedure itself, and the significance of the picture of biochemical individuality that resulted. Once the exact levels of the vitamins, nutrients, chemicals, and metals in each patient's system are accurately depicted, nutrient substances can be prescribed that will correct any existing imbalances, thereby allowing each individual to reach a level of optimum health as determined by his own analysis and particular needs. At the conclusion of each teaching series, certification as a recognized BioCybernetics counselor was given to those who had successfully completed the course. I became certified in early 1991, and continue to use BioCybernetics analyses as an important tool in my practice today.

I called Bob Santoro and spoke to him at length during the time that I was confined with my leg. I had not spoken to him since before my diagnosis with MS. His immediate response was that I should have another complete analysis done as soon as possible. Logically, he was interested in pinpointing what was out of balance in my system and then determining the best course of action to correct the conditions.

Bob Santoro and Al Weyhreter are two of my heroes. I had a real advantage over other patients diagnosed with MS as I'd already undergone BioCybernetics analyses periodically for almost four years prior to the onset of the MS. Already equipped with a basic knowledge of my biochemical composition, I had been much more dedicated than others may have been to eating what I believed to be the proper types of foods that would provide the nutrients that I thought were necessary to maintain my good health. As you will learn later, I found that I would need to make adjustments in my diet.

As soon as I was up and at least partially mobile again, I gathered the samples necessary for the analyses and sent them away to New York so that Bob and Al could evaluate them. It would be several weeks before the results came back to me, but still I felt that I had taken another positive step toward determining the cause of my affliction and therefore was that much closer to learning how to correct it.

I also made contact with the offices of Dr. Stephen O'Dell, the alternative dentist in Morrow Bay, California. Dr. Huggins had recommended him as someone who could perform the chelation therapy he was certain I needed to cleanse my system of the remaining excess mercury. I spoke with Dr. O'Dell at length by telephone before my first visit with him. Dr. Huggins had already briefed him on my case and had sent Dr. O'Dell copies of the dental repair and replacement work he had performed along with the results of the blood tests for mercury levels. I quickly brought him up to speed on the events that had occurred since my return from Colorado Springs. Less than a week after we spoke together, I was on my way to Morrow Bay to begin the treatments.

Dr. O'Dell, although a fully certified and accredited dentist performing conventional dentistry, is also an individual open to alternative dental and health practices. He concurs with Dr. Huggins that mercury and other toxic metals may cause or contribute to many different afflictions. After becoming familiar with the work of Dr. Huggins, Dr. O'Dell no longer uses mercury or silver amalgam fillings, crowns, or caps in his dentistry. He focuses on the replacement of these old fillings in his patients with biologically friendly porcelain compounds. There were still two teeth that had to have old fillings replaced, and Dr. O'Dell would do that in addition to performing the chelation.

The word chelation (key-LAY-shun) describes a process in which toxic metals are stripped, or chelated, from the body. This is done through a series of intravenous injections with a substance known as DMPS, which binds to the mercury and other heavy metals that are present in the blood, converting them to waste materials, which are then eliminated from the system through the urine. The amount of toxins removed in this way is measured by periodic urinalysis.

On my first visit, I was injected with the DMPS. I also had the two remaining old fillings removed and replaced. I was to return to Dr. O'Dell weekly until I had completed the recommended twenty-five sessions. If my mercury levels remained high after these treatments, Dr. O'Dell would refer me to a chelation specialist to complete any additional removal necessary. Each week, I would receive a new injection, and the amount of metals that were being eliminated would be measured by a urine sample I provided at the beginning of each visit. Periodically, a new blood analysis would be performed as well, to measure the amount of mercury that still remained in my system.

DMPS chelation can become a relatively expensive process, the injections and office sessions costing a hundred dollars per visit. Some of the better insurance and health plans recognize this type of chelation as a legitimate healing module, but only after referral for the procedure is made from a recognized physician or dentist. If after having an analysis performed you find that your heavy metal levels are also too high, check with your health insurance provider to be certain that you are covered for the treatment. Regardless of your coverage, I still strongly recommend this cleansing therapy to any patient who is shown to have high levels of toxic metals. As I said when I initially made the decision to undergo DMPS chelation, even if the toxic metal excesses are not directly related to MS (and I think that there is a significant amount of data that suggest that they are) your body does not need the burden of dealing with any toxic substance while it is trying to fight MS or any autoimmune disease.

While I was going to Dr. O'Dell, I began hormone replacement therapy, initially with him, and then later with the specialist that I was to see after Dr. O'Dell's portion of my treatments had been completed. Dr. O'Dell, through research and his own experience with MS patients, believed that, in female cases at least, the onset of MS was additionally associated more often than not with a drop in hormone levels, particularly progesterone and testosterone. Experienced by women, typically as they approached or began to enter middle age, or after a hysterectomy or tubal ligation, the drop in the production of these hormones appeared to be somehow related to the body's susceptibility to MS, and perhaps other autoimmune diseases as well.

Dr. O'Dell attempted to counter this tendency with hormone replacement. He began to give me DHEA supplements, the theory being that the drop in production of these hormones could be negated by the ingestion of replacements equal to what the body would be producing at healthier times in life. DHEA is another hormone, an element like progesterone and testosterone and also found in steroids. It is increasingly prescribed for women who are having a difficult time with menopause. Dr. O'Dell administered it in a liquid form obtained from Clark Pharmaceuticals, located in Washington State. I would take this supplement each day, about ten drops, mixed in fruit juice.

Through another of his ongoing studies, live cell analysis, Dr. O'Dell would check the composition of my system for the relative amounts of these elements present. A drop of my blood was placed on a microscopic slide and treated with a special dye for visibility. Dr. O'Dell could then study the composition and the structure of the cells themselves, searching for flaws in the cellular walls. By introducing other color-keyed substances to the slide and measuring the rate of absorption into the interior of the cells, he could determine the porosity of the cell—the ability to accept and expel materials through the cell membrane.

This type of study is especially important for MS patients. As we will explore in more detail in the second section of this book, the ability of the cells of the nervous system to pass substances through their membranes becomes crucial in determining the strength or weakness of the transfer of electrical energy between the protective outer layer of nervous system cells and the cells of the nerves themselves. Poor electrical energy transfer is responsible for loss of motion, lack of muscle control, and numbness or weakness in the extremities. As I was experiencing just these symptoms, I was most interested in this research.

Ever interested in healing methods that would lead me to a cure, I agreed to participate in Dr. O'Dell's experiments. My desire to become a "human guinea pig" was far from foolish, although I know it seemed that way to many of the people in my life at the time the experiments took place. I felt that I would be able to view the results from a unique dual perspective, that of both physician and patient. There would be no possibility of erroneous data or misperception with myself as the subject. I would be able to control conditions to maintain strict adherence to the protocol, judge the internal reactions of my own body, and accurately monitor the results.

Throughout the course of this healing journey, there would be several therapies that I would try. Some caused adverse reactions, and I discontinued those. Some produced either no reaction or no significant improvement in my condition, so I also abandoned those after a time. My story will address only those that I found to be either directly related to the treatment and reversal of MS, or that have had a positive effect on elimination of other conditions that impede the healing process as a whole.

Another healing module I explored during this period was ozone therapy. Ozone therapy is the addition of oxygen to all of the water in your personal environment, drinking and bathing, and introduction of extra oxygen into the bloodstream through every bodily orifice. The purpose of this therapy is to use oxygen to kill any viral organisms that may be present in the system. Many viral infections have a high mortality rate when exposed to pure or high concentrations of oxygen. Introducing these heightened levels of oxygen thereby increases the body's resistance level and lowers its susceptibility to infectious diseases.

Increased oxygen in the bloodstream also aids in the transfer of other substances between cells, not only in the vascular system, but in muscle and fat cells as well. It helps the cells to expel waste gases and materials. The bacteria killed by the oxygen are converted into a type of cellular ash that is transported from the cells and into the body's waste system, where it is removed through bodily elimination of stool and urine.

The technique, like so many others I was to discover that were relevant to MS patients, originated in Germany. I became aware of the practice through an article in a nutritional journal. Ozone therapy equipment consists of two major components: a small cylinder of O_2, pure oxygen, and a converter, or filter mechanism that converts it to O_3, ozone, much along the same lines of an air filter in a fish tank. The filter ends in a slim cylindrical adapter that is inserted into the water the patient will drink or bathe in, or it can be inserted painlessly into all bodily orifices. The entire procedure takes about ten or fifteen minutes and can be performed every other day.

So eager was I to rid my body of all types of harmful bacteria that I began to use the equipment when it arrived without delay. I oxygenated my drinking and bath water. I used the equipment on every orifice of my body, except for my nose. Using ozone therapy on the nose can produce bleeding in the sensitive sinus membranes or cause severe headaches if any material in the sinuses is pushed upward by the force of the gas.

Within a week, I had discovered that doing a thing to excess does not always mean it will produce expedited results. I experienced a healing crisis of sorts. After my first home treatment, I felt fantastic. No, my leg wasn't any stronger that I could tell, but the rest of me felt shiny inside, like a brand-new penny. I went on an ozone spree. I oxygenated everything I thought it would work on, including all parts of myself. Instead of doing the therapy as recommended once per day, every other day, I started using it a couple of times *every* day.

It worked, all right. In fact, it worked too well. I must have had more bacteria than I had imagined in my system, because the ash produced by the action of the oxygen began to build up in my nose and on the back of my throat, producing sneezing, mucus, phlegm, and other almost flu-like symptoms. I had to suspend the treatments until my body balanced itself out again. Through experience, I learned that, even though I was feeling wonderful—a natural result of the additional oxygen in my bloodstream—I needed to give my body time to eliminate the accumulated debris of dead bacteria to prevent a reoccurrence of buildup. After the flu symptoms had subsided, I began the therapy again, but did not make the same mistake twice. I followed the protocol as recommended, still feeling great, but without the adverse reactions.

I consider ozone therapy to be an important step in the treatment and eventual cure for MS. It kills bacterial and viral infections and increases the ability of your cells to absorb and expel substances and gases, and to transmit the ever-important electrical nerve impulses your body requires to maintain a full range of motion and sensation. I recommend it for virtually all MS patients. The equipment is relatively easy to obtain, and not expensive. A small cylinder of oxygen will last for some time if you use it properly, and replacement cylinders can usually be had from your local propane or welding supplier.

I consider ozone therapy to be an important step in the treatment and eventual cure for MS. It kills bacterial and viral infections and increases the ability of your cells to absorb and expel substances and gases, and to transmit the ever-important electrical nerve impulses your body requires to maintain a full range of motion and sensation.

I still oxygenate my drinking water regularly, and my bath water when I am feeling stressed or run down. I also use it in bodily orifices, though not with the frequency that I did in the beginning. My present excellent state of health does not require that I do so. Still, I like to take the treatment at least once a week, if only to guard against the buildup of any bacteria that may be forming inside of me.

I received a very positive encouragement from Dr. O'Dell during one of my visits. He had the results of my blood tests, and the mercury levels were dropping. Both he and I were excited and pleased with this important development. I was about a third of the way through my twenty-five sessions, and we were already noticing measurable reduction in the mercury, as well as in other heavy metals. In addition, he was surprised to note the high oxygen level in my blood. It was greater than normal for an average person, and far greater than that of the average MS patient. He commented upon it, and I told him about the ozone therapy. Delighted, he concurred that this new healing module I was using was a positive step. In fact, he insisted that it was "the best blood that I have ever seen." He encouraged me to continue to pursue the therapy, but smilingly cautioned against overdoing it again.

My teeth were finished by the spring of 1995, but my chelation sessions were not. Dr. O'Dell realized that the drive to his office was a lengthy one, and so, after discussing it with me, referred me to a chelation specialist located near my home, in Santa Barbara. Dr. Hoegerman would take my sessions the remainder of the way. He was also a progressive practitioner, an M.D. who used alternative medicine in his treatments. Dr. O'Dell told me that "Hogey" was a top flight doctor and quite a character, and he was certain that we would like one another right away.

Although I regretted leaving Dr. O'Dell's care, I did appreciate the opportunity to continue my treatment sessions closer to home. He arranged my first appointment with Dr. Hoegerman so that my weekly sessions could continue without interruption.

I began to see Dr. Hoegerman after completing my visits with Dr. O'Dell. There is a world of experience and a lifetime of study behind those sharply intelligent, yet kindly septuagenarian eyes. Dr. Hoegerman has spent the better part of half a century treating all kinds of patients with a range of ailments as broad as the differences between them. Unlike many older doctors who develop excellent healing skills but then remain in those modes of treatment, Hogey is always learning, searching for improvements to medicine that will treat and cure a number of human conditions.

Today, he specializes in chelation therapy. His patients are predominantly those who have undergone at least one heart attack or who suffer from arterial sclerosis. Like multiple sclerosis, this often ultimately fatal condition results when lesions, or scar tissue, build up along walls of the blood vessels leading to the major organs, especially the heart. As this scarring progresses, the inner diameter of the blood vessels becomes reduced, as does the resultant blood flow. Left untreated, arteries or veins may become permanently blocked, allowing little or no blood to circulate through them. Without circulation, poisons cannot be eliminated and new materials essential to cellular health cannot be transported. Eventually, the flow of blood is so compromised that the heart literally strangles, resulting in cardiac arrest. When the vessels to the brain become similarly restricted, stroke is the other major outcome.

Multiple sclerosis is essentially the same type of process, although it affects different areas of the body. The term "sclerosis" means "scarring." Lesions form internally on a particular area of the body, or in a particular body system. In the case of arterial sclerosis, this scar tissue forms upon the inner walls of the vascular, or blood-carrying, system. In multiple sclerosis, however, these lesions develop along the wall of sheathing cells that house the nervous system, particularly the central nervous system.

Think of this layer of sheath cells, called myelin, as similar to the weatherproof coating on a series of power cables that bring electrical current to your county. The larger cables supply the primary areas. These wires run from the power station, in your body's case, the brain, and flow into smaller substations, or transformers, that supply current to more specific areas. In the human body these would equate to the main trunk nerves that supply the limbs. Branching off from each of these stations are the cables that bring electrical power into your home. Inside of the home, even smaller wires are specific to a single area: your lamp, your toaster, your television. Your body operates along similar lines. Each main nerve cable for each limb branches off to smaller cables, sending impulses from the brain to the limbs, and eventually to the individual cells. Completing the circuit, the cells send sensory information gathered from the environment back to the brain along the same cables.

Along the miles and miles of cable from the electrical power station, many incidents can occur that can damage the clear transmission of current. Violent storms, extreme temperature conditions, broken branches, even birds nesting in the transformer box can reduce or completely eliminate the passage of current. When that happens, a brownout, or even a blackout, a complete loss of power, occurs. Your power company employs field technicians whose specific function is to check, maintain, and repair these wires.

Now, turn that picture onto your own body. There are many incidents that occur in the course of human life that can damage the electrical, or nervous system, cables. Severe illness, injury or broken bone, or the buildup of toxic substances nesting in your cells can reduce the nervous system's ability to deliver current from the main power station, your brain, to all of the other areas of your body, or to receive data from the cells that help your brain to make decisions regarding movement, sensation, and other functions.

Your body's "linemen" are your antibodies and your healing nutrients. When damage or injury occurs, these antibody linemen rush to the area to eliminate the cause of the trouble. The nutrient linemen then move into each damaged area and effect repairs, regenerating the damaged cell's structure and interior so that full electrical power can be restored.

In the case of sclerosis, it is almost as if one half of the linemen are on strike, or have been downsized out of the "company." The antibody linemen still come rushing in when illness or injury occurs. They remove the cause of the trouble by fighting the infection. However, the second half of the team, the nutrients, do not show up for their part of the job. The result is an area of dead cells that have not been restructured or regenerated, leaving scar patches, or sclerosis, along the casing cells, or myelin. Current cannot pass through these dead patches. This results in numbness and loss of movement, because the impulses from the brain cannot reach the area, and the sensory information from the cells at the end of the route cannot return to the brain. In essence, you short out.

Think of your real linemen again. A complaint comes into the power station. There's been a big storm, and the town of Left Leg has no electricity! The brave linemen leap into action, racing to locate the source of the trouble. Miles away from the power station, they find it. A wire is down, and a cow is standing on it. When the company is functioning properly, some of the linemen push the cow off of the wires and shoo it back into the field while others restring new cable and power is restored. The little town of Left Leg is happy, and the people dance.

But suppose some of the linemen are on strike. Suppose they never receive the orders to go out into the field and do the repairs. Or, imagine that they all arrive in the field, but they only have fifty feet of cable on that big wheel on their truck, instead of the three hundred feet they really need to do the job correctly. In some cases, repairs are halted entirely until sufficient materials are transported to the job site. In others, a patch can be made, splicing new wire into the old and restringing it into place. Power will still be restored in this case, but the splice, naturally, becomes the weakest part of the cable, increasing the possibility for damage to that area at a later date. The little town is still happy, but, if they all decide to turn on their air conditioners and watch TV, overtaxing the system, it is liable to break down again, exactly at that point.

Your body linemen can face similar problems. If your system is not producing enough antibody or nutrient linemen, the effects are like the real linemen on strike. No one shows up to your trouble area. Sometimes the nutrient linemen appear, but either their numbers are not great enough, or they have not been provided with sufficient resource materials to complete the job. Therefore, healing commences either slowly or not at all. The areas that remain unrepaired become dead zones, without power.

In the case of our electrical linemen, the reasons for power failure are finite and specific. No one ever stares gloomily at their home and wonders why nothing happens when they hit the light switch. The cause is easily determinable. This is not the case with MS. No one knows yet exactly why MS occurs. My story is about how I have found a way to rid my body of the disease and repair the damage already done. Later on, you will come to see what I believe are the causes of the affliction, but for now we'll concentrate on these early treatment methods.

To complete our analogy, chelation is one of the therapies that help your body linemen do their jobs by removing toxic substances that function as roadblocks or obstacles to healing. I continued to see Dr. Hoegerman weekly for the remainder of the twenty-five initially recommended injections. He treats his patients with DMPS chelation in cases where toxic metal chelation is required. During the course of my sessions, Dr. Hoegerman would order periodic blood and urine tests to measure the amount of mercury that still remained in my system and the amount that my body was eliminating. I continued to see my mercury levels drop, but he thought they should be coming down a bit faster. He began to question me about my diet.

Some of my favorite foods have always been fish and seafood. As a nutritionist, I understand the importance of the elements fish provide for the healthy human diet: proteins, vitamins, nutrients, and essential fatty acids. Saltwater fish and shellfish do, however, also contain varying amounts of methyl mercury. Methyl mercury is a natural substance similar to the mercury used in dental fillings, but in lesser density, or concentration. This substance is inherent to the fish, part of its natural biological composition. Additional, and sometimes excessive, amounts of methyl mercury can also be present as a result of the pollutants released into the water by the industrialization of society and formerly lax environmental laws. Because fish was so large a part of my diet, some of the mercury that I was eliminating was being replaced when I ate seafood, thereby slowing the reduction of mercury in my system to within the acceptable range.

Dr. Hoegerman suggested I reduce the amount of fish I consumed weekly, or change the types I ate. Freshwater stream fish like bass, trout, and sunnies do not contain methyl mercury. Where I live, these types of stream fish are hard to obtain. I do make it a point to order them whenever I travel to a place where they are offered on the local restaurant menu. Some lake fishes do not contain methyl mercury, either. However, if the lake fishes are harvested from an area where industrialization is present, like the Great Lakes area of the United States and Canada, excess mercury is likely to be found in these species due to pollution. I still undergo chelation periodically today to keep my mercury levels in the acceptable range. The process is necessary for me as I continue to eat a lot of seafood, although not as much as I did when I first saw Dr. Hoegerman.

Other important dietary elements supplied by fish are called essential fatty acids (EFA). There are several types of these EFAs, the most important to the MS patient being omega-3, omega-6, and especially EPA. EPA is found in the highest concentrations in salmon, cod, herring, whiting, kippers, and sardines. As I was to discover later, EPA provides the raw materials necessary for the production of several substances essential to cellular healing and maintenance.

Dr. Hoegerman, after learning how much fish I consumed, suggested that I have an EFA test, to determine my own essential fatty acid levels. This test would show the exact amounts of poly, mono, and saturated fats present in my system, as well as the EPA and omega acid levels. Both of us were pleased to learn that my EPA level was at 12.8. This was excellent, as the acceptable reference range is between 10 and 15 units. In fact, all of my fat concentrations were in the optimum range. He suggested that as I began to reduce the amount of fish in my diet, I should begin taking a daily EPA supplement, to keep my levels from falling into a deficient state and thereby depriving my body of the raw materials necessary to manufacture other vital substances.

Finally, after over six months of treatment, I completed the twenty-five chelation sessions recommended originally by Dr. Huggins. A final test was taken on my blood mercury levels. Although still somewhat high, they had finally dropped into the single-digit range. I could now begin to modify my diet and slow the chelation therapy. I could receive injections now every two to three weeks. We would pursue the process until my levels finally returned to the advisable levels.

While I was having these discussions with Dr. Hoegerman, I was still continuing to search for other clues to my MS. Although I did believe that mercury could be a significant factor, I did not believe that it was the sole cause of the affliction. In argument, consider the areas of the world where little or no dental care is provided on a regular basis. These people can still contract MS. Their exposure to mercury is probably minimal, if not non-existent.

Having long ago decided that conventional medicine had nothing to offer me in the way of healing, I broadened my search, including not only alternative medical practitioners, but holistic healers as well. And, even though I was a practicing nutritionist, I was to determine that diet was to play a far larger role in my eventual triumph. The next step in my recovery was to discover that my system was not as "healthy" and perfectly balanced as I thought it to be. The way that I looked at the foods I was eating was about to undergo radical changes.

5

Understanding the Imbalances—Changing Perceptions and Practices

The results of my BioCybernetics analysis were returned to me in early 1995. It had taken a little longer than usual to get this test, but I put that down to the holidays and thought no more about it. This was the first biochemical analysis I'd had performed in over a year. The last series was completed prior to my diagnosis. I was eager to learn what elements in my body were out of balance. I didn't think there could be all that many. After all, I was a nutritionist. I ate "healthy." I didn't fill my meals with fast food, candy, and other empty-calorie foods. I should be relatively okay.

I couldn't have been more wrong. Everything seemed to be unbalanced! At first I was sure that the usually infallible Santoro and Weyhreter had made a mistake. This had to be some other patient's results. After all, they didn't do the actual biochemical analysis at their facility. The sample analysis was done for them at an outside facility. Perhaps the lab mislabeled the sample.

I called Bob Santoro right away, certain that there had been an error. Shocked as I had been at the printout, it was nothing compared to the feeling that came over me when Bob assured me that there had been no error. These *were* my results. It had taken this length of time to send them to me because after seeing them himself for the first time, Bob also thought that there might be a mistake. So, he sent the second half of the samples that he had kept along to the laboratory for retesting. The results were identical.

Almost *nothing* was in the acceptable range. Some of the minerals were non-existent, or showed trace amounts only. All of the heavy metals charted much too high, their levels almost beyond the maximum measurable range. My calcium level was excessive, and my mineral ratios were entirely disproportionate. (I have devoted a chapter to BioCybernetics, the importance of the analysis, and the significance of the substance levels and ratios that are essential to optimum health.) My test showed almost freakish readings. If I was getting any better from the treatments I was presently undergoing, the test didn't seem to show it.

I felt panic rising within me, but Bob Santoro was calm and logical. He explained that some of the substances showing unacceptably high levels could be actually due to the removal of the mercury. Mercury acts in opposition to several other metals and minerals in the system. Years of excess mercury had probably caused these other substances to increase their levels as well. As the mercury left my system, the excess amounts of these substances became more apparent. Also, the substances used in the removal process might also contain elements that were affecting my readings.

Bob agreed with Dr. Hoegerman that I should reduce my intake of fish and seafood, at least for the present, as these foods were high in some of the elements my body already had in excess. He also concurred that I should be taking a daily EPA supplement, as that would keep the supply to my system at an optimum level while avoiding the other elements present in fish that I didn't need right now. As I said earlier, EPA is especially important to the MS patient, as an insufficient amount inhibits the body's ability to manufacture necessary healing substances. We will explore this subject in more detail later.

Bob suggested that I begin taking a series of nutrients and natural compounds that would replenish what I was lacking and clean my system of impurities. He promised to send me some nutrients that I should begin to take right away, including evening primrose oil (EPO). EPO is a wonderful natural source of essential oils the body utilizes and is easily digested by the human system. In a month or so, we'd do another test, to see how the levels had changed.

Another product he was insistent I begin to take right away was to become one of the cornerstones of my healing therapy. Sphingolin Myelin Basic Protein is an amazing natural substance I believe has had a direct bearing on my ability to arrest the progress of the disease. Remember how MS damages the nervous system. The sheath cells surrounding the nerves are what the disease attacks. All of the other complications and symptoms of MS are as a result of this destructive process.

Sphingolin Myelin Basic Protein is made from the spinal myelin cells of New Zealand steers. These cows are raised in a free-range, organic manner. No chemicals or pesticides are contained in their food or used on their grazing land. When the animal is harvested for human food, this substance is extracted from the spinal cord and processed in much the same manner as the raw organ concentrates I explained in the last chapter. The extract is then converted to capsule form and taken orally three times daily by the patient.

The reasons for using this myelin supplement are twofold: First, the presence of the myelin in the stomach and the digestive tract, even though it is not human, should cause the MS virus to turn and attack this new source of myelin, thereby leaving the myelin sheathing of the central nervous system alone. Secondly, the excess myelin that is not attacked by the virus will naturally find its way to your myelin cells, just as the raw organ concentrates go specifically to their corresponding organ of origin. The new myelin is fresh and undamaged by the disease. It helps to strengthen the existing human myelin and begin to aid in the regeneration of the damaged areas, eventually lessening or eliminating the lesions on the sheath.

Sphingolin Myelin Basic Protein is the brand name of this product, created by the Cardiovascular Research Company and distributed by a company known as Emerson Ecologics, located in Wisconsin. You will find the contact information for Emerson Ecologics in the resources section.

Around the time I received my BioCybernetics (BCI) analysis, Jerry and I had dinner with a good friend of ours, Dr. Jonathan Wright, a holistic medicine specialist who is a very knowledgeable healer, and deeply involved in alternative, natural therapies. After our meal, the conversation turned to my diagnosis with MS. Jonathan was interested in my condition, both as a friend and as a medical professional.

I revealed my concerns regarding my recent analysis and the number of substances that were out of balance. I relayed the recommendations of Dr. Hoegerman and Nutritionist Santoro: that I reduce my dietary intake of fish and seafood, have an EFA test, and take a daily supplement capsule to maintain the amounts of EPA I needed. Jonathan agreed with their recommendations, especially regarding the EFA test, as BioCybernetics does not test these essential substances. I had not, as yet, scheduled the test, but Jonathan's confirmation made me decide to have it performed. The EFA test would help form a more complete picture of my overall system composition.

Jonathan offered to send me a testing kit. I thanked him but declined, having decided to have the testing performed by Dr. Hoegerman's office, as I was under his care for the chelation treatments. I would have a continuous record of any changes, and using the same facility for all of the tests would serve as a data control.

Jonathan also suggested that I take a digestive enzyme supplement, an omega-3 fatty acid supplement and betaine hydrochloride, a form of hydrochloric acid (HCL), to help my body digest the concentrated EPA. HCL is naturally manufactured in the parietal cells of your stomach. HCL breaks down food fats so the body can utilize them for fuel or healing. The supplement would take some of the workload off of my system and allow my body to absorb and utilize the nutrients in my food more quickly and efficiently. It was sound medical advice, and I began to take HCL with each meal. As my condition improved, I slowly discontinued its use, and now take HCL only occasionally, particularly after eating food that may be difficult for me to digest.

I am grateful to Jonathan for providing me with an essential clue to reversing my MS. I would strongly urge other MS patients to consider adding these two supplements to their daily dietary routine. In order to arrest and begin to reverse the effects of this disease, it is crucial that your body be consistently provided with sufficient raw materials necessary to successful healing. I explore this subject more completely in the second section.

My chelation sessions were drawing to a close. I had reviewed the results of my BioCybernetics and EFA tests and I decided to take a step backward, to square one, nutrition. I needed to find out how to bring my vitamin, mineral, and nutrient levels back into acceptable range and appropriate ratios. A good friend had given me a book about nutrition and MS that was to change the way I looked at food.

Dr. Roy Lavar Swank, M.D., Ph.D. is internationally recognized for his work with multiple sclerosis patients. His clinical studies began in 1948, in the U.S. and Canada. Shortly after he began to focus on the disease, the causes and effects, he began a study in Montreal that would last for thirty-six years, following the lives of 150 MS patients. An accomplished scientist, Dr. Swank studied the effects that fats in foods that we eat may have on the disease, either positively or negatively. The results of nearly four decades of study are published in the best seller *The Multiple Sclerosis Diet Book: A Low Fat Diet for the Treatment of MS* (Swank and Dugan 1987). Dr. Swank's book (and the work of two doctors from Reseda, California whom I was to meet shortly afterwards) would become my nutritional blueprint until late 1997.

As word of my illness spread throughout our circle of family and friends, they responded with encouragement and support. I received as gifts a number of books on MS. I read many of them, touched by the personal stories, but none held clues to what I was seeking. I had decided long ago to do more than manage this disease, to find a way to live with my deteriorating condition. I needed positive actions that I could take, like chelation, that would restore my system balance and push the MS from my body.

Some of the books were medical, but interesting only if they suggested a method or natural treatment that I was unaware of or had not tried. Those that touted conventional management methods like Betaseron I tossed into a corner, unread. New Age and holistic books recommended many of the herbs, oils, healing chants, sounds, and aromatherapy I used in my own practice that would help to maintain inner spiritual and emotional balance. In the end, all of them came down to essentially the same core message: You've got MS, there's nothing that you can do about it, so now we'll teach you how to live with it.

Unacceptable. I was not going to live with my MS like a horrible tenant that you can't kick out of your house. I was going to *cure* it. I stopped reading the books. I have always believed that what you are unrelentingly exposed to, your mind will believe, sooner or later. I didn't want to become worn down enough by constant hammering to believe that there was nothing I could do to rid myself of MS.

This particular day, I was breakfasting alone. Jerry was away on business, and I wanted something to read with my meal. I wandered into the den and found my stack of new, unread books. I began to idly pick them up and scan the titles searching for some desirable morning reading. I came upon Dr. Swank's book, *The Multiple Sclerosis Diet Book: A Low Fat Diet for the Treatment of MS*. Diet and nutrition books had always interested me, and I decided that this would be fine. I returned to the table to find my favorite breakfast already waiting. Golden fried eggs, crispy bacon, home fries, buttered toast, squeezed California orange juice, and freshly brewed coffee. It smelled wonderful and tasted better. I loved breakfast at our house.

I suppose it may come as a surprise to you that a nutritionist and naturopath like myself would relish the breakfast I've just described. Because I am a health-oriented doctor, most people would think I should be eating something a bit more "natural." Interestingly, we will learn later how some of these foods are not necessarily "bad" for you. I confess that health was not the reason I was about to enjoy this meal. I was eating this way because I liked it.

I am a natural health professional, true. I am also human. Before my diagnosis with MS, my body seemed to be in excellent shape. My muscles were fit, I was not overweight, and I drank plenty of water and exercised regularly. By all appearances, I was perfectly healthy. Never one to strictly watch my diet, I had developed several bad eating habits over the years, even with my nutritional knowledge.

I have always liked to eat, a result of my Italian upbringing. It didn't help that Jerry was also a hearty eater. Jerry loves quality food, expertly prepared. His business is international and we traveled often, enjoying the cuisine of different countries. When at home, we dined out frequently with friends and attended parties and business dinners. I chose foods for taste and dining pleasure far more often than I should have done. Even with my training, I had fallen into the mindset common to many of us: If I ate something terribly rich or fattening, I would skip a meal later in the day. Or, if I consumed fried or heavy foods, I would work out longer or more strenuously the next day. I looked healthy, felt okay, took multivitamins, and made the assumption I was receiving the proper nutrition my body needed. I was about to find out how wrong my assumptions were.

I began to read the book's introduction as I ate. I was most impressed by Dr. Swank's credentials and his specific experiences with the treatment of MS. So far, so good. I took a sip of my coffee to wash down a forkful of crispy potatoes. I could live on these potatoes. I read on as Dr. Swank detailed the world-famous Montreal Study, a thirty-six-year clinical research project that followed the lives of 150 MS patients. These patients were given a nutritional program developed by Dr. Swank to replace their current diets. The results, in terms of longevity, range of mobility, and progressive severity of symptoms were measured against studies done by other researchers and facilities where the patient was given drug therapy for treatment, no nutritional counseling, and no dietary restrictions or changes.

The studies were impressive. Dr. Swank explains how fats in food affect MS. Dr. Swank believes that his clinical evidence, gathered from thousands of MS patients over nearly four decades, clearly illustrates that saturated fats compete with myelin for essential body raw materials. These raw materials—enzymes, vitamins, and nutrients—are diverted to process the saturated fats consumed by the body. The body has a finite number of these substances, and consuming saturated fats takes them away from the maintenance and repair of the myelin sheath. This diverting of materials slows the healing process and allows the disease to feed upon the weakened cells more easily. Dr. Swank recommended that MS patients immediately begin to eliminate certain foods from their diets, some permanently.

This was interesting. I finished the foreword and browsed to the fourth section of the book entitled "The Swank Low-Fat Diet: Reasons–Rules–Recipes." Turning the page, I was surprised to find that there were only eight rules. This should be relatively easy to do. I read further, and suddenly there was a different movie on the screen, so to speak. Some of the rules were no problem. I already followed a similar nutritional track. But three of the rules in particular would change the way I looked at my diet for a long time.

"You will eat *no red meat* for the first year. This includes the dark meat of the chicken or turkey." An image of my juicy grilled steak from the night before wafted before my eyes, and my mind could see Colonel Sanders waving mournfully to me as he boarded the good ship *Can't Have It*. The second rule let you have red meat after a year, but only three ounces a week. My mental image changed from a steak to a beef jerky stick. The Colonel tossed me three chicken nuggets as the boat pulled away from the dock.

"Dairy products containing one percent butterfat or more will be eliminated." There goes my buttered toast. In fact, there goes a lot of things. One of my worst eating habits was that I used butter in those days like some people use ketchup, or salt. I put it on everything, and I wasn't stingy with it either.

"All processed foods containing saturated fats will be eliminated." This can't be all that bad, I thought to myself. We don't eat much processed stuff, anyway, picturing TV dinners and boxes of macaroni and cheese. Wrong again. I would discover this edict included about 80 percent of the food in our kitchen. Flours, mixes, breads, frozen foods, desserts. I turned quickly to the "Forbidden" list of items. I might as well see how unpleasant this was going to be.

It was bad. No butter, no ice cream, ice milk, or cream cheese. No cakes, cookies, pastries, pancakes, or biscuits. No chili, no spaghetti sauce (a cruel blow to an Italian). No chips, no Ritz. Sara Lee was no longer welcome in my home. *Three olives*, and these had to be counted in your minuscule unsaturated fat intake. It's an unwritten law that Italians *have* to eat olives. We cook everything with olive oil!

The list went on. Three eggs per week, and only one per day. I stared down at my now empty, yellow-streaked plate. According to this book, I had just eaten two thirds of my weekly quantity and violated the one-per-day limit. Nestled in the Sugar category was the unkindest cut of all. "Chocolate and all products containing chocolates . . . are forbidden." My mind flashed upstairs to the night table in our bedroom.

There, a half-enjoyed box of Bavarian chocolates awaited, seductively urging me to go to the den and hurl this book into the fire.

I rose, honestly tempted to do so. As I did, I felt a slight twinge in my left leg again. My mind replaced the box of chocolate with a picture of my BioCybernetics chart. Instead of throwing the book out, I went upstairs with a fresh cup of coffee (which you may have on the Swank diet provided you don't put cream or sugar in it) settling into my bedroom window seat to read the rest of this tome of dietary doom.

It didn't get any better. I discovered that as far as MS was concerned, my lax eating habits were worse than I thought. Many foods I considered healthy were limited, discouraged, or forbidden on the Swank diet. Most of the meats I ate regularly were either eliminated entirely or allowed in such small portions that it was hardly worth bothering to eat them. Interestingly enough, the fishes listed as forbidden were ones I mentioned earlier that contained the highest concentrations of EPA: salmon, sardines, herring, tuna, and trout. Dr. Hoegerman had suggested that I eat trout instead of my usual saltwater fish choices. I made a mental note to ask him about this, as he and Swank were opposite on this point.

I didn't realize how absorbed in the book I'd become until a late afternoon lunch was brought to me. Fresh albacore tuna on a bed of crisp lettuce, cottage cheese decorated with sliced green olives and pimento, two hard-boiled eggs, a handful of Ritz crackers, fresh squeezed lemonade. With the possible exception of the crackers, most diet centers and more than a few nutritionists would consider this a healthy, low-calorie meal. Until several hours earlier, so had I.

My stomach rumbled with hunger as I tried to resolve my inner conflict. I wanted to follow any healing protocol that would bring me closer to removing MS from my body, but it was very hard to change the habits and perceptions of a lifetime, even for a nutritionally educated person like myself. I weighed the issues, staring at my lunch. I guess I could eat the lettuce and drink the lemonade. Wait. Scratch the lemonade. The frosty, inviting beverage certainly contained more sugar than this book recommended. On the other hand, what a waste of good food. In the end, I had feet of clay. I tossed the book onto the bed and ate the entire lunch, down to the last Ritz cracker. I would read the rest of the book before I made any radical dietary changes. I also decided to make a quick call to Bob Santoro and get his opinion on all of this.

I reached Bob later that day. Surprisingly, although unfamiliar with Dr. Swank's work, Bob thought eliminating some of the foods might help to bring my excessive levels back into more acceptable ranges. I told him about the forbidden fish, and he repeated that taking the EPA supplements was now imperative. He would send me some omega-3 and omega-6 compounds containing the essential oils with all other fats removed. I should add these compounds to my daily supplements.

Dr. Hoegerman and Dr. O'Dell advocate fish consumption. Dr. Huggins believes fish should be largely avoided. Dr. Swank approves only certain fishes. Hoegerman, O'Dell, and Santoro espouse the value of additional daily supplements, regardless of actual quantity or type of fish consumed. Dr. Swank does not address the value of EPA supplements at all. Which school of thought was most accurate? How could I choose?

I was to discover during my search for healing that opposing viewpoints on the quantity and type of supplements, nutrients, vitamins, minerals, and foods were the rule rather than the exception. At the present time, there is no universally accepted, standard treatment for MS. The primary reason for these differing schools of thought is that no one has been able to definitively determine the root cause of MS. Scientists have discovered the areas of the body damaged by the disease and how that damage occurs, but the why of it all still eludes the medical community. All research is essentially trial and error. Doctors and scientists pursue differently focused studies while seeking the most correct answer.

For the MS patient, these differing methodologies can become very confusing. Which protocol is most effective? What therapy will give the patient the greatest benefit? Even with my medical training, I often found myself feeling lost and uncertain. In my case, I had the advantage of access to other medical professionals for input and advice. My own best advice to the reader would be to have your own biochemical tests performed, determine what your body is lacking or has to excess, and choose a therapy that most closely addresses your particular biochemical needs. Periodic retesting will help you chart your progress. If you find a therapy to be ineffective, move to another. This book relates the healing methods that worked most successfully for me. Each of us is an individual, and although none of these protocols will harm you if followed properly, some may be more or less effective for you than they were for me.

My own best advice to the reader would be to have your own biochemical tests performed, determine what your body is lacking or has to excess, and choose a therapy that most closely addresses your particular biochemical needs. Periodic retesting will help you chart your progress.

That evening, I again ate alone, Jerry still not due back for a couple of days. I had decided that this would be my last day of eating normally. I'd finished Dr. Swank's book and would honestly try to change my eating habits and begin to follow the diet recommended. For the first time, I experienced what it was like for one of my patients when I informed them a favorite food they loved was no longer good for them. I'd always thought that the looks of horror on their faces were a bit overdramatic. Not anymore. I'd told them to avoid one or two foods. This wretched book told me to avoid practically *all* the foods I ate on a regular basis.

Still, my medically trained mind knew I could not refuse to at least try such a well-documented treatment simply because

I didn't think I was going to like it very much. I ate dinner that evening like a condemned woman with her last meal. I savored my piece of barbecued chicken, my mashed potatoes swimming with butter. I went overboard with dessert: vanilla ice cream, brandied cherries, chocolate hot fudge, and a huge dollop of fresh whipped cream.

I took a walk after dinner to gather my thoughts. Why was I reacting so strongly to this dietary change? Was this another one of my MS mood swings? No, I had to be honest with myself and admit that my eating habits had lapsed from the conscientious to the convenient over the past several years. If I were another patient with my medical condition and came to myself as a doctor for treatment, wouldn't I recommend the same changes? Certainly. Perhaps not as restrictive, but definitely excluding a majority of the foods I had been regularly consuming. Besides, the real issue was not whether or not I could ever eat cheesecake again. It was far more serious. How determined was I to be healthy again? What was more important, reversing this disease or a stack of pancakes? Of course there was only one answer. This land was so beautiful, and I realized how many things in my life there were to be thankful for, despite this all-consuming illness. If this new diet would help me to achieve my goal, then I would do my best to follow it closely. I returned to the house with a renewed determination to try this new protocol.

Jerry came home that weekend, full of news of the latest products and developments that he had seen at the trade show. His stories were amusing, as always, and we enjoyed each other's company for the rest of the day. Jerry had eaten after landing at the airport and went upstairs early. Still on East Coast time, the next morning he was up long before I was and breakfasted before I came down. He was seated at the table, reading the Sunday paper when I appeared with my new Swank breakfast of Irish rolled oatmeal, flax seed oil, and raisins. Jerry hardly noticed. Wistfully, I glanced at the remains of the steak and eggs he'd eaten. My oatmeal tasted like wood chips in comparison. This was the third day I'd eaten this for breakfast. The flax seed oil tasted strange, nothing like butter. Raisins are tasty, but not exciting three days in a row.

One of the nicest activities Jerry and I enjoy together is our Sunday movie outing. We have a late brunch and drive into Santa Barbara to see a first-run movie. We sit in the darkened theater like two teenagers, eating huge tubs of popcorn and sharing that too syrupy, nearly flat soda that seems to be sold only in theaters and bowling alleys. We did this almost every Sunday, and we loved it. Jerry had already chosen several movies we might like to see. I finished my unremarkable breakfast, told him which films I liked, and went upstairs to change into casual clothes.

We always enjoyed our drive. We could stop and walk along the ocean, check out an antique sale, or generally just putter around as we pleased for most of the afternoon. We arrived at the theater early, as usual. Neither of us liked to miss the beginning of the film. We made our usual stop at the refreshment counter, and my heart sank as Jerry ordered our usual massive bucket of popcorn with extra butter. He grabbed the tub with our huge soda and headed toward the seating section. Suddenly struck by an idea, I told him I would catch up to him. He went to choose our seats, and I motioned to the girl behind the refreshment counter.

"Excuse me," I said pleasantly. "Do you know if this is real butter on the popcorn?"

Thinking was evidently not a job requirement in her case. Blinking her large blue eyes from beneath puffy blonde bangs, she just stared at me uncomprehendingly. I repeated the question, more slowly. This time she did reply, in a manner of speaking. "What? Well, it says 'Buttered Popcorn.' See?" She pointed to the popcorn machine with its gaily colored marquee, her logic being that perhaps I had simply failed to notice the sign. "It *says* 'Butter.' So I guess, well, like sure, it must be butter." And then, her eyes lighting up, she delivered her final stroke of brilliant, irrefutable logic. "Like, well, if it was something else, it would say it, right? Like, it doesn't say, um, 'Cheese' or anything."

God, I wanted to laugh. "No," I agreed, fighting to keep a straight face, "it certainly doesn't say 'Cheese.' But," I continued, "maybe it says 'Butter' but it's not really real butter. Maybe it's margarine, or something else."

I was beginning to confuse the poor thing. She wrinkled her forehead, her skin obviously unaccustomed to a thoughtful expression. "But, like why would it say 'Butter' and be, like, margarine? Wouldn't it say '*Margarine* Popcorn'?"

This was priceless. She had no idea what I wanted to know. I tried another tack. "Well, maybe it says 'Butter' when it means 'Margarine' because people like butter better. Maybe they use margarine, though, because it's," I couldn't help it, "like, way cheaper, you know?"

Suddenly, a light bulb went on all over her face. "Wow! I never thought of that!" (Or probably much else, either.) "Maybe we do. The boss," she looked over her shoulder toward a door marked 'No Admittance' and dropped her voice conspiratorially, "he's pretty cheap, you know?" Furrowing her brow, she was struck by another thought. "You know, come to think of it, our butter comes in a big can. It doesn't usually come in a can in the *store*. Wait a sec. I'll like, investigate."

I wanted to howl until tears streamed down my face. Whatever movie we saw that day couldn't possibly be as funny as this. Sherlock Barbie disappeared below the counter, rummaging under the cabinet. She emerged triumphantly moments later, holding a five-gallon can with two holes punched into the top. "Here it is!" She thumped it onto the counter. "Let's see what it says on it."

She read the front of the label while I quickly scanned the back. Just as I'd suspected, the stuff wasn't butter at all. It was artificially made of oils and flavoring. As far as I could tell, it didn't contain any measurable amount of saturated fat. I could eat this! I raised my eyes to the face of my assistant to find her looking concerned. "You know," she said, "this doesn't even *say* butter on it. It says 'Popcorn Flavoring.' *As if.* It doesn't taste at all like *popcorn.*" She glared over at the "No Admittance" sign again. "You know, he's like, *lying* to people. That's like, so bogus and rude. I knew he was, like, *so* uncool, but I really needed the job, you know?"

She was really the best, this kid. "Yeah, I know. We've all got to have a job."

She wasn't finished, though. Once the rusty wheels of that little brain started turning, there was no stopping them, it seemed. She looked at me closely, leaning in to ask me in a lowered voice, "How did you know it wasn't butter? Did you, like guess, or are you like a food inspector or something?" I shook my head negatively. "Can I get in trouble for telling people it's butter?" Again, I shook my head, fighting hard to keep my mouth from turning up at the corners. And then, finally, "You won't tell anybody, will you? I mean, like, that it's not real butter, it's this bogus non-butter stuff? I don't want the boss thinking that I was telling people. They might, well, you know, like not eat it, and I don't want him blaming me or anything."

I had to get out of there. My movie was starting, and my head was beginning to hurt from this conversation. I promised I would never reveal the secret of the bogus can of non-butter. It would be *our* secret. She thanked me so profusely I almost ran to the seating section, eager to get through the doors before I burst into laughter. We saw her many times on future visits. Although we never had another long conversation, she never failed to wink at me conspiratorially each time she handed the big tub to Jerry.

Like many MS patients, the decision to radically change my diet would affect the people around me. It can be very difficult to maintain a new dietary regimen when living with others who are eating normally and have no interest in altering their own food intake. The temptation for the patient to "cheat" is always strong when she is surrounded by people eating "regular" food. Even if self-discipline is maintained, the patient can feel isolated and "left out" while those around her enjoy unrestricted meals. Inevitably, the patient attempts to involve other family members in the new diet. It rarely succeeds, as my own example will illustrate.

Dinner that evening was the first time Jerry was exposed to my new Swank diet. I chose a vegetable stew recipe from Dr. Swank's book, and it was served with a plate of fresh rolls and a crock of butter for Jerry and some wheat crackers for me. The stew was delicious, with large chunks of potatoes, carrots, onions, rutabagas, turnips, and parsnips in a seasoned, savory sauce. I had enjoyed several spoonfuls when I noticed that Jerry, after buttering a crisp French roll was just pushing his stew around in the bowl. Aware of my look, he asked me, "Hey, Celeste. What kind of stew is this?"

I answered him, taking another bite of the hearty mixture. "It's called 'Sunday Stew,' Jerry. It's part of my new diet and nutrition plan. I found the recipe in a book by Dr. Swank. He specializes in the proper diet for MS patients."

He continued to turn over and examine the contents, looking puzzled. "If this is stew, where's the meat? And," he continued, holding aloft a yellowish chunk of vegetable, "what exactly is this thing?"

"It doesn't have any meat, Jerry. And that's a rutabaga."

"Excuse me? It doesn't have any meat? You can't make stew without meat. And what the hell is a rutabaga doing in here? Who eats these? What *are* these?"

He looked so perplexed, I had to laugh. "Of course you can make stew without meat. And rutabagas are turnips. I eat them. And tonight, so do you." I waved at his bowl encouragingly. "Go ahead. Try some."

He examined the vegetable steaming gently on the end of his fork like a scientist who has discovered a new form of mold. He slowly brought the fork to his mouth. I watched as he chewed and analyzed the taste. Selecting a second chunk of vegetable, he examined it carefully, attempting to identify it. He couldn't. He looked across at me, waving the laden fork. "What's . . . " he began, but I answered before he had finished.

"It's a parsnip. They're good. See?" I found a piece and ate it heartily.

"For whom?" He stared at the contents of his bowl in growing dismay. "Celeste. What the hell else is in here? And, more to the point, *why* are we eating this?"

I finally had the chance to tell him about my decision to try and follow the Swank diet and the reasoning behind it. To his credit, he listened carefully to everything. I explained the evidence of Dr. Swank's long-term testing of his patients in Montreal. I saw his eyes widen when I listed what I could and could not eat. I told him that this new diet would be a difficult change, but I was determined to try it as a viable protocol. He said nothing until I was completely finished speaking. Looking at me earnestly, he offered,

"Celeste. I give you a lot of credit for trying this, I really do. And I think that you should, especially if you feel it will help you. But, please understand," he leaned forward for emphasis, "*I don't want to do it with you.* I don't mind trying reasonable dishes once in a while," his withering look clearly indicating tonight's menu did not fall into that category, "but I don't have anything wrong with me. I don't need this diet."

"But, Jerry," I said, very gently, "everybody could use less fat in their diets, don't you think?"

"Well, trim the lamb chops, if you want. But I want meat. I want *regular* food. Food I can recognize. Food I *like*. This," he jabbed at a white chunk, "does not qualify."

"Don't you think that it's tasty?" I thought the stew was delicious.

"No. It's at best a side dish. This," pushing the bowl away, "is *not* a main meal." He was trying his best to be reasonable and I appreciated it. "Do whatever you need to, but from now on, unless you ask me first, include me out, okay? Are we agreed?"

"Yes, Jerry, we're agreed," I replied. I didn't think that he'd eat it, but I gave it a try. He went into the kitchen, returned to the table, buttered and munched on a roll. A few minutes later, our cook appeared with a grilled steak, tossed salad, and French fries.

From that night on, we ate two separate dinners. Sometimes he did try little tastes of the dishes I was eating, and once in a great while he would eat a serving of one of them. But, he never really embraced any of it, and I never again tried to make him.

I followed the Swank diet for just over a year. Although extremely difficult in the beginning, it became easier when I reintroduced meat to the meals. Dr. Swank recommended adding a daily multivitamin. I was already taking one each day, as well as the Sphingolin Myelin, the EFA supplements, and the HCL digestive enzyme. A new BioCybernetics analysis showed my excessive mineral levels were beginning to drop. I was concerned that some of the nutrients I had been lacking were not accumulating. My calcium remained very high, even though Swank restricts calcium-rich foods, largely dairy products.

There were certain aspects of the Swank diet that I could not reconcile as a nutritionist and in light of the biochemical imbalances I was attempting to correct. My body needed the natural EPA from fish, and the omega oils, for instance. The natural sources of these substances were largely restricted or forbidden on the Swank diet. Other nutrients lacking in my system could not be obtained in sufficient amounts to erase the deficiencies by strictly following the Swank diet. I explain more about these specific substances in the second section. Despite these specific difficulties, the diet was helping to cleanse my body and I began to feel more energetic. So I continued to follow the Swank diet closely until I was introduced to two acupuncturists who were to change my outlook on diet once again.

6

Ancient Answers, Rude Awakenings

My left leg, finally, had almost returned to normal as 1996 was just beginning. I had been following the Swank diet for almost a year, and continuing to take the myelin, nutrient, digestive, and hormonal supplements prescribed for me by the healers that I had seen. The imbalances in my body were slowly being corrected. Substances that were present in excess were leaving my body. Others that were deficient were slowly starting to rebuild their resource levels. I wouldn't term my overall condition a remission. That would imply the disease would manifest itself more virulently at sometime in the future. I would say instead that I had arrested the progression of the MS. Although I had not yet found a way to reverse the condition, I believed it no longer dominated my system. I did not possess all of the answers I needed, but it appeared I was on the right track.

I had moved out of my office in Solvang when my leg became very weak, but continued to see patients at my home. I suspended my practice for several weeks while I was in Colorado Springs, and again while recovering from the night club disaster. At this time I had resumed practice out of my home, but it was becoming inconvenient as the number of patients was growing.

I went looking for a new office. I considered expanding the scope of my practice to include education sessions for patients afflicted with multiple sclerosis. I wanted to develop a "wellness center" where people with all sorts of complaints, not necessarily chiropractic, could come and be educated on the importance of proper nutrition in helping their bodies to heal themselves. Patients could be treated with my "Heart Songs" technique (which I explained earlier), have BioCybernetics analyses, begin a nutrient program, and be treated with advanced chiropractic non-force techniques. I explain more about this type of chiropractic treatment later.

I viewed several potential facilities over the next few weeks, but all of them proved to be unsuitable in one way or another. I declined most of them because they were not ADA compliant. The Americans with Disabilities Act requires that commercial buildings used for medical purposes be handicapped accessible, equipped with entrance ramps, elevators if necessary, handrails, and special sanitary facilities. This was especially a concern in my practice because it is very difficult for MS or chiropractic patients with certain complaints to navigate stairs, outside or inside of the building. I got a call from a real estate agent who had something she thought might be suitable. Located right in Solvang was a multi-acre piece of property with two buildings, an inground pool, spa, and sauna. There was ample space for parking. The buildings were single storied, so ramps or elevators would not be necessary.

I visited the property with the agent later that day. I thought it would make an excellent treatment center. The place had been empty for some time and needed substantial repairs, but other than that it was ideal. I wanted Jerry's opinion. Jerry has always had a keen eye for equity. He pointed out that it was in a very good location, near our home and close enough to Santa Barbara to attract my patients, but far enough away to avoid traffic and competition from other chiropractors with more established practices. I'd own it, which increased my future options. He suggested we take another look at the place together. After examining the property, Jerry thought it would be a sound investment if the price were right, and we made a counteroffer.

The seller accepted and the sale was completed quickly. Workmen arrived shortly afterwards to restore and renovate the buildings and grounds. The bathrooms were completely redone, adding special handicapped-accessible features. The second, smaller building became the treatment rooms. The larger housed a patient lounge, conference room, consultation offices, staff lounge, and administrative office. The large center room would be for conferences, seminars, and teaching sessions, conducted by either myself or knowledgeable guest speakers. I planned to ask Dr. Huggins, nutritionists Santoro and Weyhreter, and other excellent alternative medicine healers, educators, nutritionists, and chiropractors. The work was completed by the spring of 1996. Finally, the Healing Valley Health and Wellness Center was open for business.

My patients loved the new complex, and word soon spread about this new facility that treated patients with care and concern, using natural remedies and the latest chiropractic techniques. We are able to help many people, and I still consider it one of my most successful ventures.

The new treatment center had been open for a couple of months when I had an interesting conversation with my good friend Leanore. She asked if I'd ever considered acupuncture for the remaining areas of numbness in my left leg. I said no, but conventional medicine had nothing to offer me, so I was always eager to explore alternative avenues. She gave me the name of an acupuncturist in Reseda who also provided nutritional counseling. I still felt that I was being divinely led through this healing process, and I visited Dr. Matthew Van Benshoten's office the next day.

The doctor had a full practice and was only accepting new patients on a limited basis. I gave the nurse a brief medical history. She added my name to the waiting list, and after the call, I put the idea to the back of my mind. My own practice was time consuming and I figured it would be weeks before I got a return call, if at all. The call came less than a week later. I believe the fact I was a fellow medical professional with MS had a lot to do with moving my name to the top of the list, but I didn't care. I was given an appointment for the following week.

Dr. Van Benshoten's office surprised me. New Age music whispered softly throughout the suite, and soothing smells of fragrant herbs filled the air. I was presented with the standard medical history forms to complete and an information packet concerning the practice. Evidently, his treatments were not conventional. The packet contained strict patient instructions, appointment and billing procedure reminders, and several articles by Dr. Van Benshoten and his colleague, Dr. Joseph McSweyne. These articles discussed acupuncture, holistic techniques, and Chinese herbal remedies the practice utilized.

Another lengthy article was included that discussed dairy products and the adverse effects they may have on human health. Citing case studies of patients with diabetes, mental illness, and behavioral disorders, this article postulated that each disease or disorder may be linked to the consumption of dairy products. The article did not address MS specifically, but I began to wonder how dairy products might relate to my condition. Were they helpful, harmful, or completely without influence? I knew I would have to investigate the subject more thoroughly. I include a complete discussion of the role of dairy products in the diet of the MS patient in chapter 13, "Dangerous Dairy."

Dr. Matthew Van Benshoten is an energetic, lively person, passionate in his convictions and an expert in the art of acupuncture. He was interested in my own medical and nutritional background, especially the fact that I was a fully accredited naturopath. He specialized in Chinese healing arts, and combined acupuncture with healing herbs specially selected for each patient. He suggested that more might be needed in my case, as the nerve damage I had sustained was not as a result of injury or trauma. Dr. Van Benshoten asked if I had read the article on dairy products while I was waiting. I said I hadn't finished it. He suggested I do and consider changing my diet to one that he advocated for his patients, a diet that eliminated all dairy products and all refined sugars.

This was a radical step, and I asked why he recommended it. He explained that his practice had a great deal of success with autoimmune patients by eliminating these products from their diets, and it might help me as well. I had just mastered life on the Swank diet. I wasn't looking forward to eliminating more food choices. "But," I protested, "I've eaten these foods all of my life. Eggs used to be my favorite breakfast. Wouldn't I show some sort of symptoms if I were allergic? Like hives, nausea, or flu symptoms?"

"That's exactly the problem," he replied. "Most people don't show symptoms like the ones you describe. That's why it's so difficult to convince them these foods may be at the root of their problems. We've found that hidden allergies to dairy, eggs, wheat, and other substances can account for many symptoms of the autoimmune afflicted. Patients who have followed this diet experienced a reduction or in some cases complete alleviation of symptoms. It's entirely up to you, but I think you would benefit if you gave it a try."

I told Dr. Van Benshoten I would read the rest of the dairy article. At the conclusion of my first visit he gave me Chinese herbs that aided in digestion of foods to which I might have hidden allergies, a copy of the diet he and his colleague Dr. McSweyne termed Zero Dairy, Zero Sugar, and a list of products I could substitute for the restricted foods. During a follow-up appointment, Dr. Van Benshoten gave me the results of his initial examination. He had concluded that an overgrowth of intestinal bacteria was triggering antibody formation and autoimmune inflammation of my muscles and joints. I do not now believe this was strictly accurate as my mobility problems were more directly related to the lesions on my nervous system. By that time, I had finished reading his material on the toxins that may be found in dairy, and the problems that hidden food allergies may cause.

I decided that before I made any further radical changes to my diet I would order an allergy test for myself to determine any sensitivity to dairy products or eggs. The test came back positive for both dairy products and eggs. This test and its significance to the MS patient are explained in detail in chapter 13, "Dangerous Dairy."

I decided that even though it would be extremely difficult, I would adopt the new dietary guidelines. The list of substitute products was largely of a soy and tofu nature. The next time I was in Santa Barbara, I visited a good local health food store and purchased many of the products on the list, to see which ones I would like. I bought several cookbooks on vegetarian and health food recipes, written by everyone from famous actresses to vegetarians and nutrition experts.

I followed these additional diet restrictions for almost another year, incorporating them into the principles of the Swank diet. I continued to structure my meals in the Swank portions and food combinations, but crossed all items containing dairy or refined sugars off of my allowable foods list. The new recipes were an exercise in trial and error. Some, like Moroccan Chicken, sounded great and tasted awful. Others, like Tofu Turkey Patties, looked revolting, but were the most delicious things. I used to take them to work in a plastic baggie. One thing was especially nice about their very unattractive appearance: I never had to worry about people helping themselves to my lunch.

I visited Dr. Van Benshoten's several more times. Often I would consult with his office by telephone as I found that driving the considerable distance between us caused my weakened leg significant discomfort. Many times I would speak with his associate, Dr. Joseph McSweyne. He is a talented and open-minded healer, constantly studying and exploring new treatment methods, expanding upon his already considerable knowledge of Chinese herbal healing. I continue to consult with Dr. McSweyne about once a month. He prescribes my herbs, changing the mixture as my condition changes and improves.

The treatment center was running on a full schedule. I felt that more than two years after my diagnosis, my health had improved greatly. My BioCybernetics analyses showed my excess levels continued to drop, and ratio imbalances were also falling into line, although some of them still remained very unequal. The alternative medications and therapies had not produced any noticeable side effects other than a moderate loss of weight due to the diet restrictions. I wanted to share the steps I had taken with others who were suffering with MS. Perhaps I would be able to help them achieve some improvement in their own conditions. I decided to contact the National Multiple Sclerosis Society (NMSS) to see if I could arrange a meeting and present my information and results to date.

The motto of the NMSS states that the organization is "dedicated to ending the devastating effects of multiple sclerosis." They purport to be interested in any and all research or treatment methods that will determine the origin and find a cure for this disease that affects over 300,000 persons in the United States alone, over four times that number worldwide. MS cuts across racial, gender, geographic, and economic lines. Although certain groups have proven to be statistically at higher risk, it attacks the prominent and the obscure, the beautiful and the homely, the innocent and the corrupt. Nobody knows, to this day, what causes MS. Researchers and scientists continue to study the problem, but no clear, definitive answer has been found. Nobody offers the patient any other choice but ways to "manage" or live with this disease that ruins lives.

I reached the NMSS by contacting the local office that served my area, the Channel Islands Chapter. The national headquarters of the NMSS is located in New York. I attended a meeting of a local chapter in Los Olibos, but was disappointed in what I found there. It seemed that most of the "support" offered was in the form of sympathetic commiseration. I was more determined than ever to introduce these suffering people to the alternative treatment methods that I had already explored and found successful.

I had what I thought to be the perfect way to introduce both my treatments and the Wellness Center to fellow MS patients. I decided to invite some people from the NMSS to visit our facility and talk with me about my healing progress. I called the chapter office, explained my credentials and the purpose of the proposed meeting. Shortly afterwards, I received a return call accepting my offer. Unfortunately, this potentially productive meeting resulted in disaster.

I was very excited and spent days arranging my notes for the small lecture I had planned. I gathered my series of BioCybernetic analyses, my blood mercury tests, my fatty acid tests, and anything else that I thought would show the progress that I had made using alternative therapy. I contacted Bob Santoro, who willingly sent some samples of beef protein nutrients and the Sphingolin Myelin to distribute to my visitors.

The day of the visit I was up with the sun, arranging my carefully prepared information packets, checking my notes one last time, making sure that I looked perfect. I deliberately chose to wear heels, to emphasize the improved strength and mobility of my leg. I drove myself, not wishing to give the impression that I could no longer operate a motor vehicle. I packed my usual lunch of tofu-turkey patties, a piece of fruit, and a container of soy milk, and was on my way.

I arrived early to be certain that everything was in order. Newly decorated with an Egyptian theme, the facility was stunning. I set some aromatherapy candles into fragrant water bowls to burn, filling the lecture room with subtle, relaxing scents. Speakers whispered with the sounds of the ocean, courtesy of a hidden CD player. I laid out the materials that I had so carefully prepared and took a deep breath. Everything was perfect.

They arrived on time. There were eight guests altogether, all female, four in wheelchairs. I'd like to say that this is the moment in my story when my guests and I looked at one another and realized that this was an historic occasion. Nothing could be further from the truth. Three of the ladies were from the NMSS administrative offices, three were community volunteers, and two were volunteers working at the local chapter office, providing counseling, information, and comfort to callers and visitors.

I should have seen trouble on the horizon when two of the ladies wrinkled their noses as they encountered the first wisps of scent from the aromatherapy candles. I didn't. I'd seen patients react that way, on occasion, but soon begin to like the subtle therapy. One woman kept looking at the bowls and then pointedly at me throughout the entire lecture, hoping that I would take the unsubtle hint and blow the candles out, or at least open one of the glass doors leading to the patio.

I had arranged the lecture chairs in a semicircle. Lecture chairs are the kind that have those little tables attached to them so that the audience or students can take notes if they wish. I moved quickly to position four of them for my wheelchair bound guests so they could utilize the little tables. I sat in a chair facing the semicircle. After the introductions had been made all around, I began to talk.

"When I was forty-two years old, I took my daughter, Sara, on a hiking trip in Hawaii . . ."

I spoke for almost three quarters of an hour, referring to my notes and to the information packets that I had given to each of them. They had brought me their own information packet, which I had placed on the floor beside me. I am an experienced teacher and lecturer, and have learned to observe my audience, much as a stand-up comedian or politician might when appearing before a crowd of strangers, although eight would hardly be considered a crowd.

While I was speaking, I noticed that the two nose wrinklers barely glanced at the materials I had provided, even when I referred to specific passages or charts during the presentation. Some of the others complied politely, but I could see that they were not absorbing what I was saying. Only two of the guests in wheelchairs got into the lecture, and soon, as was natural, I was directing most of my remarks to them, making the eye contact that would let me gauge the level of their understanding.

Concluding the prepared portion of my remarks, I said, " . . . and, so, ladies, I wanted to share my experiences with you today in the hopes that what I have discovered will be able to help others afflicted with MS. Does anyone have any questions or comments?"

There was silence for a moment. All of the guests looked to the two in the front as if waiting for them to deliver any pronouncement that they might have before interjecting their own remarks. Finally one of the women spoke, and I knew then that this discussion was not going in the direction I had ideally imagined.

"Chiropractor. That's not a *real* M.D., now, is it?"

"Well, ah, not in the sense you mean, I suppose," I replied, caught slightly off guard. "We do, however, attend several years of college and earn a degree. In addition, we must be licensed to practice by each individual state."

She nodded as if I had confirmed some unknown, but negative fact. She continued, flicking the corner of her materials packet, "Are any of the other people that you went to for treatment *real* doctors?"

This was not what I had expected at all. "Why, yes," I answered, still off balance. "All of them, except Bob Santoro, and he's a clinical nutritionist and brilliant scientist."

Stuck for a rejoinder, she tried a new line of inquiry. "Are all of the drugs that you have taken legal?"

I was becoming a bit frustrated. My answering tone was not quite as warm as it could have been. "First, I don't take drugs. That's exactly my point. These are natural substances, made from living organisms, human, animal, and plant. Nothing I have taken during my therapies is synthetic."

"And what are these natural substances supposed to do for you, exactly?"

Hadn't she been listening at all? Exasperated, I burst out, "Well, *look* at me!" I stood up in my high heels and did a little spin for their benefit. In retrospect, it was probably one of my worst moves. "*This* is what they can do for you, for anyone!"

The two sour ladies became even more so, and I saw, too late, envy in the eyes of the rest, including my two best listeners. I thought my actions would inspire them, show them what I firmly believed was possible. Instead they saw it, I think, as an attempt to show them up, or show myself off.

"Well, *Dr.* Pepe," the second sour sister sniffed. "*Some* of our members obviously have a higher Kurtzke rating than you so obviously are fortunate to have."

"Kurtzke rating?" I echoed.

She got that "see, you're not so smart" expression on her face. Condescendingly, she explained. "Yes. Dr. John Kurtzke, *M.D.*," the emphasis present to clearly define her evaluation of my own credentials, "developed a ratings scale for MS severity of disability that *doctors* use to measure a patient's level of affliction. Yours was obviously low, and you have learned to manage your symptoms so that you can appear almost normal."

This was bizarre. It was bad enough that they were obviously not open to what I was telling them, but now she was making it seem as if I were trying to perpetrate some hoax, some scam for my own hidden purposes. My voice intense with passion, I replied.

"Excuse me, but, with all due respect, that's crazy. I can show you my MRI. My brain and my spine showed multiple numerous lesions. I couldn't use my left leg normally for almost two years!"

I should have chosen a better word than "crazy," because it didn't help matters. After a long, pointed, and disdainful look around the room, especially at the now regrettable candles, my antagonist responded. "Have you ever had another MRI performed?"

"Why, no," I replied, surprised at the change of topic. "New research is beginning to indicate that repeated MRIs can exacerbate the MS patient's condition."

"Then you don't *know* if your MS is indeed improved, do you? You could be in remission of whatever symptoms you *may* have originally had. They could return at a later date, or even grow more severe." That last was delivered in a tone that said she couldn't be happier if that was indeed the outcome.

I didn't bother to answer. It was pointless. She obviously wouldn't listen to me anyway. The first lady took up control of the conversation again, in her best Mother Superior tone. "We have proven treatments for MS that thousands of patients use daily to fight the disease. Why should we recommend your methods?"

"Because they work. And they do it naturally, without the risk of side effects that your 'treatments' can cause." I seized the information packet they had given me, flipping the pages until I found what I knew would be there. I think that was the moment when "socially correct" left the room. This wasn't fair! It wasn't as if they had considered what I had to offer and then decided they preferred their existing solutions to mine. They weren't even listening. In fact, it seemed as if they resented the fact that I had even suggested these methods to them. Finding the page I sought, I pointed to a paragraph and read it aloud, my voice sarcastic.

"Clinical Name: Interferon beta-1b. Brand Name: Beta-seron. Betaseron is injected subcutaneously every other day. Flu-like symptoms are common, so Betaseron should be taken at bedtime with Tylenol or Advil. Swelling, redness, discoloration, and pain are common after injections. Betaseron should not be used when pregnant. Women taking Betaseron should use birth control at all times. During the clinical trial, there were four suicide attempts and one successful suicide by patients taking Betaseron."

I paused and scanned my audience, some of whom were beginning to look somewhat uncomfortable. Returning to the typewritten sheet, I read on. "Possible side effects: fatigue, chills, fever, muscle aches, sweating, swelling, redness, discoloration, pain, depression, suicidal tendencies, sadness, anxiety, loss of interest in daily activities, irritability, low self-esteem, guilt, poor concentration, indecisiveness, confusion, eating and sleep disorders."

I looked at each one of them in turn. "And now, you want to tell me with straight faces that what I have told you here today is a less viable method of treatment than *this?*" I waved the drug information sheet. "I'm sorry, ladies, but I'm not buying what you have to sell. I don't intend to put my life at risk with a drug that causes all of these changes in the body, adverse conditions, and 'possible' side effects while it does absolutely nothing to improve or repair the condition!"

"But, it most certainly does!" The head sour sister flashed back. "Patients who take these excellent medications do experience a lessening, or even in some cases disappearance of their symptoms when using Betaseron properly."

"And, if they stop using it, then what? The symptoms return, probably far worse than before. It doesn't cure the disease. It only masks the problem, like a shot of Novocain. And the poor souls who take it, especially women, are doomed to a childless lifetime of needles, swelling, and side effects. It doesn't even halt the progression of the disease, does it?"

"No, it doesn't. You get worse anyway." All heads turned toward a woman named Rosie, one of the attentive listeners in the wheelchairs, speaking for the first time. "I did."

"I did, too." This from Marcia, the other wheelchair-bound visitor who had paid strict attention to my lecture. "I wasn't in this wheelchair before I started taking Betaseron." I noticed the other two women in chairs nodding silent agreement. My heart went out to all four of them.

If she had dared, I'll bet the head lady would have liked to have slapped them. She stood up abruptly, terminating our discussion before any more of the troops defected to the enemy, namely me. In a voice that would have frozen a bonfire, she addressed me down the length of her nose.

"Well, thank you for your time, *Dr.* Pepe. We appreciate your interest, but we have approved treatments for our members and see no reason to make any alternate recommendations at this time. Besides, the NMSS does not endorse or prescribe any product to our members."

"Then why do you include this information sheet on Betaseron in your literature?"

"To provide MS patients with *viable* methods of treatment." She sniffed audibly.

"Management, you mean," I countered, losing heart. I was never going to convince them, at least not today. It was futile to try. She didn't bother to answer me and I didn't much care, anyway. I never wanted an argument. I only wanted to help others discover what I was learning, that there were indeed alternatives to this unacceptable life sentence. The meeting was over. I had prepared a coffee and tea service, and motioned to it now politely. The two most opposed to me didn't even bother with the courtesy of declining, stating abruptly that they had other appointments. I offered to escort them to the door, but was informed that they could find their own way out, thank you. Without further comment and without taking the information packets, they left, their heels clicking on the mosaic in the atrium as they departed.

I was startled to notice that Rosie and Marcia had lingered behind. Some of their companions paused at the door and called to them to come along. They had come together, however, and told the others to go ahead, they had some questions. Ignoring the disapproving looks launched in their direction, they turned their chairs away from the departing women and smiled at me tentatively. I returned the smile, kicked off my shoes, and offered them some refreshments.

"Dr. Pepe, there are some things we'd like to know, if you don't mind," said Rosie. She was quite lovely, tall and thin, with short brown hair cut stylishly and frosted attractively with blonde highlights. She was about my age, and I couldn't help thinking what a horror her life must be. My voice full of warmth and compassion, I responded that, of course I didn't mind, I was entirely at their disposal.

We spoke together for another hour. They were interested in the nutrients I had brought in as samples, particularly the Sphingolin Myelin Basic Protein. Both of them quizzed me intensely on the use and results of taking the substance. Both of them also shared with me their horror stories of a life lived with Betaseron. Both of them suffered from bouts of severe depression. Betaseron caused Rosie to lose quite a bit of weight from her already thin frame. Marcia had experienced noticeable weight gain. Neither of them held out much hope for a brighter future. In addition, Marcia was beginning to experience vision problems, another sign of the growing progression of the disease. Both were frustrated, hopeless, and more than a bit afraid.

I tried to offer what comfort I could to these two wonderful souls with shattered lives. I gave them each a good supply of the Sphingolin Myelin and the beef protein extract, and the contact information for BioCybernetics and Emerson Ecologics. They took them gratefully, if a little timidly. Was I certain that the myelin, in particular, wouldn't interfere adversely with their drug therapy? I responded that I didn't see how it could, as the drug they were presently taking was supposed to shield myelin, or at least leave it alone. As a healer, I did advise that as I was not familiar with their medical histories, they should contact these excellent companies and consult with their doctors, who I hoped would be more open to considering the substances than my recently departed visitors.

I walked them to the parking lot after we had finished our refreshments and discussion, inviting them to contact me any time that they had a question or just wanted to talk. Thanking me warmly, they got into Marcia's specially equipped car that she operated by hand controls on the steering wheel, having lost most of the use of her legs by the time that I met her. I waved as they drove away. I have never again heard from the members of the NMSS that visited the Spa that day, including Rosie and Marcia. I don't know if these two lovely ladies are still with us. If they should obtain copies of this book, I hope they will have the courage to try these therapies, before it is finally too late. I don't know if all of the damage their bodies have suffered can be reversed, but I do know that the alternative healing methods I presented to them that day and ones I was shortly to discover will prevent them from getting any worse.

7
Righting Viral Wrongs—
Vitamin Therapy

The unpleasant meeting with the NMSS representatives haunted me for several weeks afterward. Although I didn't doubt the effectiveness of the treatments I was undergoing, I did begin to question whether or not anyone would believe in them, no matter how well I became. I was determined to continue on my course of action, however. Now that it seemed that I had the disease at least under control, I wanted to move on to the next level. I wanted to find a way to push it out of my body entirely.

I have said more than once throughout this story that I felt as if I had been divinely led on this journey. I was struck by this feeling once again when I received a telephone call, seemingly out of the blue, that was again to change the direction of my investigation and my efforts to find a cure. One morning, as I sat in my office at the Spa, a call came in from a doctor in Alabama who wished to speak with me about BioCybernetics. Always eager to educate someone new on this procedure, I gladly took the call.

The voice on the other end of the line was friendly, warm, and educated, with a distinctive and charming Southern accent. It belonged to William Crawford, N.D., head of the

Crawford Center in Mobile, Alabama. Dr. Crawford is a naturopath like myself. I liked him instantly, and soon we were deep in conversation about our various methods of treatment and nutritional counseling. He contacted me because he was interested in including BioCybernetics as part of the diagnosis and treatment program at his facility. I explained the procedure and said he could learn how to interpret the data and develop the individual nutrient counseling needed by becoming a counselor himself. He was most interested, and went on to become certified through Santoro and Weyhreter's course.

The conversation turned to myself, and I told him that I had been diagnosed with multiple sclerosis in 1994. He inquired as to my current condition, and I summarized all that I had done since the initial diagnosis. The Crawford Center treats patients with a variety of ailments, but for the last few years has been primarily devoted to those with autoimmune complaints. Dr. Crawford had done quite a bit of work with MS patients, and had seen good success with nutritional and vitamin therapy. I told him of the dietary restrictions I had been following. He asked if I had seen a marked difference in my condition afterwards. Not radically, I told him, although I felt more energetic and alert. The imbalances in the minerals and metals in my body were slowly decreasing, but they were not, as yet, corrected. Also, some of the essential substances in my body that were below the acceptable level still were not increasing. However, I wasn't experiencing any new symptoms, and the Swank book counseled that eliminating dietary fat prevented the nutrients needed by the myelin from being utilized to digest the fat in the food.

He agreed that this fact might be relevant, but the fortunate lack of new symptoms could also be a result of taking the Sphingolin Myelin Basic Protein and the other substances I used daily. Then, he said something that surprised me.

"Well, I think it's to be expected that you didn't see more improvement in your charts when you altered your diet. Food plays an important part in treating a virus, but not in that way."

"The damage done by multiple sclerosis is a result of a viral infection. In fact, I firmly believe there is scientific evidence that MS is not even a new virus; it is instead a mutation, a reoccurrence of an old one," said Dr. Crawford. "... In actual fact, the old virus has remained dormant in their system for an extended period of time. Then, a series of conditions, which I believe may be nutritionally, traumatically, or virally related, triggers the old virus, and it mutates, changes form according to the trigger mechanism, and re-manifests itself as MS."

"Excuse me?" I stopped him. "Did you say that MS is a virus?"

"I did, indeed. The damage done by multiple sclerosis is a result of a viral infection. In fact, I firmly believe there is scientific evidence that MS is not even a new virus; it is instead a mutation, a reoccurrence of an old one. Something from the patient's childhood or adolescence from which they never fully recovered, although they seemed to have become perfectly healthy again. In actual fact, the old virus has remained dormant in their system for an extended period of time. Then, a series of conditions, which I believe may be nutritionally, traumatically, or virally related, triggers the old virus, and it mutates, changes form according to the trigger mechanism, and re-manifests itself as MS."

I said nothing for so long on my end of the line that he had to ask if I was still there. My mind flashed back through my life. The bout with the measles, the mono, the various accidents and broken bones. This guy could be on to something that I had not even considered. "But I thought research was showing that it may be genetically, or even geographically related."

"Both of those factors may indeed play a part, but I believe only as is related to the susceptibility of contracting the disease itself. The genetic link may determine who is more likely to have the mutation occur. No, something within the body itself causes the old virus to reawaken and grow. That's why your myelin supplement has been working. The virus feeds on it instead of your spinal cord. I also believe the trigger mechanism that causes MS, or indeed any autoimmune disease mutation, is to be found within the cells themselves. There is a doctor in Germany, Hans Nieper, who has not only treated MS patients with vitamin and mineral therapy, he has cured thousands of them completely."

I was stunned. You mean, there already was a cure? A *natural* cure? Why didn't anyone tell me about this? Why didn't anyone know? I saw nothing on this treatment, no mention whatsoever, in anything that I had been given or researched on my own. I said this to Dr. Crawford, who replied, "Well, Celeste, I guess you've just been looking in the wrong places."

We both laughed, and he went on to tell me about the world-renowned and widely respected chemist from Hannover, Germany. Dr. Nieper had spent almost thirty years studying the effects of vitamin and mineral substances on the body at the individual cellular level. He had successfully treated over 1300 patients with MS by the time he had written his landmark work, *The Treatment of Multiple Sclerosis.*

Over the next few months, I was to learn a great deal more about the amazing work of Dr. Hans A. Nieper. In fact, after reading the article Dr. Crawford sent me and other published reports by Dr. Nieper, his findings and his treatments were to become one of the cornerstones of my victory. I explain the findings of this brilliant medical man in chapter 12, "Achieving Balance Through Vitamin, Mineral, and Supplement Therapies."

I spoke to Dr. Crawford again once I received his materials and he had received mine on BioCybernetics. Additionally, Dr. Crawford wanted to see the results of my most recent BCI analysis and EFA tests. He also requested that I send him a hair and blood sample for special analysis that he and his colleagues used at the center. This analysis would determine the presence of viral concentrations in my system and if any pattern of infections existed. The actual testing would be done by a laboratory known as Trace Elements, headed by another outstanding clinical physician and researcher, David L. Watts, D.C., Ph.D.

I was most happy to comply. This new line of thought was so exciting. I asked Dr. Crawford if he thought I should go to Germany, to experience Dr. Neiper's treatments for myself. He responded that it might be an option, but the treatments were very expensive and almost certainly would not be covered by U.S. health insurance. The treatments could also take from three to six months to complete, depending upon my rate of progress. I was still very interested in going, regardless. Dr. Crawford gave me the contact information for Dr. Neiper's clinic, and after considerable thought, I placed a call to Hannover, Germany.

The nurse who answered was charming, full of good-natured Old World courtesy. She spoke English flawlessly with just the slightest trace of a German accent. She thanked me for my interest, but explained that Dr. Nieper had not been taking on any new patients recently. His colleagues were accepting new cases, however, and she was certain that they would be able to find a spot for me as well. She said that she would send me all of the information on the clinic and the procedures, and I could review it and decide if indeed I wanted to come. She asked how I had heard of their facility, and I replied that Dr. William Crawford had introduced me to the work they did there. The nurse was familiar with Dr. Crawford and the Crawford Center. He had been in contact with Dr. Nieper several times in regards to the Calcium-AEP treatments Dr. Nieper pioneered and instituted. We ended the conversation with her promise to send me the literature.

I was to find out later that when I first contacted Dr. Neiper's facility he had been ill. At that time, in late 1996, his health was beginning to fail. Dr. Nieper passed on in 1998. I regret that I never had the opportunity to meet him personally. By all accounts, scientific and personal, he was truly a great man.

I spoke to Jerry about going to Germany for three months to the Nieper clinic, but the idea of so lengthy a visit out of the country caused him some concern. He agreed that if it was the best way to finally rid myself of the virus, then I should go. However, he also suggested that I wait until the results of these new tests of Dr. Crawford's were completed before I made any final decision. This sounded sensible, and I agreed.

I was thrilled by the Nieper protocols, especially after reviewing the articles sent to me by Dr. Crawford. My mother called me a few days after I had spoken to the German clinic and I excitedly relayed the information to her. My mom and I had begun to grow closer over the last two and a half years and spoke to each other regularly. That day, she was silent for a minute, then had some of her own news to offer. She'd found a very interesting article in the local Victorville, California paper about herpes and MS patients.

The Institute for Viral Pathology in Milwaukee, Wisconsin had made two interesting discoveries. In a group of eleven MS patients examined, eight of the eleven were found to have some form of the herpes virus present in their brain tissue. Additionally, out of twenty-five MS patients studied, fourteen were shown to have a form of the herpes virus present in their bloodstream. The article did not note the race, age, or gender composition of the study subjects, nor whether these analyses were done on live patients, or postmortem by autopsy.

The article further stated that it was now the opinion of the "research authorities" at UCLA that if MS was a virus, or a mutation of an old childhood illness never fully eliminated, by treating the old virus with modern viral technology, the onset or progress of MS could be slowed or prevented entirely. These were the same "authorities," mind you, who two and a half years earlier had told me there was nothing that I could do about MS. The piece concluded by saying that if MS was proven to be a virus, and if further research confirmed these probable origins, then the findings could lead to an entirely new type of treatment for a disease formerly thought to be incurable.

I was very impressed and excited by the article. I placed a call to Dr. Meyers, the UCLA specialist whom I had seen on referral from Dr. Curatalo. I wanted to speak with him personally, but he was unavailable. I left a message and asked the nurse for his fax number. I faxed him a copy of the article and contact information for Dr. Crawford and Dr. Watts, who were involved in similar lines of research. I never received a return call from Dr. Meyers or anyone else at the facility. I am not aware of anyone from UCLA contacting either Dr. Crawford or Dr. Watts, though I faxed UCLA on more than one occasion.

The hair and blood analyses that Dr. Watts performed were completed within a couple of weeks. Dr. Crawford called me at home one evening with Dr. Watts also on the line. It was Dr. Watts who first broke the news to me that there was definitely a viral record in my hair analysis, and certain concentrations of telltale substances in my blood as well. Dr. Watts was of the opinion that I had at one time been afflicted with the Epstein-Barr Virus, or EBV. I found this surprising, as I had never been diagnosed with that illness.

Dr. Watts asked me what major illnesses, if any, I did have as a child or young adult. I told him about the measles. Dr. Crawford urged me to tell Dr. Watts what illness I'd had as a teenager. I thought this a bit odd, as I'd already told Dr. Crawford, but I didn't mind repeating it. I said that I'd had mononucleosis when I was about seventeen.

"Well, there you go, Celeste," said Dr. Watts. "There's your Epstein-Barr."

"But," I protested, "they told me, and my parents, that what I had was mono."

"That's also entirely correct. Mononucleosis, especially twenty years ago when diagnostic testing was nowhere near as advanced as it is today, was often commonly cross-diagnosed as Epstein-Barr, and is in fact, entirely similar. In fact, they are probably one and the same thing, with infinitesimal differences. Not only did you have it, but, by the looks of this analysis you never really got rid of it."

"But, how is that possible? I recovered, went on with my life. It took a long time, granted, but I did get over it!"

"No, you got *better*. Your body reduced the virus to a harmless level, but never eliminated it entirely from your system." Suddenly, I remembered the words of Dr. Crawford during our first conversation: "MS is not even a new virus; it is instead a mutation and reoccurrence of an old one, something from the patient's childhood or adolescence they never fully recovered from."

"So," I continued, "what you're telling me is that my MS is EBV resurfaced to attack me again because my body never got rid of it the first time?"

"In a word, *yes!*" Dr. Watts's response was immediate and emphatic.

I was silent. It was as if an idea that whispered in the corners of my mind had swung round to face me at last. Everything was clear in an instant. The reason that the patients on the low-fat Swank diet did so well was apparent. In the cases of most MS patients, the raw materials needed to attack and eliminate the virus were utilized instead on digestion and absorption of dietary fat. When fat was eliminated from the diet, these resources could concentrate on the disease. Dietary sugar is processed by many of the same vitamins and enzymes that metabolize fats. Eliminate sugar and you accomplish much the same result. The reason I did not see any new symptoms was because I had eliminated these foods from my diet and the virus was attacking the myelin supplements I took every day. Dear God, something *finally* made sense!

"Celeste, are you there?" Dr. Crawford inquired after my long silence.

I answered him with a simple question. "So, what do I do now?"

Dr. Watts answered. "Seems to me that we need to treat the EBV. Eliminate that from your system, and the MS no longer has raw materials from which to create itself. Then, restore your system to a natural balance, and the MS itself should finally die."

This was incredible. This was an *answer*. Even if it was not to prove to be *the* answer, it was a fine place to go next. Now, I wanted to start right away.

"What do you need from me so that we can start this right away? Do you need me to fly down there? I can be on a plane in the morning."

Dr. Crawford answered. "No, I don't think that you need to come all the way down here, Celeste, although you are more than welcome to, of course. The first thing we need to do is to get you started on a vitamin B protocol. It was first used by a very learned man named Dr. Linus Pauling on his own seriously ill patients. This is a series of injectible vitamin compounds that I want you to take daily in the specific concentrations that I will send to you. I assume that you are familiar with the procedures of self-injection?" When I answered in the affirmative, he continued. "I will express a supply to you tomorrow. You'll have it in two days. Follow the instructions that I will send with it to the letter. In fact, call me when you receive the package and we'll do your first injection together."

I felt my spirits soar as I realized that, at last, I was led to something that might be the answer I had been so desperately seeking. I asked Drs. Crawford and Watts about the advisability of going to Germany to Dr. Hans Nieper's clinic. Crawford, as I knew, was particularly familiar with Nieper's protocols. Both of them agreed I should first pursue the vitamin B injectibles, then have another system analysis to see what imbalances remained. When the EBV had been reduced to trace amounts or eliminated entirely, I could begin Dr. Nieper's protocols with Dr. Crawford, if I wished, as he was familiar with the procedures and additionally could obtain the substances used by Dr. Nieper in his treatments.

The kit from Dr. Crawford arrived two days later. It contained a supply of syringes and the injectible compound, along with preparation instructions. I called him as planned, and he walked me through the first injection. There were no problems of any kind, and soon I was using the vitamin injections daily as a firm part of my treatment routine. The protocol Dr. Crawford prescribed contained a mixture of B and B-family vitamins in specific ratios. I explain in greater detail about each of these substances in chapter 12, "Achieving Balance through Vitamin, Mineral, and Supplement Therapies."

I spoke with Al Weyhreter a few days after my conference call with Dr. Crawford and Dr. Watts. He, too, found the conclusions of these two medical men to be extremely interesting. He recommended that I supplement the Crawford therapy with some of the BioCybernetics nutrients that were specifically designed to combat viruses.

Distributed by BioCybernetics as the Virus Protocol Pack, it is actually a series of five natural substances to be taken on a rotational basis. Each one is taken two or three times daily for four days, then discontinued and another in the series takes its place. After twenty days, the cycle repeats itself. The protocol is continued until all symptoms are gone, or in my case, until a system analysis showed that the virus had left my system. The five substances in the protocol pack are distributed as Monolaurin, Virusin, Astragalus, Echinacea, and Aracadonic Acid. Some of them may be familiar to you, especially if you are conversant with natural healing substances. Most of them are obtainable in better health food stores and nutrition centers.

Be aware of what you are buying, however. Concentration per dosage of these healing substances can vary widely between manufacturers. Read the labels carefully to be certain that you are receiving more than trace elements of each substance from the over-the-counter products available. I recommend you purchase your nutrients and natural healing substances from a recognized natural food or vitamin supplier to be certain you are receiving the highest-quality supplements mixed with a minimum amount of inert or filler substances.

After learning of this new outlook on the classification and cause of MS, I began to rethink my dietary restrictions. As I reasoned it, the positive effects of the Swank and Zero Dairy, Zero Sugar diets were essentially replicated by the myelin supplements that I took daily. I had done some nutritional research since beginning these diets, and especially into the article given to me by Drs. Van Benshoten and McSweyne regarding the dairy controversy and the food group's effect, if any, on the MS patient. Disturbingly, I found that some of the claims made in the article were not entirely supported by factual data. I explore this subject in chapter 13, "Dangerous Dairy."

Now that I had the new information from Drs. Crawford and Watts, I began to explore the vitamin and nutrient content of foods in more depth. The low levels of some nutrients in my system still concerned me. Deficiencies could be just as harmful as excesses, especially if the deficiency of one mineral was in direct contrast to the excess of another mineral involved in a chemical ratio. In other words, if I had too little iron in my system, this could cause or leave me at greater risk for a number of conditions. If I also had an excess of copper, that too would create its own set of problems. But, as I was learning, the ratio of iron to copper was equally important to proper cellular function, and presented another set of difficulties when incorrect. I provide further explanation of the various minerals and their relationships or "ratios" to one another in the chapter 11, "BioCybernetics–Vital Analyses You Should Undergo."

I began to realize that some of the nutrients my body needed I could not get from my present dietary intake. I needed to make a decision. I could either continue with the restrictions and continue to take the vitamin injections and nutrition and essential oil supplements, or I could consider allowing a broader range of foods back into my diet. I decided to stay with my present regimen until something better presented itself. I was, however, running out of recipes using food that I could eat and also liked. Though I did find several good recipes in each of the books that I read, sometimes you have to wonder if the people who wrote the books actually ever ate some of the dishes.

In the latter part of 1997 I began to shop around for some new healthy menu choices. I came across a book that seemed to be just what I was looking for. Written by learned biochemist Dr. Barry Sears, *The Zone: A Dietary Road Map* (Sears and Lawren, 1995) was a completely new way of looking at food. Dr. Sears's research into the functions of substances at the cellular level was exhaustive, spanning decades. He was instrumental in the development of several new methods of treating cardiac conditions, motivated by the fatal heart attack of his father at an early age, and his own genetic predisposition to be at the same high risk. An explanation of Dr. Sears's findings is included in the chapter 16, "Making the Right Choices: Understanding the Role of Food in Creating a Nutrition Program That Works." Suffice it to say here that the breakthrough treatments and medications he developed were the forerunners of even more valuable later work that was to save the lives of millions.

During his research into the effects of basic food components—the proteins, carbohydrates, and fats that make up every edible item on the planet—Dr. Sears noted that optimal performance and cellular health were achieved when an ideal balance of these foods was ingested as part of a daily nutrition program. This biochemical state of optimum performance is routinely referred to by athletes as "the Zone," the physical place where the athlete's personal best is achieved, competitions are won, and records are broken. Dr. Sears adopted this term as the name of his nutrition program. He began to look at food in a very unique way—as a drug.

His perceptions are entirely correct. Food *is* a drug. The amounts and concentrations of the foods that we eat and the proportions of those foods that we consume have a direct bearing on our present state of health, just as do drugs. Foods can cause us to gain muscle, gain fat, or lose either. Foods can stimulate us, cause mood swings, or when eaten in the wrong combinations, depress us. Foods can make our elimination system too loose, or too sluggish. They can cause us to urinate more frequently, or to retain water. They can give us energy, or they can make us sleep. In short, foods can cause all of the reactions that medications can cause. Food, therefore, can be accurately viewed as a drug.

Dr. Sears breaks these food "drugs" down into their individual components. Viewing these basic components in the same way that a chemist does when mixing a drug compound to treat an illness, he reassembles them in specific mathematical measurements to provide those nutrients needed to achieve maximum cellular health, and therefore maximum physical performance. The amounts of proteins, carbohydrates, and fats are measured in units called "blocks." Dr. Sears teaches the readers to calculate their own height, weight, and body fat percentage. The number of food blocks needed at each meal to provide the individual with the maximum nutrients can then be determined.

Correlating this information into a precise mathematical table of values, Dr. Sears formulates a high-performance nutrition program, using not only natural foods but others commonly found in the daily diet, including some fast food choices. Far from writing the work as a purely clinical trial, Dr. Sears put his new high nutrition diet into practice. He convinced the coaches of the Stanford University Men's and Women's swim teams to try his program, following the diet strictly over a period of several months. The results? The Stanford swimmers medaled eight times at the 1992 Barcelona Olympics. Pretty impressive. Dr. Sears also explains the function of one of the most basic elements in our system, the eicosanoid (ee-KAY-san-oyd). An explanation of the significance of eicosanoids is included in chapter 16,"Making the Right Choices: Understanding the Role of Food in Creating a Nutrition Program That Works."

Using Dr. Sears's worksheets, I calculated my measurements, and from them my percentage of body fat. I was then able to easily calculate the "blocks" of proteins, carbohydrates, and fats I should eat at each meal to provide my body with the maximum vitamin and nutritional benefit, as well as optimum food balance. I was pleased to note that the proper number of blocks could be combined in a variety of ways to create a satisfying portion of food at each meal. This was not a starvation diet by any means. The best news is that almost all of the foods you could think of are allowed.

I can't impress on you enough the valid scientific information contained in Dr. Sears's book. I believe that it provides an almost complete nutritional plan that anyone can follow and achieve excellent results. One interesting side effect of the Zone diet is that overweight persons tend to naturally shed the excess pounds. And, as your body fat percentage changes, so do the number and combination of food blocks, thereby always keeping your system in nutritional balance.

Once again, before deciding to entirely scrap the Swank and Zero Dairy, Zero Sugar diets, I made a quick call to nutritionist Santoro and Dr. Crawford. Both of them saw no harm in switching to the Zone diet, although they agreed that I should continue to avoid or limit dairy until my excess calcium levels were brought down into the acceptable range and I tested negative for allergy. Dr. Crawford was already familiar with Dr. Sears's work with AZT (a breakthrough drug used in the treatment of AIDS), as he saw many autoimmune patients regularly. He knew the quality of any research with Dr. Sears's name attached. Bob Santoro was especially pleased, as he had been concerned with the failure of some of the deficient vitamin and nutrient levels in my body to increase over the course of my following the other diet protocols.

Once I had received this dual positive confirmation of my proposed changes, I drove down to the fresh seafood markets that line the Santa Barbara waterfront. I bought two of the biggest lobsters I could find. I picked up some fresh vegetables, fruit, and wild rice. I felt like a paroled prisoner. I had faithfully followed the Swank diet for two years and had further limited my diet for the past year by incorporating the

Zero Dairy, Zero Sugar regimen. I never lost my love of good food, but was determined to make quality decisions regarding my health and the best course of treatment for my MS. I was fully prepared to eliminate the foods these protocols specified forever, if necessary, and resign myself to tofu-turkey patties. So, it should come as no surprise that upon discovering sound medical facts not only lifting the restrictions but recommending I consume a wide variety of foods again, I was immensely pleased.

I returned home and thumped the bag of groceries onto the work island in front of our startled cook. With a smile on my face, I gaily requested that she prepare these enormous crustaceans for the evening meal.

"But, Dr. Celeste," she questioned, in the careful tone of one who isn't sure if she is indeed speaking to a crazy person, "aren't you supposed to do your tofu diet thing?"

"Not anymore, my dear! It's a whole new world now!" I fairly danced over to her with the book in my hand. Handing it over with a dramatic flourish, I presented it to her, exclaiming, "It seems that I now have permission to enter, ta-da, the Zone!"

She laughed, and I went on to explain the new diet rules. I had already figured out what my blocks would need to be for each meal, and how much protein, carbohydrates, and fat made up a block. I would prepare a weekly menu of the meals I'd like to eat with the portion sizes. Although I would still be severely limiting most dairy foods, I could begin to eat regular meals with Jerry again. This, of course, would cut her work load in half. There was joy in the kitchen from all parties present. I was leaving the kitchen as she called out a final question. "So, Dr. Celeste, you can have eggs again, yes?"

The memory of legendary breakfasts came to my mind. "No," I replied wistfully, "I still can't have eggs." Then, I brightened. "But, I *can* have pancakes!"

Dinner with Jerry that night was a celebratory affair. It seemed that all of my disjointed pieces were finally beginning to fall into place. I was finally obtaining the answers that I needed to win this all-important fight. I had found new therapies and a new nutritional program that seemed to offer what I searched for. Things were definitely looking up. Grinning at Jerry, I wiped the trail of non-bogus, real butter from my chin.

With the Zone diet, I continued to follow the Crawford and BCI protocols throughout the remainder of 1997 and well into 1998. Periodic BCI analyses showed that, at last, my deficient levels were beginning to rise. My excesses continued to drop, but more rapidly. The combination of myelin supplements, B injectibles, and the Zone diet was working. It would be well over another year before my therapies would change. At that time I would begin the protocols of Dr. Hans Nieper, entering the final stage of the treatments that would rid my body of the virus completely.

Though my overall health and energy levels steadily improved, I still could not rid my left leg of the persistent numb areas. Sometimes, especially if I was on my feet for several hours during a full day of patient treatment, my ankle would begin to twinge and become slightly unstable. I didn't want to consider the lack of sensation might be permanent. I continued to search for a way to reverse the damage and restore my leg to full health and normalcy once again.

The Divine Hand guided once more. This time, I was to discover that my search was not to take me into some far distant land. In fact, my next step on the journey was right under my nose, smiling in the warm sun of a California Christmas.

8
Replenishing the Losses, Restoring Mobility

The rest of 1997 spun itself out relatively uneventfully. The dietary changes that I had made with the introduction of "the Zone" were beginning to show. I had more health and vitality than I'd had in years. The vitamins and nutrients that my body was so severely lacking were beginning to be replaced through a combination of this new diet regimen and Dr. Crawford's vitamin B injectibles. I felt that I was well on my way to beating this virus.

Still, there were other issues that I was anxious to see resolved. The nerve damage that I had suffered with the first manifestation of the MS was still present in my left leg and ankle. Before the illness, my left leg had always been the stronger of the two, ever since that car accident, years ago now, when my right ankle was broken so severely. A broken bone was much preferable to a fatality, of course, no matter how severe the injury. But, since that time, I had a tendency to develop a body stance that threw most of my weight onto my left leg, especially on occasions where I needed to stand for long periods of time. After the onset of MS, I was no longer able to make that weight adjustment. And so, on days that were physically stressful, I found myself unsteady on my feet at the end of the day.

I needed to find a way to strengthen my bone structure again. My calcium levels were still charting way too high, so the idea of taking an additional supplement to support my bones did not seem to be the most sensible course of action. The excess calcium was already throwing some of my mineral ratios into an unbalanced state, and, although I was working with the BCI team and Dr. Crawford to correct these conditions, adding additional calcium at that time might have exacerbated the problem and set my progress back several months, which I certainly did not want.

I was put in mind of this need to correct and strengthen my bone structure while in London, England, in the early fall of 1997. I was with Jerry, attending an annual international vitamin and nutrient trade show and convention. At the show, we met up with our holistic friend from Seattle, Washington, Dr. Jonathan Wright. One evening we fell into a discussion while at dinner with him and his wife that would lead to another key to my eventual victory. We had not seen Jonathan since our dinner together the year before. During the meal, we discussed his current projects, and he and Jerry talked about the trade show while Jonathan's wife and I enjoyed our own conversation. After a while, the conversation turned to my affliction, and my current state of affairs.

Jonathan and his wife were most interested in the protocols that I had tried and the steps that I had taken. Jonathan especially was excited by the news that Dr. Crawford and Dr. Watts believed that MS was a new, mutated form of an older virus that had never left the system. As a holistic healer, this made sense to him, as did the new prescribed therapies. He thought they were an excellent way to restore balance to my system.

In fact, he was of the opinion that all of these protocols placed me firmly on the right track. He was certain that I was finally on my way to ridding myself of this disease, which had dominated my life for over three years. I told him about the problems that I was still having, the lack of muscle stability at times, limited mobility at others, and the numbness that still refused to leave me. Last, I told him about Dr. Barry Sears's Zone diet and the new outlook it had given me on food.

Jonathan agreed that perhaps the weakened condition of my leg might be due to existing damage that might be difficult to rectify, and he was very interested in my work with the Zone diet. By this time I had become proficient at calculating the proper number and combination of meal blocks. Using the food in front of me to illustrate, I explained how these combinations result in optimum nutrition, allowing the body to manufacture the substances needed for correct metabolism and the production of other essential elements and enzymes necessary for overall system function.

Besides the general, though important feelings of additional energy and well-being, Jonathan asked me what concrete improvements I had seen while following the Zone. I replied that the BCI analyses performed since I had altered my dietary intake showed the elements out of balance in my system were beginning to fall into line. Vitamin and nutrient levels that had charted as deficiencies were gradually rising toward more acceptable ranges, and those in excess were slowly dropping. It was an incremental process, however, with no immediate gains or losses. I found it frustrating, because I was anxious to have my inner system return to a harmonious state.

Jonathan had a most interesting thought. The purpose of the Zone was to give the body a supply of optimum nutrition at each meal, correct? I agreed. The Zone does this by allowing the proper manufacture of eicosanoids, the building blocks of all cellular function. I also agreed with this assessment.

"If all of this is correct, and is taken as a given," he reasoned, "then the amount and combination of foods is calculated to produce optimum conditions in the human body. However, the Zone program is structured to maintain this condition of optimum nutrition for perfect system *maintenance*. It includes no protocols, or you are not aware of how to calculate the combinations that *rebuild* the system when elemental deficiencies or excesses exist at the basic cellular level. Perhaps your own personal reserves are so depleted that although you are ingesting the ideal combination of nutrients, your body cannot manufacture enough of the substances you need in order to correct the deficiencies more quickly.

"In essence," he continued, "it's almost like having a high credit card balance. You make enough money to pay off the current charges, but not enough to pay off the old outstanding debt except for a little at a time. In your body, even though you're working hard and moving in the right direction, the deficiencies that still exist limit your present condition as they allow the root cause, the virus, to maintain a foothold in your system. You need to find a way to replenish the losses you've already suffered on a more timely basis. Then, I think, is when you'll see real progress.

"Look, Celeste," he concluded, seeing my thoughtful expression, "I'm not an expert on eicosanoids, but I know someone who is." He grabbed a pen from the breast pocket of his jacket and a trade brochure from the pile on the table. Scribbling a few lines onto the white space where the mailing label would go, he said, "Look this guy up, or at least call him when you get back to the States. He's done a lot of work with hormonal and system imbalances, and he may be able to help you find something that will restore what you've lost more quickly so that you can go forward, maintaining your levels once you've brought them back into line."

I thanked him sincerely for the contact and his educated opinions. I felt fortunate to have such a caring friend who was also a learned medical professional. Although I was never his patient, Dr. Jonathan Wright had now provided me with what would prove to be another valuable avenue of investigation. I glanced at the number before stashing it in my purse. Dr. Bradford Weeks. I made a mental note to call him when I got home.

When I did return home, I found a ton of work waiting for me. There were patient cases to review, files to update, new cases to schedule. While organizing some of the growing pile of materials on my desk, I came across some notes that I had made during the trade show trip. In amongst the brochures was the telephone number of the doctor that Jonathan Wright had recommended to me. I decided to contact him, never realizing just how important this brilliant physician was to become in my eventual victory.

Bradford S. Weeks, M.D., is a world-renowned physician recognized for his many contributions to medicine. His long and distinguished career encompasses many diverse fields of study, including extensive research on the human cellular system and the role of hormones in system function, autoimmune dysfunctions, and the research and treatment of MS. He was also a past President Emeritus of the AAS, the American Apiary Society. This fact was to become particularly significant to me. I contacted Dr. Weeks at his Clinton, Washington office.

Dr. Weeks often consults with patients via telephone. These telephone consultations are recorded and transcribed, becoming part of the patient's permanent file. He listened carefully as I reviewed my medical and family history, interjecting questions on topics that required further clarification.

Dr. Weeks is involved in the treatment of the autoimmune- and MS-afflicted patients. The focus of his therapies concentrate largely on the restoration of body imbalances through hormone replacement. He requested that I send him a blood sample so that he could perform specific testing on my hormone levels. As soon as he received the results, we would discuss them and begin to plan a course of treatment for me.

We spoke again about two weeks after our initial consultation. My results definitely showed that several of my hormone levels were indeed excellent. Dr. Weeks recommended that although I was producing the correct amounts of these essential substances, I was in my middle forties, and it would be natural for these levels to begin to drop with the advancement of age. Statistics indicated that this was the time that women were especially susceptible to the onset of MS. Those already afflicted often experienced an exacerbation of existing symptoms or the manifestation of new ones of greater severity. In an effort to prevent this from occurring, first Dr. O'Dell and now Dr. Weeks recommended that I begin to take hormonal supplements to maintain the correct levels.

Dr. Weeks prescribed progesterone and HGH, Human Growth Hormone. HGH regulates more than just the growth of the human body. After an adult has reached full height and adult bone mass, HGH begins supporting other systems in the body. Progesterone is another hormone important to several system functions. I was beginning to understand the role of hormones in the production of the correct amounts of substances essential to proper cellular function. Now that I was familiar with the work of Dr. Sears, I knew that cellular health promoted the proper manufacture of good eicosanoids. Cells in poor condition produced excessive bad eicosanoids, resulting in overall system instability and increased risk of complications. At the least, the failure of my body to maintain sufficient amounts of the substances needed for production of good eicosanoids would certainly allow the disease more fertile ground for growth and further damage to my system. I discuss this topic further in chapter 16, "Making the Right Choices: Understanding the Role of Food in Creating a Nutrition Program That Works."

I added these hormonal supplements to my daily routine. Dr. Weeks also sent a supply of nutrients specifically formulated for women. These contained several vitamins, minerals, and extracts from healing plants such as aloe. During this time, Dr. O'Dell relocated, moving his practice outside of the United States, and I began to get the DHEA supplements from Dr. Weeks instead. I would continue the hormonal therapy with Dr. Weeks over the next several months.

The holiday season had arrived. I spent hours on my feet, walking, standing, shopping. There were presents and decorations to obtain, social invitations to accept and decline, meals and parties of my own to plan. About the middle of December, my left leg began to ache again, no doubt encouraged by the unkind demands I was putting upon it. One day while shopping in nearby Santa Maria, I decided see a chiropractor, as my lower back was beginning to twinge. I was the only chiropractor in residence at the Spa, and had not been treated chiropractically at all since my diagnosis with MS. The Divine Hand was surely upon my shoulder again as I found my way to the offices of Dr. Wayne Miller.

Wayne Miller, D.C., and his father, Robert Miller, D.C., are chiropractic healers with extensive knowledge of the human skeletal and nervous systems. Their techniques are non-force, and they specialize in a technique known as "The Activator." This adjustment protocol realigns the bones and opens the neural pathways so that proper sensation, mobility, and function can return to the skeletal area or limb affected. They have used this technique successfully on a number of trauma injury patients and elderly patients affected by arthritis or osteoporosis.

I felt immediately at home in their offices, and although they had other patients awaiting treatment, they graciously welcomed a walk-in visitor. I was given the standard form by a cheerful receptionist, and I completed it hastily. I skipped over most of the medical history sections, as I was only seeking a simple adjustment that would reduce the strain on my back and perhaps allow my leg to be a bit more stable until I had finished my holiday madness and could enjoy a few days of uninterrupted rest.

I liked Wayne Miller the moment he entered the treatment room, characteristic broad smile on his pleasant face. A few years younger than I, Wayne, although not tall, is able to easily manipulate and adjust patients several times his own size. His hands are sure and strong, and he is, quite frankly, knowledgeable as hell. We spoke for a bit about the complaints that I was seeking to correct, and then he examined me. He glanced over my chart, and then looked at me questioningly.

"I don't see anything here that indicates that you ever sustained any serious injuries in the past. Did you just not complete this, or were you never injured?"

I had to admit that I had only cursorily completed the form. I told him that I was a walk-in appointment, and a chiropractor myself. I had just wanted a quick adjustment, so I didn't think that a full explanation was necessary.

"So, basically, what you're saying is that the thing you hate most for your own patients to do, you have now done cheerfully to me?"

We both laughed. He had me there. I *did* hate it when my patients didn't complete their forms. It made decisions much more difficult when considering what course of treatment would most benefit them. I only wanted a one-session visit, however, so I asked him what had prompted him to refer to the chart before adjusting me anyway. His reply really startled me.

"Well, I believe that a lot of the difficulty you are experiencing on your left side actually stems from old injuries you sustained on the right side of your body. Your left side compensated for these injuries, and you were never adjusted properly after those old right-side traumas were healed. Now, your leg is still trying to compensate out of old muscle habit. It's this old instinctive compensation that probably made your left leg the most susceptible to the attack of the MS. You've always thought of it as your 'stronger leg,' but it's more accurate to think of it instead as the one that bore the brunt of activities and your weight when injuries occurred."

I was surprised by what he had to say. I proceeded to fill him in on all of the injuries that he couldn't possibly have known about. I told him about breaking my ankle, sacrum, and coccyx, which had deviated to the left when I was sixteen. He nodded knowingly. "See, Celeste? Your left side has been compensating for your injuries for most of your life."

"Well, what can I do about it? I've been told that the only way to correct the problem is to re-break the coccyx and let it heal again, correctly. Frankly, there is no way I'm going to put myself through that. I didn't want to before I contracted MS, and I have no inclination to do so now."

"I agree with what you are saying. However, I believe that there are adjustment techniques that we can use to align you properly, even with your tailbone permanently out of position. I can't do it all today, though, and I don't know how you feel about starting a series of treatments with me."

I smiled at him. I already trusted him completely. As a fellow practitioner, I readily recognized competence. "Actually, I feel very good about it. I don't treat myself in the area of chiropractic. Is there anything that you can do about my leg today?"

Even though I chiropractically adjusted people all of the time, it never occurred to me that my own injuries could be so interconnected. I suppose when things happen in your own life, you naturally just handle them. You think you're healed, or healed the best you can be, and you just go on.

"Sure, I think so. I think that we can ease the back strain as well, because I really think that's all it is. Let me excuse myself for a minute, and I'll be right back to you."

Left alone in the treatment room, I thought about the discussion I'd just had. Even though I chiropractically adjusted people all of the time, it never occurred to me that my own injuries could be so interconnected. I suppose when things happen in your own life, you naturally just handle them. You think you're healed, or healed the best you can be, and you just go on. I honestly never considered that all of the injuries to my right side could have weakened my left side by carrying my weight as I healed. Dr. Miller was right. I had considered my left to be the "stronger" side because it always managed to compensate whenever I needed it to.

Dr. Wayne reappeared a few moments later with his father, Dr. Robert Miller. A genial and knowledgeable man, Dr. Robert has nearly four decades in clinical practice. They often consult one another on cases and routinely share new techniques or refinements in treatment. Periodically, both attend neurological and osteopathic seminars to remain versed in the latest developments and chiropractic techniques. While Dr. Wayne worked on my lower back and left leg, Dr. Robert discussed several topics with me, including my extensive exercise routine. I had continued my workouts daily, with very few exceptions, pushing it to the limit each time, doing repetitions until my leg could not continue. I mentioned the Jimmie Huega Center and the advice they had given me.

Dr. Robert agreed that exercise was key to maintaining health and mobility, but he disagreed with my practice of taxing my leg on a daily basis. "Celeste, I understand your desire to strengthen the weak limb, and I agree with you. But, you are not giving your leg a chance to rebuild itself. When you exercise extensively, you are actually destroying muscle tissue, tearing it down to rebuild stronger tissue in its place. This rebuilding process takes time, however. When you exercise strenuously every day, you do not give your tissues a chance to complete the rebuilding of a previous section before tearing it down again in another area. I'd instead recommend that you reduce your routine. Limit the treadmill to twenty or thirty minutes, work out every other day, and by no means utterly fatigue your left leg."

This was most interesting. Although I had exercised for years, I had never been what you would call a body builder. I understood basically that carefully planned exercise routines would tone your body and build muscle, but now I had a much clearer picture of how the process actually worked. I hadn't given my muscles, already weakened by MS, a chance to rebuild themselves. I readily agreed to make the changes he recommended. The session was over, and, not surprisingly, I felt much better. The discomfort in my lower back was gone, and I could complete my shopping. I decided to begin treatments to realign my skeletal structure with the Miller team, and made an appointment for the next session before I left that day.

I continue to see Dr. Wayne and Dr. Robert once a week. In fact, we have even discussed a possible professional association, an option I have been considering. After several months of treatment, I have found my body to be more supple and flexible than it has been in years. I still schedule regular visits, as the demands on my time and my physical self continue to increase the stronger I become.

Even though I was now undergoing regular chiropractic treatments as the spring days of 1998 lengthened into summer, I still could not get rid of the nagging numbness in my left thigh and isolated spots on my calf. I was beginning to think that the damage was irreparable. I didn't like the thought, but considering how I could have ended up, I had almost come to accept it. It was at this point that Dr. Bradford Weeks was to step to the forefront of my story once again. He would introduce me to the most radical treatment yet, in an effort to finally restore my leg to full, undamaged function.

9

Exploring the Alternative Edge, The Final Phases

Spring of 1998 found me feeling better than I had for years. I had experienced no new occurrence of fresh symptoms, my BCI analysis levels were continuing to come into line, and I found that even though I had thought that my body was in fairly good shape, after regular visits with Miller Chiropractic, my body was more supple and flexible than I could ever remember it having been.

I was continuing to follow my other protocols, taking the vitamin, mineral, and nutrient supplements daily. My team of doctors was pleased with my progress in each of their selected areas as well. However, no one seemed to have any concrete answers as to how I could get my leg to feel again; it was still numb. Even with surgery, there was no guarantee that the dead zones would ever come to life again.

I had this on my mind when I called Dr. Weeks for our monthly teleconference. During the course of our conversation, I mentioned to him that I wished I could find a way to finally restore my leg to normal. I thought that perhaps he would also tell me that the nerve damage was permanent, and all things considered, there were worse reminders that I could have been left with after this was all over.

Dr. Weeks was silent on his end of the phone for a moment. Then, slowly almost, he made a suggestion that was to change my perspective on truly alternative treatments. "Celeste," he began, speaking as if choosing his words carefully, "there is something that I may be able to recommend to you that might indeed be able to restore your leg to full function. I'm not certain that it's something that you would want to try, however."

Me? Good old "Try Anything Celeste"? Though he didn't know it, he was speaking to a woman who had tried just about everything in this quest for healing, from coffee enemas to oil suppositories, from fasting to spiritual prayers and chants. There were other suggested remedies that I had witnessed and not actually tried for myself, as well. I considered myself to be game for almost anything, especially after some of the things that I had already gone through.

"Sure, I would!" My voice was positive. "Look, if it will help this damn leg of mine, I'm definitely interested, no matter what it is. Lay it on me, doc!"

"Celeste," he continued, and I sobered somewhat at the sound of the seriousness in his voice. "This is not a decision to be made lightly, especially before you have heard all of the particulars. The treatment that I am about to explain to you is considered extremely radical by most of the medical community. Even some alternative healers won't touch this, and they are usually a pretty open-minded group, as a whole."

I was still intrigued, but I admit that his manner was causing me more than a bit of concern. What could this possibly be? I was about to find out.

"There is a treatment method that could indeed restore the feeling and the function in your leg. It's part of an ancient practice known as apitherapy. The specific protocol is called BVT, which stands for Bee Venom Treatment."

"Bee Venom Treatment?" I echoed. This was well beyond the scope of anything that I had ever experienced or had heard of before. "What *is* that?"

"Well, quite simply, it's the systematic injection of the poisonous venom of the common black and yellow honeybee, *apis mellifera.* This is accomplished in one of two ways. Either the pre-collected venom is injected into the affected areas of the patient or multiple live bees are placed upon the patient and allowed to sting the same regions."

Open minded as I was, this notion caused me to instinctively recoil. I'd been stung by bees before. In fact, I had been stung every summer since I came to live on the ranch, including just a week or two before this conversation. Bee stings were painful. They swelled and hurt for quite some time after the actual sting. The bees, it seemed, always managed to sting me along my injured left side, too, a fact that I certainly did not appreciate. And now, this learned doctor whom I trusted as much as I have ever trusted any healer was suggesting that I deliberately put bees on myself and encourage them to "do their thing."

"You can't be serious!" I exclaimed.

"I am," he assured me, "entirely serious. I told you, this is not the therapy for everyone. Although very few people actually experience adverse reactions, many simply cannot get over the very natural fear of the insects themselves."

With good reason, too. A new thought struck me. "Can't you get the same elements from other forms? Does the stuff in the bee venom come in pills, or maybe in a liquid form?"

"Unfortunately, at this time, it does not. Bee venom is extremely difficult to collect, and a small amount can be very expensive. It is far easier to obtain the venom from its natural container, so to speak. That is why live bees are used for the procedure. The venom is fresh, and in the proper proportions for each sting to be the most effective."

I was still intrigued, although the idea was revolting. "So, how is this accomplished? Do I have to let a bee a week sting me? Does the sting have to be in a specific spot, or do I just go out into the meadow and throw a rock at the hive?"

Dr. Weeks laughed heartily. After a moment, he continued his explanation, laughter still in his words. "No, I really don't suggest that you do that! I don't think that you are understanding this procedure. It isn't just a matter of finding a bee and letting it sting you. It also isn't a matter of placing a single bee on any one spot. This is a series of stings, several per session. And, it takes several sessions to complete the treatment, or even in some cases to notice lasting improvement. This is not something that one should enter into frivolously, or begin without the intention of completing."

A *series* of stings? Over a *period* of time? This was an entirely different affair. I might have been able to brave one sting once a week or so, but several? I wasn't sure that I was up to that, and said so. Dr. Weeks, bless him, was completely understanding.

"I know how you feel, and I understand. I told you that this was not for everyone, by any means. It takes a great deal of courage to go through with this, because it is not pleasant. It does involve a certain amount of pain, and other side effects could possibly occur."

"Like what?" I might as well hear it all.

"Common side effects are swelling, redness, itching, pain around the sting area, possibly nausea, dizziness, or light-headedness. There are several other minor complications that may arise. Of course, on rare occasions, more serious side effects are felt. In very rare circumstances, a patient may even experience anaphylactic shock."

"Anaphylactic *shock*? That's fatal, isn't it?"

"It certainly can be. That is why BVT should never be administered at any time without an antidote kit close at hand. Both the patient and the therapist must also be familiar with how to use it, if necessary."

Ooh. I didn't know about this. Open-minded was one thing. Reckless was entirely another. I asked, "Is this a new treatment discovered recently? I've never heard of it."

"Actually," he responded, "it's an ancient art practiced by human healers as long ago as the days of ancient Greece. BVT is only a portion of the healing art of apitherapy, which the Chinese have practiced for thousands of years, and it is still used in modern Asian nations today as a viable healing protocol for all sorts of ailments. If you're interested, I can send you some information about the procedure before you decide. I'll also send you some contact information for someone here in the States who probably knows as much about the treatment and the administration of it as anyone I know."

"Well, I'll certainly be glad to read anything that you want to send to me, of course. It's still a very alien idea, but I'm willing to at least explore the possibility."

"Good for you! I thought you might at least want to consider it, that's why I even bothered to mention it to you. I'll send you the information first thing in the morning. Call me when you've reviewed it, and we can discuss it further."

"That sounds great," I lied. It sounded pretty far from great, but this wonderful doctor had done so much for my healing already that I felt that I owed it to him, if only out of common courtesy, to at least look at what he had on the subject. I was getting ready to hang up, when another question suddenly struck me.

"You seem to be pretty well versed on the subject. If you don't mind my asking, how did you come to know so much about it?"

He laughed, and then answered me. "Of course I don't mind if you ask. Always feel free to ask me anything. The reason that I know quite a bit about apitherapy and BVT is that because until recently, I was the president of the American Apiary Society."

You could have knocked me down right there. I was stunned; the only rejoinder that my brilliant mind could formulate was a humble sounding, "Oh."

He laughed again, but kindly. "I'll let you go now, Celeste. Give me a call when you've read the materials I'm sending. Don't wait for your next scheduled conference. I'll instruct my nurses to be expecting to hear from you."

I didn't know what to think when I hung up the phone. Up until this point in our doctor-patient relationship, Dr. Weeks had always been the calm voice of reason. Every therapy, every protocol that he had recommended made sense and proved to be beneficial. I couldn't imagine that he'd ever prescribe or recommend anything that would be harmful to me. But this . . . BVT was something entirely different. I decided not to mention this to Jerry or anyone else before I at least looked at the materials Dr. Weeks would send.

During the last four years, my search for a cure for MS had taken me down many unfamiliar roads. I was introduced to several alternative treatments that I never knew existed, like BVT. Although, as you know, I am a chiropractor and a naturopath, that does not mean that I spend my life reading medical journals or that I am conversant with every alternative medical development. I try to remain well versed in treatment and nutritional options that address the focus of my practice, which before the onset of my own MS was chiropractic. BVT, although proven to be helpful in the treatment of arthritis, is not largely applicable to chiropractic healing. Therefore, I had no knowledge of the protocol. Of all of the treatments that I had experienced or would undergo, the decision to try BVT caused the greatest personal conflict within me. I was determined to thoroughly research the protocol before making that choice.

Dr. Weeks's materials arrived a few days later, and included information on several topics. There was a complete explanation of the ancient art of apitherapy, which is the use of all of the products of the bee hive in nutrition and healing. There was also quite a bit of information on the American Apiary Society. The AAS is the American affiliate of a larger global entity known as Apimondia, the International Federation of Bee Keepers Association. Each organization is devoted to promoting the awareness and education necessary to recognize apitherapy as a viable and legitimate healing protocol, and to advance the quality of the bees and products from the hive for nutrition, healing, and further scientific research into the benefits of the use of bees and their byproducts. Dr. Bradford Weeks was formerly the president of the AAS. The current president, world-renowned psychiatrist and apitherapist Dr. Theodore Cherbuilez, also serves in an executive capacity with Apimondia. I have included a wonderful in-depth interview with him in chapter 14, "Deadly Savior—Bee Venom Treatment."

There was a wealth of information on Bee Venom Treatment, or BVT, itself. The practice didn't look any less gruesome than it sounded on the telephone. Apitherapists, using live bees, place the insect on the skin of the patient and allow the bee to sting, releasing the venom. The stings are precisely planned, either placed directly on the affected area, or along specific acupuncture points. I had become familiar with these points in my treatments with Dr. Van Benshoten and Dr. McSweyne. Either one of these sting patterns is followed, or a combination of both. The most disconcerting aspect of the treatment was the number of stings per session recommended. A far cry from the one or two stings I thought would be applied, the protocol called for as many as twenty to thirty stings per session! I didn't know if I was up to this.

I had a strong desire to repair my leg, to be sure, but this was a *very* big step. The literature made no effort to sugarcoat the fact that bee venom was a poisonous substance. Great. I'd spent the last four years trying to take poisons *out* of my system, and now I was thinking about deliberately placing fuzzy little bugs on my body with the intent to put more poison *into* it. That couldn't be good. But, this was also a recommendation from Dr. Weeks. I really trusted this doctor. I didn't know what to do.

The final piece of information included was a flyer from a woman on the East Coast named Pat Wagner. Mrs. Wagner, it seemed, was not only an apitherapist, she was also an MS sufferer. Known as the "Bee Lady of Waldorf" because of her extensive use and subsequent promotion of the treatment, she claimed to have been severely bedridden and almost blind when she was introduced to BVT. Today, she says that she has been cured of MS and lives a normal life. She credits this miracle recovery to the use of BVT. This was fascinating but somewhat difficult to believe.

Mrs. Wagner had written a book detailing her experiences, *How Well Are You Willing to Bee?* (Wagner 1997). I thought the use of 'bee' in the title was a cute touch, but the title made me think. Just how well *was* I willing to be? Enough to try *this*? The flyer had a contact number that you could call to buy her book. I was interested in learning all that I could about BVT, so I called and purchased a copy.

Anyone who is seriously, or even timidly considering BVT as a healing option should obtain a copy of this excellent book. *How Well Are You Willing to Bee?* is a wonderful self-help resource written in an easy, conversational style and absolutely packed full of information on apitherapy, the care and keeping of the bees, and the practice of BVT itself. Charts of the human body are included, illustrating the proper location of acupuncture points on the various parts. From these charts, the new BVT practitioner can learn where to apply the bees, maximizing the effectiveness of each sting. There are also session schedules, detailing how many stings to apply in each area, and the period to wait between each treatment for any given area. In short, this book is actually a teaching manual, a home study course, in effect. After carefully reading the book, one should be able to administer treatment safely and successfully.

Pat Wagner has also shared with her readers the amazing story of her own battle with multiple sclerosis. Diagnosed as a young girl, still in her teens, Pat was treated by conventional medicine, given a nightmarish array of drugs, including beta blockers of the same type as those later to become Betaseron, Avonex, and Copaxone. At the time she was introduced to apitherapy and BVT, she was bedridden, almost completely immobilized, and nearly blind. She tried BVT, driven by one last, desperate hope. And this time, hope did not disappoint her. Today, this deeply spiritual woman is a fully mobile grandmother, her faculties, and her life, restored and whole once again. Because Pat is internationally respected as an apitherapist and has first-hand experience with BVT in the treatment of MS, I have included an in-depth personal interview with her in the second section chapter, *Deadly Savior–Bee Venom Treatment.*

I was still undecided, even after reading her excellent book and reviewing the medical and acupuncture charts several times. In my life, I had endured a great deal of pain at various times. During the mercury removal, my mouth was tender and sore in at least one or two spots for weeks. I'd undergone dozens of blood tests, injections, and therapies that were at times uncomfortable or unpleasant. BVT, however, held the promise of a type of pain I didn't know if I could handle. And, even though I'd tried many different nutrients and supplements that could become toxic, the danger in those was minimized by the close supervision of trained professionals. Somehow, allowing oneself to be stung with fifteen to thirty bees over various parts of one's body seemed to be far less precise a protocol and carry a far greater risk.

I needed assurance. I had questions that went beyond the scope of the book or the other materials. In short, I wanted to speak to someone who had been through this. In the back of Pat's book, she lists her contact information and invites anyone who is interested in BVT to contact her. I have listed Pat's contact information in chapter 17 for those of you who would like to obtain Pat's book or perhaps have other questions for her. I decided to call her.

The instantly likable, warm voice that answered belonged to Pat Wagner herself. I introduced myself, told her that I had recently purchased a copy of her book, and asked if she would mind speaking with me for a few minutes; I had some questions. Gracious and friendly, she assured me that she indeed had the time to spend. She also asked me why I was interested in BVT. I had introduced myself as Dr. Celeste Pepe, so she was curious to learn if my interest was professional or personal. I paused for a moment, and then I told her that I had MS.

"Oh, you poor thing!" She sympathized. "You're not taking Betaseron, are you?"

"No!" I replied with resounding emphasis. I filled her in on the highlights of my journey toward a cure for the last four and a half years. She listened intently, expressing both interest and surprise at some of the treatments that I had used and found effective. She asked about my present condition, and I told her of the numbness that I couldn't seem to shake from my left leg.

"Well," she enthused confidently, "that should be easy to fix! When do you want to start?"

"That's a big part of the reason I'm calling you," I replied. "I'm not sure if I *do* want to start."

She was silent for a moment, and when she spoke, her voice was gentle and kind. "Let me tell you about my own experience, and you can decide for yourself when I've finished if you'd like to try BVT for yourself."

She proceeded to tell me a horror story I will never forget. Every experience that I had feared was in store for me if I followed the dictates of conventional medicine had actually happened to Pat. She was subjected to numerous MRI's, and pumped full of an endless and terrifying array of drugs while all the time her condition worsened. It was heartbreaking. Finally, when she was completely bedridden, her vision became so bad that she could not determine the gender, much less the identity, of any visitor to her room, which had become a virtual prison. Then, a series of circumstances she attributes to Divine intervention caused her to learn of apitherapy and BVT. She determined to give it a try.

"Weren't you terrified?" I interjected.

"Actually, yes and no," she responded thoughtfully. "I wasn't looking forward to anything that would cause me more pain, certainly, but I definitely did not want to live another *minute* the way that I was. Besides," she laughed, "at that point I was so numb that I figured I probably wouldn't feel much of it anyway."

"And, did you?"

"Of the two first test stings, which everyone does before seriously beginning treatment, I felt one, but not the second. I put a piece of ice on the sting, and before I left there that day, the pain, which wasn't *terrible* to begin with, was gone. And, for the first time in many years, I could move the area that was stung! For me, that was enough to convince me that no matter how much discomfort BVT caused, it was insignificant compared to the gift that I received in return, life flowing back into my limbs."

Looking at her circumstances, I could see the validity of her perspective. After all, didn't I do essentially the same thing? I wanted to find a cure for my MS, to try new protocols in order to accomplish my goal, even if they were unknown and seemed strange to me. I was willing to take those courses of action although even at my worst, I was nowhere nearly as debilitated as Pat had been. I told her as much, and then I asked another question that had been on my mind.

"Why live bees, Pat? Couldn't you use extracted venom? Or is this just another natural healing substance the government won't approve?"

"Actually, the government doesn't object to BVT at all. But it could never really be prescribed on a regular basis as a serum because it's so hard to collect. There is a special process that is needed to harvest bee venom. It would cost far too much for the government to train technicians to collect the venom and process it for human medical use. The process is time-consuming, and it takes several dozen bees to produce just 1cc of collected venom. The price anyone would have to charge for the labor just to break even would be astronomical. Besides, they would never keep up with the demand, no matter what they charged."

She continued. "Live bees are so much less complicated to use. They are relatively easy to keep, and after you've mastered the technique of catching the bee in a tweezers and placing it on the area you want to sting, it is really so much simpler than using collected venom anyway. Live bee venom is always fresh, always perfectly mixed, and always just the right dosage. Believe it or not, using live bees eliminates most of the margin for error."

Again, viewed from her perspective, everything made sense. But I still wasn't certain that I could deal with the idea. "I'm still not sure I'd be able to handle the bees. Especially by myself."

"In the beginning, I worked with a certified apitherapist who applied the bees. My husband learned the technique, and now we both assist others who want to use BVT themselves. Do you have someone close to you that could do the treatment with you?"

Jerry flashed into my mind. There was no way I could picture him holding a bee in a tweezers, waiting to put it someplace on me. I hadn't even told him about this. "No," I answered honestly. "I don't think so."

"Well, there is collected venom available. You said that Dr. Weeks recommended you explore this treatment. I think that he could certainly get some for you. You're a doctor, so I'm sure you know how to give yourself injections. Besides, you told me that you were already doing vitamin B therapy through intravenous injection."

"Actually, I'm a chiropractor and a Doctor of Naturopathic Medicine rather than a conventional M.D., but, yes, I do know how to do self-injection."

"Well, why don't you ask Dr. Weeks to send you some collected venom and a prescription for a shock kit, which you can get at your local pharmacy. Then, you can give me a call, if you like, and I'll walk you through your first time and help you to get comfortable with it."

"I think I'd like that, Pat. How kind of you to offer. In fact, I think that it's probably the only way that I would be able to go through with this, to have someone to talk to while I was actually doing it."

"Okay! We'll call it a date, then. When you've got everything, give me a call, and we'll get you started. Trust me,

Celeste. You'll really be glad that you decided to do BVT. You won't believe how much better you are going to feel."

I thanked her again for her time and caring concern for a complete stranger. I resolved to contact Dr. Weeks and get the collected venom. I was still more than a little afraid, but I was determined to at least give BVT one session. Before I went any farther, however, I felt that I had to tell Jerry. I wasn't at all sure how he'd take the news.

At first, he didn't take it well at all. I was so much better than I had been. He didn't see the need to take the additional risk, or the logic in injecting poison into my system when I had been trying for so long to remove the existing toxins. So what if I had a couple of numb spots on my leg? I could live with that, couldn't I?

Actually, I couldn't live with it. I didn't want to stay damaged, even if it was only relatively slight, especially if there was a way to reverse it. I wanted to be *whole*. I didn't see why he couldn't understand that. We appeared to be heading for an argument, which I certainly didn't want. I put Pat's book and the materials from Dr. Weeks on the coffee table in front of him, and said I was going to bed. I'd appreciate it if he'd take a look at the information, but whether he did or not, I had already decided that I was going to do this. I left him downstairs before the conversation became any more heated.

I probably should have anticipated his negative reaction. Like many patients diagnosed with severe illness, some treatments which I considered caused my loved ones understandable concern. Naturally, Jerry did not want to lose me to some potentially dangerous procedure, even if it could benefit or improve my overall condition. During the course of my research, many MS sufferers related similar experiences, as did cancer and AIDS patients. Chemotherapy, radioactive suppositories, and AZT are all approved treatment options. They are also potentially hazardous, even deadly. Many times the families of the afflicted person will object vociferously. Although they are reacting out of love, their negative response creates additional stress for the patient. Those not afflicted with a serious ailment cannot readily understand why the patient would want to expose herself to further risk. They do not realize that to the patient, any symptom of illness is intolerable. It is not enough to be content with the fact that one is not dead or an insentient vegetable. Every patient wishes to be restored to health, for all traces of the ailment to be permanently eradicated.

Those close to a person afflicted with a major illness or medical condition must realize that the patient suffers mentally and emotionally, as well as physically. The loss of function, sensual perception, and mental clarity is as devastating to the individual's self-image as are the physical complaints, causing severe emotional trauma. Anger, fear, frustration, desperation, and despair are common. Emotions cause a biochemical reaction in the human system. When the patient experiences these natural responses to the enormity of her situation, the biochemical substances produced by those responses negatively affect the body's ability to produce healing substances. Therefore, those closest to the patient should strive to view the ailment from the patient's perspective, offering emotional support and positive reinforcement. A patient with a determined and confident outlook can participate proactively in the healing process, mentally and biochemically. Friends, family, and others should remember to voice their opinions on new or different treatment options based upon the probability of real benefit to the patient. They should never allow their own fears of losing a loved one color their advice.

In the end, Jerry acquiesced. He knew that I had decided to pursue this course of action and would do so, regardless. He respected my medical abilities and my judgment. My choices of treatment had proved to be valid to date. He knew I had thoroughly researched the subject, and my decision was not an impulsive one. Once his concerns had been reconciled, he became supportive of my choice.

Dr. Weeks was pleased that I had spoken to Pat Wagner and subsequently chosen to try BVT. He understood my reluctance to use live bees in the treatment, and concurred with the opinion that if I was going to have to do this without a treatment partner, at least in the beginning, then collected venom would probably be a more easily controlled scenario. Pat was correct in her assessment that the collected venom was far more expensive, but all things considered, it still seemed to me to be the way to go, at least at the start. I did have one important question for Dr. Weeks. I wanted to know about the dangers of anaphylactic shock. His answer was honest and direct, and I was reassured by the explanation.

"I am pleased to see that you are concerned with the possibility of anaphylactic shock. To me, that indicates that you are going to be a responsible patient who views this treatment with the respect and serious attention that it deserves. Bee venom stimulates the adrenal system, along with providing the healing benefits. Any time that the system is stimulated in that way, the possibility of shock exists. Also, although very few people who have undergone the treatment have proven to experience allergic reactions to the venom, the time to find out that you, too, are prone to adverse reaction is not while you are alone and unprepared."

"The shock kit that I prescribe contains, primarily, a preloaded syringe of epinephrine," he explained. "Should the symptoms of allergic reaction or shock begin to manifest, this injection will counter the effects. When properly used, it will stabilize your condition, allowing you time to be transported to the hospital for further treatment. Before you begin the protocol, in fact, before you administer the test injections, I strongly urge you to practice the procedures necessary for use of the kit. Once you have become familiar with the steps, and are comfortable with them, then you can safely proceed to complete the test injections, and later the complete protocol."

Now that I understood more about the kit, and had discussed my concerns with both Pat Wagner and Dr. Weeks, my trepidation was beginning to subside. This was not the haphazard treatment I had initially considered it to be. No, it was a precise protocol, with specifically delineated steps. Although completely natural, it was not at all a new science or experimental procedure.

The bee venom arrived about a week later, along with the prescription and a listing of the additional materials that comprised the shock kit and completed the safety precautions. I have included a detailed list of these materials in chapter 14, "Deadly Savior—Bee Venom Treatment." I filled the prescription at a local Rite Aid pharmacy. I was provided with a preloaded syringe of epinephrine that was marketed under the brand name of Epi Pen. This precautionary safety protocol was prescribed for several other purposes besides BVT, including diabetes. I doubt if the pharmacist had any idea that I was planning on using this as a BVT safety net.

I obtained all of the other simple but necessary materials needed to complete the shock kit, and took them home with me to begin the practice sessions before I administered the actual injections. I took out the instructions and read them thoroughly several times, memorizing the steps. Epinephrine needed to be administered within a specific time frame when allergic or adverse reaction to the venom occurred. I performed a series of practice drills, repeating the emergency procedures until I felt that I would be able to execute them correctly in a crisis situation.

Finally, I felt that I was ready. All of the materials were at hand. I had the venom, clean syringes, and needle points, and the emergency kit on standby. The moment had come. I called Pat Wagner, and as soon as I heard her cheerful voice on the other end of the line, the nervousness that I had been feeling began to subside. I joked with her that if BVT stimulated the adrenal system, perhaps just threatening patients with the treatment would be enough to recharge their adrenaline without them actually having to undergo the procedure. Pat has an excellent sense of humor, and we both laughed, breaking the tension I was feeling.

With Pat standing by on the speaker, I carefully withdrew a tiny amount of venom with the syringe from the specially topped medical bottle. Beads of nervous perspiration forming on my upper lip, I made the first injection, right above my left knee. Immediately afterward, I made the second directly into one of the numb spots farther up on the front portion of my left thigh. Aside from the sensation of the needle penetrating my skin and the muscle beneath, initially I felt nothing else. Pat provided a running commentary of information and encouragement as I waited, tensely, for some reaction to occur.

And then it came. Slowly, at first, and then more rapidly, I felt a fire begin to envelop my knee, radiating outward from the injection site, similar to the shock wave from a powerful blast. Excitedly, I communicated this to Pat, who cheered me on, saying that this was exactly what I was supposed to feel. There was some pain, yes, but by no means excruciating pain. The injection site began to swell, and the flesh became an angry red color, raising a small welt. This was also entirely normal, said Pat. The firelike feeling radiated outward, fading into insignificance about three or four inches away from the area.

I was so concentrated on observing the first site that I had entirely failed to notice the second. It, too, had begun to turn red and swell. I realized with sudden disappointment that I didn't feel the second area at all. Although, physically, the results appeared to be the same as those of the first site, in essence it was as if I was observing the body of another person. I couldn't feel a thing. It had not penetrated the numbness. The experiment was a failure.

My voice leaden with disappointment, I spoke my thoughts aloud. "Well, that's it, I guess. I've failed, Pat. My knee has all of the reactions that you say are to be expected. My thigh looks the same, but I can't *feel* it. I guess it doesn't work on me, after all." I honestly wanted to cry. I thought of all of the mental anguish I had suffered over the last few weeks, deciding whether or not to use this treatment. And now, after all of my preparations, expense, and angst, my dead leg couldn't have cared less, it seemed. All of this was for nothing. I could hear the gentle kindness of this suburban grandmother as she reached out to me in my disappointment. Speaking with infinite patience, she simply said, "But sweetie, that's only the same as one little sting. You didn't really expect that one little sting would cure you, did you? If it was going to, then why did Dr. Weeks send you such a nice amount of venom? I don't think that he thought you would spill any, so he'd better send you extra."

The warmth and wisdom of her words began to open the curtain of hope that I was disappointedly trying to close. The way that she said them brought a smile to my face, just as it probably had to hundreds of other new patients she'd seen and helped. Although outside of her certification as an apitherapist, Pat Wagner has never received any other former medical training, she is a true healer. Slowly, I responded, "Perhaps you're right. I may have been a bit unrealistic. I suppose, deep down inside, I was secretly expecting some major event to occur. I'm not even sure what, but something. And, I really thought that my leg would feel it, too. As a doctor, I should know better, but I admit I really was expecting something bigger."

"Well," she replied, understandingly, "of course you did. Everybody does. It doesn't matter if you're a doctor. You're a *person*, too. Everybody wants most of all to be well. We're always looking for a 'miracle cure.' BVT is a miracle, honey. It's just not an instant one." She paused for a moment, and then continued brightly, "You've already had your first step toward a miracle today. You *have* accomplished something, after all."

I wanted so desperately to believe she was right, but I couldn't see at all what I could have achieved. My leg was still numb. Looking down at it in disgust, I could see that a nice little welt had made its appearance. "What's that? What have I done that's so wonderful?"

She laughed. "Look at the clock, Celeste."

I did, but still didn't draw the meaning for a moment. "It's 2:15, my time. So?"

"*So*," she replied, her words deliberate. "You injected yourself at 1:53 your time, right? Well, that's twenty-three minutes ago. You're still sitting there, talking to me, aren't you? You are not allergic to the venom. You can begin the treatments!"

Stunned for a moment, I stared blankly at the clock. Then I realized that she was correct. It *had* been over twenty minutes, the standard window for allergic reaction to occur, if it was going to. I *was* fine. I wasn't allergic! I felt my spirits begin to rise again, and I agreed aloud with her. She continued to offer encouragement.

"There, see? I told you that I thought you'd be fine. God created bees to help heal us, Celeste. When we use them properly, real miracles can occur. I know. I see proof of it every day, whenever I look into the mirror. You can have a miracle, too, one that God has planned just for you. But, you have to start the treatment in the proper way, and not hang all of your hopes on these two little stings. They were only meant to test for allergy. It looks like you passed!"

"Yeah," I laughed, my perspective restored, "I did, didn't I? Okay, I passed. Now, what's next?"

"You call me back in two days, and I'll walk you through your first real session. I know that you already have my book, so it will be easy for you to refer to the acupuncture charts I will teach you to use."

I felt a rush of warmth and gratitude for this wonderful person who had selflessly taken time out of her own life to be there for a stranger. "Pat, I can't thank you enough for all of this. I realize that I am taking up a good deal of your time, and I can't express how deeply I appreciate it. Thank you so much for your wisdom, and your kindness."

"There's no need to thank me," she replied sincerely. "I feel that God created the bees to heal me, and they did. My helping patients who come to me, and passing along the knowledge and technique to others is my way of thanking *Him*."

"And, I know, as surely as I know my own name, that He looks down from His Heaven and smiles, Pat. God bless you always. You are truly one of His lights unto the world." She thanked me graciously for my sincere statement, and we ended our conversation with my promise to call her in two days' time.

I did call her again at the time we had agreed upon. I was to begin my first real session with the equivalent of eight stings, the injections administered to various points on my upper and lower body. I didn't sting the numb areas during that session. The process took about a half an hour. After it was completed, I felt the fire sensation begin to flow throughout my body. The injection sites swelled, and some of them itched. Pat told me not to scratch them, and recommended a couple of simple remedies for relief should the itching become intolerable, like applying an ice cube to the irritated area.

We also mapped out a treatment schedule. I would repeat the procedure in two days' time, increasing the sting equivalent to twelve, and then again after the same time interval with the equivalent of fourteen, sixteen, and finally, the injection of a full 1/2cc of venom, comparable to twenty stings. Once I had reached that plateau, I was to continue at that level every other day, following a specific rotation of points of treatment. In addition, I was to use some of the injections to treat the affected areas directly, shooting the venom into the numb spots on my upper and lower leg.

I followed the Bee Venom Treatment protocol for the next six weeks. I began to notice changes in my body. All traces of minor joint or muscle stiffness disappeared. I was able to stand on my feet for far longer periods of time, without fatigue. I had continued my workouts, and realized my repetitions now ended as strongly as they had begun in all of the exercises, even the ones for my left leg. My energy levels were as high as I could ever remember them having been. My senses appeared to be heightened: smells, colors, and tastes were more vibrant than ever. Even Jerry commented upon how much more alive I seemed. He was now completely comfortable with my use of the BVT.

A good friend of mine, Christa, is a registered nurse. I discussed the treatments with her about two weeks after beginning the full schedule of sessions. She was fascinated, but questioned my ability to inject all of the recommended acupuncture points as some were located on my back and spinal areas. She offered to come and help me with those, and I quickly accepted. I shall always be grateful to Christa. A true friend, she went out of her way to arrange her life around mine because she cared.

About five weeks into the treatment, we had completed a session and were enjoying a cup of tea and conversation in the sun room. Suddenly, Christa leaned forward and stared hard at me.

"Celeste, what are you *doing?*"

I had been absentmindedly scratching my left thigh while we were talking, and answered her without thinking. "I'm just scratching my leg. It's really itchy.

I followed the Bee Venom Treatment protocol for the next six weeks. I began to notice changes in my body. All traces of minor joint or muscle stiffness disappeared. I was able to stand on my feet for far longer periods of time, without fatigue.

I guess I should probably go and get a piece of ice, huh?" I looked over at her, startled to see her grinning at me as though her lovely face would split in half. "What are you laughing at?"

She fairly jiggled in her chair, her eyes bright with excitement. "Repeat what you just said to me. Except, this time, think about it, dummy!"

I didn't get it. "I said, 'My leg is really itchy. I think I should go get some ice.' So?"

"So," she echoed, drawing the word out like a contestant on *Password*, trying to get her idiot partner to guess the damn clue. "*So . . .* "

"So, my leg is itchy from the venom. What . . ." Suddenly, like a thunderbolt from God Himself, it struck me. My leg was itchy. *My left leg was itchy.* I shot from my chair like a million volts had just raced through it. I screamed in delighted understanding. "Oh, God! Oh, *God!* My left leg is *itchy! I can feel my left leg!*"

She had jumped up as well, and we fell upon each other, laughing, crying, and screaming delightedly. We proceeded to do this mad dance of joy. Anyone who saw us two adult medical professionals in that moment would have bet all the money he had on the fact that we were crazy. That was probably one of the single best moments in all of my search for a cure. I had come so far in beating this disease, had successfully completed so many therapies. The numbness was the only symptom I hadn't been able to shake, no matter how hard I tried. Until now. Pat was right. I *did* get my miracle, after all.

I rode the emotional high of first feeling my leg again for about another week and a half. Extreme emotions are common to MS patients, caused by the biochemical imbalances in the body. This feeling, however, was the true joy that came from obtaining what I had desired for so long. I continued my sessions, and, each time, more and more feeling returned to the areas that had been numb for over four years. The day came when the injection actually hurt, immediately, and I knew the BVT therapy had finally restored full sensation to the area. I was elated. And, then, one morning, I received a letter that was to drop the bottom of my safe little world right out from under me.

The letter came from the Rite Aid Corporation. I had purchased my epinephrine syringe there. I had included it in my shock kit, practiced using it, and taught the procedure to Christa. It was always kept handy in case something went wrong during the BVT. The letter itself was brief, impersonal, and to the point. The message, however, made me weak in the knees for the first time in weeks. Fear began to rise within me as I read,

Dear Epi Pen User:

The manufacturers of Epi Pen and Epi Pen Jr. have voluntarily instituted a program to withdraw specific defective lots and replace them with new product.

The reason for this withdrawal is that specific lot numbers, distributed between July 1997 and April 1998, may contain a sub-potent dose of epinephrine which may be ineffective in a medical emergency . . .

Dear God. All those sessions. All of that venom! I was miles from the nearest hospital. I performed the treatments alone before Christa came to help me. If I had gone into shock, I never would have been able to receive emergency treatment in time to prevent permanent damage, or death. *Jesus.* I just sat there, shaking, for a long time. The thought of what could have happened was terrifying. Then I recalled the moment that I'd heard the Voice in our car, over four years ago, and remembered the words, *Trust always, for I will never fail you . . .*

"Thank You, God," I breathed, fervently. *"Thank You!"*

The letter concluded by listing the defective lot numbers, and offered to exchange the syringe for a new one. The shelf life of this medication is several years. Therefore, an exact duplicate of the letter that I received from Rite Aid in June of 1998 is included in chapter 14, "Deadly Savior—Bee Venom Treatment."

The more I thought about it, the more two things struck me, in addition to the fact that the Lord had graciously watched over me. The first was anger. The letter, which I received in June of 1998, referred to Epi Pens that were manufactured between July 1997 and April 1998. That means that *some* of them could have been on the shelves of the pharmacy, and in the medicine cabinets of unsuspecting patients for almost a year before anyone was notified! I'd hate to think that someone died before the defective medications came to the Epi Pen company's attention.

The second feeling that came over me was one of enormous relief. BVT was considered to be a radical, dangerous protocol. I was initially terrified at the thought of it. Now, understand me clearly. I believe firmly that used improperly, BVT can be very dangerous. Any medication, when improperly used, can be dangerous and even fatal. But, live bees are a natural product, made by God. Bees are never defective or out of stock. They never pass their expiration date. When using either the live creatures themselves or the collected bee venom properly, the procedure is entirely safe. That does not mean anyone considering BVT should ever "fly without a net." Use the "buddy system"—treatment with an experienced partner—and keep your shock kit handy.

I continued with Bee Venom Treatment until I exhausted my supply of serum. By that time, my leg was completely restored. No numbness remained, and my mobility was as good as it was prior to my illness. Bee Venom Treatment had made a permanent difference. When I had finished the protocol, I felt wonderful.

I went to the Rite Aid that afternoon. I was angry at what I considered to be the negligence of the corporation in not expeditiously notifying prescription holders of the defective medication. I said as much to the pharmacy attendant on duty, but also realized that to direct my anger at him was futile. He had no part in the incident other than to hand me my filled prescriptions. I did communicate with the Rite Aid Corporation itself in the form of a strongly worded letter, but, not surprisingly, never received either an acknowledgment or response of any kind.

I continued with BVT until I exhausted my supply of serum. By that time, my leg was completely restored. No numbness remained, and my mobility was as good as it was prior to my illness. BVT had made a permanent difference. When I had finished the protocol, I felt wonderful. Jerry decided that we should go out to dinner to celebrate. I suggested we go back to the restaurant we had gone to the night my leg crumpled under me. Jerry had not suggested it, concerned it might hold bad memories for me. I had other ideas, however.

Once again, I dressed carefully. This time, however, I made certain to wear very flat shoes and comfortable clothes. The meal was wonderful. We were not out with friends this time, and after we ate, Jerry asked if I wanted to get going.

"Yes," I laughed, "I *do*. Right out on the dance floor!"

"Celeste, are you sure . . . " he began to caution me, but I had already slid out of my chair, leaving his warning, and this time my shoes, behind me. I danced to everything that night. Ten minutes passed, then twenty, then an hour. I danced on, my legs sure and strong, my back supple, my body fluid with the sounds of the music. My face shone with the inner ecstasy I felt. More than the bees, more than the protocols, more than the BioCybernetics analyses, this was the real test. This was what I had lost. And now, at last, after five long years of searching, this was what I had regained, once again. I danced on, oblivious to everything but the joy of my whole, healed body.

10
Year Five: Into the Clear—
Whole, Healthy, Cured!

I am nearly at the end of my story. I was to make one more change to my nutrition program, completing the method I use today. Late in the fall of 1998, I came across a nutrition book by Dr. Peter J. D'Adamo and Catherine Whitney, *Eat Right 4 Your Type: The Individualized Diet Solution to Staying Healthy, Living Longer & Achieving Your Ideal Weight* (D'Adamo and Whitney 1996). Its principles became the last refinement I made to my personal nutrition program.

I explain the work of Dr. D'Adamo in chapter 16, "Making the Right Choices—Understanding the Role of Food in Creating A Nutrition Program That Works," so I won't go into detail here. Suffice it to say that this well-researched book explores the origins of the human race, and the subsequent development of the four main blood types as we moved through prerecorded and recorded history. Each type appeared after the people adapted to specific environmental conditions, to optimize the nutrients they got from the available food supply.

For instance, the blood type known as O is the oldest, the type from which all of the others originated. Type O people were primarily carnivores. They were hunters, killing their food source. Their diets were mainly meat. As people settled down, they began to cultivate grains and fruits, developing an agrarian culture. The diet of these type A people became largely vegetarian as the wild animal population was used up, and domesticated animals were still a thing of the future. A third kind of people were nomads who traveled from location to location, some of them raiding parties that attacked the domesticated agrarian communities. Their diets consisted of a mixture of wild animal meats and cultivated grains. These people became blood type B. The newest type, AB, appeared less than one thousand years ago, and shares the qualities of both its A and B ancestors.

Dr. D'Adamo has proved through scientific and clinical research that our bodies are genetically predisposed to more easily digest certain kinds of foods, depending on our individual blood ancestry. Type O persons do much better when their diets consist of mainly animal proteins and fats, with a few vegetables. They do not do as well with grains, breads, and pastas. Type A persons, like myself, are far more successful eating a largely vegetarian diet, with occasional animal meats. They also do well with fish. Type B's thrive on a diet that is a mixture of the two, and AB's have their own set of special rules.

I believe that both Dr. Sears and Dr. D'Adamo are correct in their assessment of the principles of optimum human nutritional intake. Most of the people who followed the Zone plan experienced success. Some, however, did not do as well. The Zone diet seems to be primarily developed to be blood-type-O-friendly, high in protein and animal meats. As type O is found in the largest population group, of course the diet would be successful with a significant percentage of patients. I decided to combine the principles of Sears and D'Adamo, and tweak the Zone to build my meal blocks from foods that were blood type A friendly. There I found my last key.

After following my new modified Zone/Eat Right diet, my BioCybernetics analysis showed that my levels of vitamins and nutrients were quickly moving back into optimum ranges.

My deficiencies were increased, my excesses decreased, and my ratio imbalances were beginning to right themselves. Moreover, I felt satisfied at every meal, and I no longer experienced cravings for food or gnawing hunger pains, no matter how long it was between meals. I was pleased with the results, as were Drs. Weeks and Crawford, and nutritionists Santoro and Weyhreter. Only one thing remained to correct: my calcium imbalances.

Throughout the five years I was afflicted with MS, my calcium levels had remained consistently high. No matter what protocol or nutritional plan I followed, I couldn't seem to get the calcium to fall into line. Finally, Dr. Crawford suggested that I try the Nieper protocol. We had this discussion in early 1999. Unfortunately, at that time, Dr. Nieper had just recently passed away. However, Dr. Crawford had been using the Nieper protocols for a couple of years by this time, and he was well versed in their administration. The B vitamin injectibles had worked very well for me, so I was very open to adding this as a last and final step.

I explain in detail the protocols and valuable work of Dr. Nieper in chapter 12, "Achieving Balance through Vitamin, Mineral, and Supplement Therapies." His treatments are specifically designed not only to destroy the living MS virus inside of the patient, but also to eradicate all traces of the lesions that have already occurred in the brain and central nervous system. Dr. Nieper had been successful in treating large numbers of MS patients in this fashion. Almost all of them had seen their symptoms and existing disabilities lessen, and in some cases disappear completely.

Dr. Nieper, and now Dr. Crawford, used a substance known as Calcium-AEP in the treatment. In orotate, or oral pill form, this calcium and nutrient supplement would help to remove the remaining excess calcium from my system. You would think that the exact opposite would be the result. In fact, that was the concern voiced by Dr. Watts, Dr. Crawford's associate, when Dr. Crawford discussed it with him. Both Dr.

Crawford and I wanted to give it a try, so Dr. Watts agreed that a short trial, closely monitored, would probably not cause too severe a setback if it didn't work. Besides, I was so healthy at this point that my body could probably tolerate the excess without any adverse effects, provided that it wasn't continued for too great a length of time.

I began to take the orotates at the end of January 1999. By March, my calcium levels had decreased by over one third of what they measured before taking the Nieper protocol. By June they were reduced by almost half. My levels continued to drop rapidly, entering the high acceptable ranges (at the time this is written).

In closing this section, I'd like to review those protocols and healing therapies that I found to be most useful on my journey to recovery. Although all of them may not work for you, or may work with differing degrees of success depending on the other factors in your life such as age, gender, or ethnic origin, I believe that any and all of them are preferable to one day of Betaseron, Avonex, or Copaxone. The therapies that I have used are all of natural origin. When used properly, they will not hurt you. I cannot make the same guarantee for any of these drugs, or for any treatment commonly prescribed by conventional medicine.

The first, and most important, step is to determine your current internal composition. I strongly urge you to have a BioCybernetics analysis, an EFA, or Essential Fatty Acid test, and an IgG RAST test. (I will cover this test in detail in the second section.) These tests will illustrate your inner system balance, and reveal what, if any, hidden allergies may be present. Periodic retesting will allow you to chart the progress of all of the therapies that you will undergo in your own quest for healing.

After receiving the results of your tests, consult with a dentist. Determine the types of fillings and dental devices currently in place in your mouth. Investigate the possibility of replacing mercury and silver amalgam fillings or devices. Present evidence may not completely support mercury toxicity as the primary cause of MS, but the poison cannot possibly do your system any good, and your bodily resources do not need to fight additional biochemical enemies while you are trying to achieve healing.

If your BioCybernetics analysis shows that you have excessive mercury or other heavy metals present in your system, you should consider DMPS chelation therapy to cleanse your body of these unwanted excesses.

Exercise is most important. If you do not develop a regular routine to strengthen and maintain muscle tone, you risk losing mobility. Once it is lost, it can become a slow and painful process to restore your range of motion once again.

Women especially should consider hormone supplementation. Science has proven that when hormone levels drop with advancing age, women are more susceptible to the onset, manifestation, and exacerbation of the disease.

MS is indeed, in my firm opinion, a mutation of an old virus. Search your own medical history for any serious illness or injury during your childhood or adolescence. Whether you can recall ever being seriously ill or not, you should consider a virus protocol like the one prescribed for me by nutritionist Weyhreter.

Begin vitamin and nutrient therapy to provide your body with the substances that it may be lacking. In my case, I took the beef protein extract and the Vitamin B compound injectibles. Your therapy should be tailored to your own specific needs as defined in your test results by your enlightened medical professional, certified nutritional counselor, or clinical nutritionist.

Do seriously consider Bee Venom Treatment. Since I have experienced it for myself, I can assure you firsthand that it works to restore lost movement and sensation, even after years without feeling or function. Find a certified apitherapist and a reputable apiary to supply you with the correct type of bees. Do not forget to take all of the necessary safety precautions. I have included contact information for the AAS, certified apitherapists, and reputable suppliers of live bees in the resources section.

Dr. Neiper's Calcium 2-AEP treatments worked very well for me. In fact, it was the only substance that successfully brought my excessive calcium levels back into line. Dr. William Crawford is well versed in the therapy. Contact information for the Hans A. Nieper Clinic in Hannover, Germany, and the Crawford Center in Mobile, Alabama, is included in the resources section.

The single most important supplement you should be certain to take is the Sphingolin Myelin Basic Protein from Emerson Ecologics. This pure concentrated supplement will divert the focus of the MS, causing it to attack the myelin in your stomach and leave the myelin in your spine and nerve sheathing alone.

Regardless of the therapies or protocols you utilize, remember to build a solid foundation on nutrition. Whether you begin with the Swank low-fat diet, or move right into the Zone as modified for your blood type with the Eat Right principles, you must formulate a specific plan for your daily diet. This will ensure your body is receiving the optimum nutritional benefits from food, especially during your healing period. Proper nutrition will keep your body in balance, strengthen your system, and make it resistant to progression of the disease or the contraction of new illness in the future.

Finally, never give up hope! Remember, if you are ever diagnosed with a life-threatening disease, you must pursue, with all of your might, every doctor, of all varieties, with every healing modality known to them, and never give up, until you find the ones that heal you. God bless you on your own quest. Faith will light your way, and perseverance will bring you success. If you would like to contact me personally about any part of my story, my practice, or in my capacity as a certified BioCybernetics counselor, you will find my information listed in the Resources chapter.

If you do follow my path and are cured of your own affliction, I'd love to hear from you. Knowing that I have helped at least one person by writing this book would make all of my efforts worthwhile. And, when you're healed, if you are ever in California, look me up. Maybe we'll go dancing!

The following section contains detailed explanations of the scientific research behind each therapy or treatment, and some background on those who developed each of them. I also include information on the vitamin and mineral content of different foods, and show you how you can plan nutrition programs and chart your own progress on your personal journey to wellness. God bless and good luck!

Section II:
Finding the Facts—
Fighting the Fiction

11
BioCybernetics—Vital
Analyses You Should Undergo

Everything that occurs in the body of any living organism, including and especially human beings, occurs first at the cellular level. Analyzing the levels of substances within your cells is the first step to determining where the imbalances are and enables you to begin to correct those imbalances to restore your optimum health.

The tests that were performed on me during the course of my pursuit of a cure for MS should be of paramount importance to those afflicted with any number of illnesses, from arthritis and AIDS to cancer and heart disease. I strongly urge every reader, especially those suffering from these ailments, to have these tests performed as soon as possible. They will determine imbalances that exist in your system and hold the keys to righting those imbalances and curing your affliction.

Even prior to the onset of my illness, I had understood the importance of this analysis of life functions and actively pursued the mastery of the medical protocols necessary in the analysis of cellular composition and function. Several years prior to the appearance of my MS, I had become a fully accredited BioCybernetics counselor, trained to interpret the cellular composition tests known as BCI analyses. BCI stands for BioCybernetics Inc., the company that created the testing procedures.

More than just a simple determination of the levels of vitamins, minerals, essential amino acids, and toxic materials that may be present within the body, BioCybernetics illustrates the relationship of those materials to the glands, organs, and their attendant functions within the human system. Additionally, the BCI system educates the patient on the steps necessary to correct those imbalances, including which substances to eliminate from the diet or environment, and the supplements to add that will restore the system's balance and promote optimum cellular function.

In this chapter, I will give you a practical overview of the three most common types of cellular analysis, and a "crash course," if you will, on the use and implications of the BCI system. We will walk through the practice together so that you may come to an understanding of the importance of these analyses. I will explain the three major types of analytical tests performed—blood, urine, and hair—and illustrate through a series of simple charts and graphs both the optimum range of elemental ratios, and the imbalances as detected in my system after diagnosis with MS.

We will examine each section carefully, as I translate into lay terms exactly what is occurring inside your body every second of every day that you are alive. As with many aspects of life, these functions, actions, and reactions go largely unnoticed until something goes wrong and your system is so inwardly out of balance that you begin to manifest outward signs of the malfunctions.

Knowing the Score: Important Biochemical Analyses

As I've stated previously, all the functions of your body begin at a cellular level. The BCI system interprets the data gained from three basic and vital cellular substance tests performed on the patient: blood, urine, and hair. Let's first examine these tests, and what each entails.

Blood Testing: Probably the most common and widely pre-scribed test for determining the human condition. Blood samples can be tested for a vast number of specific ailments, to obtain a marriage license, or to detect a variety of substance abuses or other abnormal physiological conditions. Specimens are commonly collected by either a registered nurse or a hematologist. Blood samples are drawn from the vein of the patient, or by pricking the tip of a finger.

Blood testing is a long-established practice in the field of elemental analysis. In fact, blood testing has become so detailed that individual genetic characteristics can be obtained that uniquely identify the person. This has become increasingly important in the field of criminal investigation. Since the data obtained are so reliable and contain such exact-ing details, they can be used as evidence in a court of law for either a criminal or civil suit, as we've seen in major criminal trials and political scandals in recent years.

Major cities across the United States are proposing that every baby born in city hospitals have a blood sample taken shortly after birth. This sample would be analyzed for various inherited conditions, such as drug addiction, AIDS, sickle cell anemia, and other blood abnormalities. When detected early, many conditions can be immediately cared for, and, in some cases, completely cured before the infant has reached six months of life. If ongoing research proves that certain persons may have a genetic susceptibility to viral infection, early blood testing can alert parents and medical professionals to a child at risk. Steps can then be taken throughout the child's life to neutralize this susceptibility, reducing or eliminating the onset or severity of serious illnesses like EBV, Type 2 diabetes, MS, and other neurological disorders.

Urine Testing: Also known as urinalysis, a sample is obtained from the patient for a variety of purposes. Specimens are collected in sterile containers, and testing is usually performed by an off-site laboratory associated with your physician or hospital. Your practitioner will either ask for an interpretation from the laboratory, or have the results returned for his or her own interpretation.

The data obtained from a urinalysis have become a key factor in many areas outside of disease detection and diagnosis. For example, athletes, human and equine, are regularly tested for the presence of performance-enhancing substances such as steroids and Lasix. Government and municipal employees are screened through urinalysis for evidence of substance abuse involving drugs or alcohol. The test is used for the same purpose by the penal system, in the areas of parole and probation of convicted criminals. Additionally, many large corporations in the private sector are regularly using urinalysis to prescreen a prospective employee for substance abuse. In the arena of health, urinalysis can detect the presence of sugar, protein, or yeast in the sample, indicating the possible presence of diabetes, kidney malfunction, or bladder-related infections.

Hair Analysis: This is the least known but perhaps most exact analysis that can be performed to determine the elemental levels within a patient's system. This test is performed by gathering a section of hair, approximately an inch in breadth from the base of the neck of the patient. The testing is always performed by a laboratory specifically equipped for the purpose. Human hair can best be viewed as a timeline, an accurate historical record of events, illnesses, and substances that have entered, are present in, or affect the body. For instance, hair analysis is crucial when determining the length of time a person may have been exposed to a toxic substance. Heavy metal toxicity is a gradual process. Repeated exposure to elements such as mercury, or poisons such as arsenic will be reflected in the hair sample. This permanent record helps the medical professional determine the period of time involved in the exposure, the amount of the toxin or poison present, and the appropriate treatment for the patient based upon that information.

The BCI System and You

BioCybernetics, or the BCI analysis system, is the extrapolation of the individual patient's data obtained through the three tests I've just described. The data's relationship to the patient's metabolism and glandular and organ function can then be interpreted by a medical professional. BioCybernetics determines the ratios involved in the levels of elements present, and details a prescription of nutrients and supplements that must be added to the patient's system to correct the imbalances present and restore optimum system function. The BCI system is optimally effective with periodic retesting to chart the progress of balance restoration and adjust the supplements necessary as that balance is restored.

When a patient orders the BCI tests, the process can become somewhat involved. Tests are performed and returned to the referring physician for analysis. After diagnosis has been made, a certified BioCybernetics counselor will subsequently meet personally with the patient to further explain the results, and the steps necessary to correct the imbalances found. The program's true value is maximized only when the patient, working in concert with the counselor, adheres strictly to the regimen prescribed by the BCI tests, including periodic retesting and the ingestion of nutritional supplements necessary to correct the imbalance of conditions present.

Although the initial analyses are not cost prohibitive, the series of treatments and purchase of nutrients necessary may become expensive. In some cases, the nutrients prescribed may be costly. Some health insurance plans may cover the expense when referral for testing and nutrient prescriptions are made by a recognized health care provider or plan-approved medical professional. Review your health insurance documents or consult with your plan provider. However, and I cannot stress this enough, the cost of undergoing the BCI series is more than offset by the price the patient will pay for ineffective or experimental medical treatment, not to mention that the patient may end up paying the ultimate price: life itself. The upside to the situation is that by correctly utilizing the BCI system, a patient can correct the imbalances present and restore optimum health.

By determining the imbalances present in a human system and introducing a prescribed and regulated regimen of nutritional supplements to correct the deficiencies and eliminate those substances that contribute to an overabundance of undesirable elements, conditions that exist within the patient and that are manifested by outward symptomatic illness can be arrested, reversed, and, in many cases, completely cured. This includes those conditions thought by the majority of the medical profession to be incurable, including heart disease, cancer, multiple sclerosis, and AIDS.

Now, let's look at how BioCybernetics is applied to an actual patient: myself. I have arranged the data gathered through the tests performed upon myself into three sections: Metabolism, Glandular/Organ Function Ratios, and Elemental Analysis. Each section contains charts and graphs that illustrate the data, showing the normal ranges necessary for optimum health and the levels present in my system after my initial diagnosis with MS. As I pursued the courses of treatment you read about in the first section of this book, these elemental levels changed, slowly returning to normal ranges.

BCI analysis of my present condition would show that almost all of my data fall within the normal range. I am healthier today than I was *before* I was diagnosed with MS. I assure you that I am not unique. Anyone can change the elemental composition of his or her cells, with either positive or negative results. Although some patients may have progressed in their illnesses beyond the point of realizing complete recovery, further progress of the particular condition can be arrested. Optimum health means that repair has taken place if damage was previously present. I cannot guarantee that following the BCI system regimen will cure your condition. I can assure you that employing this protocol will certainly not make you any worse and will probably improve your quality of life by significantly reducing your present level of suffering.

What's Your Type?
Determining your Metabolic Rate

Metabolism is the process by which your body engine burns the "fuel" it is fed. Metabolism is affected by all substances introduced into the system, by eating or drinking, inhaled through breathing, or absorbed through the skin.

Eating and drinking are the most obvious ways in which we give our metabolism fuel. Let's compare your body's metabolism to the fuel system in your gas-powered automobile. Your car will run on any grade of gasoline. The metabolism will attempt to process all fuel, regardless of the nature of the substance. If your car is a high-performance vehicle, or is expected to work harder than usual, a higher grade of gasoline is

I cannot guarantee that following the BCI system regimen will cure your condition. I can assure you that employing this protocol will certainly not make you any worse and will probably improve your quality of life by significantly reducing your present level of suffering.

necessary for optimum performance. Lower-grade gasoline may cause your car to backfire, run roughly, or break down. When food fuel is ingested in the proper combinations, your metabolism processes it efficiently, utilizing the elements it needs and eliminating excess or unnecessary portions. When the wrong combinations, or excess amounts of a particular type of food fuel are consumed, your metabolism begins to malfunction.

Elements inhaled can affect your metabolism, positively or negatively. Pollen, smog, coal dust, asbestos, and cigarette smoke are just a few well-known examples of toxins which can be inhaled and adversely affect the body's health. On the opposite end of the scale, fresh, clean air provides oxygen and other essential elements to the cells, promoting metabolic efficiency. Other olfactory stimuli are equally important. The smells of food, for instance, stimulate the metabolism, creating the sensation of hunger or triggering stored food processing.

Perhaps the least known method of introducing substances into the body is osmosis, absorption through the skin. Your skin is a porous organ, allowing elements to exit the body through perspiration, and external elements to enter. Again, this process can effect the metabolism either positively or negatively. A classic example of toxicity caused by osmosis is the mercury poisoning that affected hatmakers in eighteenth- and nineteenth-century Europe, known as "Mad Hatter's Disease."

Individuals engaged in hat manufacturing routinely used mercury as a part of the process. Mercury is a highly volatile and reactive substance. It is also deadly when absorbed in great quantities into the system. Medical science of the era had no knowledge of the toxicity of mercury or the skin's ability to absorb the substance. Constant daily exposure, unprotected by gloves or sanitary conditions, caused these individuals to receive excessive quantities of mercury. The resulting toxicity led to a breakdown of internal systems, specifically brain function, resulting in insanity, and often death. Modern manufacturing methods and the increased use of synthetic materials have virtually eliminated this cause of mercury poisoning. Skin osmosis can also be used to positively affect the system. Nicotine addiction can be broken through the use of medicinal patches placed on the patient. These slowly release medication absorbed through the skin, controlling the craving for nicotine until the addiction has diminished to the point where the patient can overcome the desire without the need for medication. Some allergies are also treated in this manner.

Now that we see how our world can affect our metabolism, let's look at metabolism itself. Through his breakthrough research, George Watson, Ph.D., was able to identify two main classifications of metabolism. His research focused on cellular oxidation, the process by which oxygen is absorbed into the individual cell, and its relation to the deficiency or excess of essential nutrients present in the system that determine the body's ability to convert raw materials into usable energy. He discovered that human metabolism can be classified as either "fast" or "slow," depending upon the rate of this oxidation process.

Building upon the work of Dr. Watson, David Watts, Ph.D., discovered that metabolic rate can additionally be determined through the presence of certain mineral patterns, specifically the calcium-to-phosphorus ratio present in the system. I will discuss element ratios in more detail later. These patterns additionally determine function dominance of certain organs and glands, resulting in distinct personality types. Each classification has distinct characteristics and resultant nutritional requirements. Let's look at an overview of each type.

"Fast" metabolizers process fuel ingested quickly, are more able to break down and utilize complex foods like proteins and fats, and require a higher number of calories to maintain their metabolic rate. Persons with type O blood are statistically more apt to be fast metabolizers, although this metabolic rate is found in persons of all blood types. Fast metabolizers are more likely to be sociologically classified as "Type A" personalities.

Type A personalities prefer "life in the fast lane." They are more ambitious, spontaneous, and impulsive, possess strong leadership qualities, and are subject to intense bouts of positive and negative emotions. They respond well to, or may actually thrive on, stressful situations, as they are quick thinkers and adapt well in crises. Type A persons often insist on performing more than one task simultaneously, such as reading a book or report while using the exercise bicycle, or completing a craft while watching television. Conversely, Type A persons have difficulty relaxing, and can be egotistical and impatient with others. They are more susceptible to high blood pressure, stroke, and cardiac arrest if the stress levels become too great or prolonged in their lives, or they fail to eat properly.

"Slow" metabolizers are in direct contrast to their fast counterparts. Their bodies do not utilize complex foods as efficiently. They fare better with a diet high in carbohydrates and some simple proteins like those found in fish and legumes. Persons with blood type A and type B are more likely to be slow metabolizers, although again, all blood types may produce this metabolic rate.

Slow metabolizers are often sociologically classified as Type B personalities. Type B's are methodical, careful, determined, and persevering. They possess excellent research and analytical abilities, are not prone to emotional outbreaks, and dislike stressful or confrontational situations. They relax more easily and rest for longer periods of time than do their type A counterparts. Type B persons often become diplomats, teachers, counselors, or scientists as they are patient, well-organized, and show an exacting attention to detail. Type B individuals can be dogmatic, stubborn, and resistant to change or new ideas. They can become susceptible to obesity, osteoporosis, and chiropractic disorders if they fail to maintain a proper exercise routine or ingest insufficient protein and calcium or an excess of sugar. The following two charts will illustrate the differences in each metabolic type.

Chart 11-1 shows the specific indications of each metabolism class, and the areas of your system most affected by each.

Chart 11-1 Metabolism Types

Metabolic Type	Oxidation	Calcium-Phosphorus Ratio	Personality
Fast	Fast	2.6 or lower	Type A
Slow	Slow	2.7 or higher	Type B

Chart 11-2 illustrates the diet and nutritional requirements of each metabolic type. Metabolism is determined most accurately through hair analysis as described earlier in this chapter, because hair samples contain a chronological history of system function.

Chart 11-2 Nutritional Requirements
for Metabolism Types

Metabolism Type	Oxidation	Carbohydrate	Protein	Fats
Fast	Fast	Low	High	High*
Slow	Slow	High	High	Low

* Obtained optimally from vegetable and fish oils

The presence or absence of mineral concentrations in the system directly affects the function of essential organs and glandular systems. Understanding these relationships helps us to further comprehend the inner workings of our systems, and how the relationship of these elements and functions can result in chronic disease or debilitation. Furthermore, once the abnormalities are detected, steps can be taken to correct the condition and restore the patient to health.

Chart 11-3 illustrates each gland or organ and the mineral that solely, or in combination with others, affects proper function. The consequences of imbalance in these elements or in their relationship to one another are explained more fully later in this chapter.

Chart 11-3 Glandular/Organ
to Mineral Relationships

Gland/Organ	Mineral
Parathyroid	Calcium/Phosphorus
Thyroid	Iodine
Anterior Pituitary	Magnesium
Posterior Pituitary	Potassium
Pancreas (tail)	
Islets of Langerhans	Zinc
Pancreas (head)	
Enzyme Secretion	Chromium
Spleen	Iron
Prostate/Uterus	Selenium
Thymus	Copper
Gonads	Manganese
Adrenal Cortex	Sodium

The body's physiology is a complex composition of elemental relationships and integrated reactions. In addition to these singular relationships, the ratio of elements and minerals present in your system to one another affects organ-to-gland interaction and physiological and biochemical systems. When glands or organs are paired together in functionality, usually with opposing duties that maintain system balance, they are referred to scientifically as an axis pair. This term denotes their opposite or reciprocal functions.

Chart 11-4 details specific mineral ratios linked to the function of these axis pairs.

Chart 11-4 Mineral Ratios to Glandular/Organ Axis Pairs

Mineral Pairs	System Affected
Calcium/Magnesium	Blood Sugar Balance
Calcium/Phosphorus	Parathyroid (Fast/Slow Oxidation)
Calcium/Potassium	Thyroid
Sodium/Potassium	Post Pituitary/Adrenal Axis
Magnesium/Potassium	Hypothalamus
Zinc/Potassium	Post Pituitary/Pancreas Axis
Zinc/Copper	Pancreas/Thymus Axis
Copper/Iron	Liver
	Thymus/Spleen Axis

Blood testing is also an essential method for determining mineral excesses or deficiencies in addition to hair sample analysis. Presence of mineral concentrations and the ratio of red to white blood cells in the bloodstream are indicative of glandular/organ function or malfunction.

The relationship of several of these mineral or elemental concentrations and their respective ratios to one another when combined as a whole may additionally result in a manifested condition. For example, low hemoglobin in the blood may be the result of liver, bone marrow, or spleen malfunction, iron or copper deficiency, or a combination of these factors.

When the test results are obtained, the physician or clinical specialist now has a specific collection of data from which to draw a conclusion and pronounce diagnosis. After diagnosis is given, a bioanalyst, specially trained in these procedures and relationships, can determine which ratios, excesses, and/or deficiencies are responsible for any given condition. After the areas responsible for the manifested condition have been identified, the bioanalyst can then recommend a specific regimen of supplements and concentrates that bring the abnormal ratios and relationships into harmony in order to effect repair of bodily systems and thereby achieve optimum health.

Chart 11-5 illustrates mineral and blood composition ratios as related to specific bodily system, organ, and gland functions. I have included all elemental relationships in this chart to give a complete picture of how each substance in the blood affects a specific area of the body. A complete explanation of each elemental term would be overly complicated and is not essential to our discussion, except to show that any number of imbalances in the blood can produce or exacerbate malfunction in a number of physiological areas.

Chart 11-5 Blood Composition and Mineral Ratios Affecting Glandular /Organ Systems

Blood Elements	System/Gland/Organ
Calcium/Phosphorus	Parathyroid
Carbon Dioxide	Lungs
Chloride	Intestinal Tract
Alkaline Phosphates	Adrenal Glands, Prostate, Uterus
Sodium	Adrenal Glands, Kidneys
Lactic Dehydrogenase	Pancreas
T-4 by RIA	Thyroid
White Blood Count (WBC)	Spleen, Thymus
Total Bilirubin	Spleen
Lymphocytes	Lymph Glands
Lymphocytes/Poly SegmentedNeutrophils	Immune System Functions

Blood Elements	System/Gland/Organ
SGPT	Gonads, Liver
Mean Corpuscular Volume	B-12, Folic Acid
Mean Corpuscular Hemoglobin	B-12, Folic Acid
Mean Corpuscular Hemoglobin Concentration	B-12, Folic Acid

When elements in your system are out of balance, your body's ability to repair damage and prohibit or fight off existing diseases is inhibited. Review all of these charted illustrations carefully, keeping in mind three important points.

First: The proper level of nutrients, minerals, and essential elements will vary with each person tested. These illustrations are meant for example only. The data contained in these charts are a reproduction of my own analyses while afflicted with MS. After testing, persons with similar levels of these substances should not necessarily view the results as indicative of the presence of MS, or any other condition or disease in the system.

Second: Understanding the individual elements displayed in these charts and their relationships to one another is not necessary for the purposes of illustration of system imbalance. Even a general explanation would be far too complex for the untrained individual to comprehend. This is why it is essential to have the services of a fully certified counselor or bioanalyst to assist you in understanding the amounts of these elements present in your own body, and what those levels and ratios may indicate.

Third: As a practicing medical professional, I must stress the following: All testing and analyses performed on your body should be recommended and supervised by a licensed physician or medical professional, in addition to the interpretation given by the counselor or bioanalyst. If your regular physician is not familiar with these procedures, find one who is! Become an educated consumer. Choose your physician at least as carefully as you choose a mechanic for your car or a contractor for your home. Find a physician who is familiar with hair analysis, glandular/organ to mineral ratios, and BioCybernetics and its importance in fighting disease or correcting chronic conditions. Testing done independently without benefit of medical support, or without instituting the recommended nutritional and supplemental support is ill-advised and may be dangerous.

BCI counselors are trained to interpret your results and recommend the protocols necessary, as well as regulate future tests and adjustments to your requirements, and you can follow their recommendations with assurance of their validity. However, you should not forgo periodic examination by a medical professional trained in the field related to your condition or disease who places a value on BioCybernetic analysis. These periodic re-examinations will verify the progress you have made toward regaining a state of optimum health and alert you to any additional developments that may be occurring within your system.

Charts 11-1 through 11-5 have shown how elements of your body interact with one another as your living machinery functions on a daily basis. In the next series of charts, we will examine specific elements and minerals present in the body and discuss how they relate or contribute to a number of common body problems. The charts you will see next depict the results of actual tests performed upon me at the Crawford Center in March 1999.

When the tests were conducted, I had already experienced all of the treatments and therapies I outlined for you in the first section of the book. Although my health today is better than it was before my affliction, you will notice that some of the levels of minerals present are still elevated, or in some cases below normal. These elevations and deficiencies are partially due to ongoing therapy and the dietary and supplemental intake necessary for me to battle MS and maintain the health I now enjoy. Others are elevated or deficient due to imbalances that still exist within my system that may have had nothing to do with multiple sclerosis, but which do affect the overall function of my body. As the therapies I undergo become more complete and treatment progresses, and as I further refine my diet after each condition is corrected, these abnormal levels and ratios should return to the acceptable ranges.

My condition is a perfect illustration of why periodic retesting is so vital in achieving optimum results. When periodic testing is conducted, changes in each individual elemental level or combination ratio can be charted as the process of correcting these abnormalities is refined by dietary adjustments or an increase or reduction in additional supplements. This "fine tuning" continues, with the ultimate goal being for all levels of elements and ratios within my system to fall regularly within the reference ranges normal for my body.

> *When periodic testing is conducted, changes in each individual elemental level or combination ratio can be charted as the process of correcting these abnormalities is refined by dietary adjustments or an increase or reduction in additional supplements. This "fine tuning" continues, with the ultimate goal being for all levels of elements and ratios within my system to fall regularly within the reference ranges normal for my body.*

Therefore, it becomes plain that people having these tests performed should make every effort to follow their personal retesting schedules. Whether you are an athlete seeking to better your physical condition, or a patient afflicted with a chronic or serious disease, charting the progress of your mineral elements and ratios will ensure that you achieve optimum results in the minimum amount of time. Once your optimum level of health has been achieved, and after you and your medical professional have determined what nutritional supplements, mineral concentrations, ratios, and dietary intake are essential to maintain this state of health, periodic retesting remains crucial to long-term success. Although the time period between tests may be increased, retesting ensures that should any condition or imbalance begin to manifest itself, it will be detected early, at a stage when it may be more easily corrected and restored to normalcy.

Periodic retesting additionally begins to build a database of readings specific to your own personal inner workings. Just as you would retain the service record of a well-maintained car or boat, or a record of your pet's veterinary visits, periodic BCI analyses become your "service record." Should an adverse pattern begin to develop, it is more easily detectable and subsequently correctable when a larger amount of data acquired over a longer period of time has been obtained and stored for comparison.

One fact that is important to remember when viewing these charts is that they are a depiction of *my* results. These were the steps that I followed, and, yes, they were successful for me. Your physical condition, genetic composition, height, weight, age, gender, and medical history will vary from mine.

Before beginning the same protocols that I utilized, I urge you strongly to obtain a knowledgeable physician, specialist, or health care professional that will work with you through your healing process. I am certain that the successful results I realized would not have been possible had I not worked closely with my own physicians and medical professionals. Your system is delicately balanced. It must be monitored closely and subjected to repeated testing to track the imbalances as they are corrected. The tests that you will see here I still undergo periodically, to refine and adjust my healing regimen and maintain proper system harmony.

The following series of charts is for illustration only, and is presented to give you some familiarity with their appearance and the reference ranges of each element considered to be normal in the average human body. Reference ranges have been established for the purposes of these analyses by extensive scientific study of the levels of each element found in "healthy" individuals. Effective as a benchmark in determining the imbalances that may be present in an individual patient, they should be viewed as guidelines as opposed to the absolute limit for determining excess, deficiency, toxicity, or acceptable levels. Keep in mind that each individual's actual reference ranges will vary slightly, even in those who are considered "perfectly healthy." Again, race, age, gender, physical condition, dietary intake, medical history, and additional individual factors will all contribute to the determination of each person's acceptable levels of any given element, mineral, or ratio relationship.

Chart 11-6 shows the level of nutrient minerals present in my system in March 1999. Each individual element level is shaded differently for visual presentation only. The shading itself has no other significance.

Chart 11-6 Hair Analysis—Nutrient Mineral Range Test Results

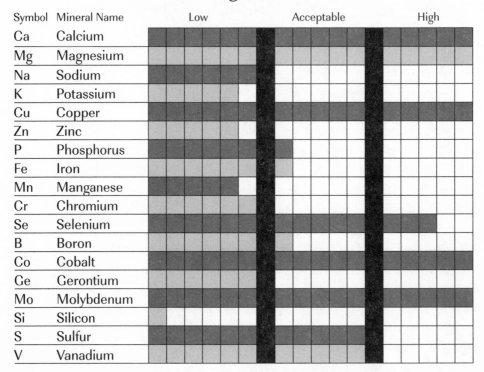

Symbol	Mineral Name	Low	Acceptable	High
Ca	Calcium			
Mg	Magnesium			
Na	Sodium			
K	Potassium			
Cu	Copper			
Zn	Zinc			
P	Phosphorus			
Fe	Iron			
Mn	Manganese			
Cr	Chromium			
Se	Selenium			
B	Boron			
Co	Cobalt			
Ge	Gerontium			
Mo	Molybdenum			
Si	Silicon			
S	Sulfur			
V	Vanadium			

Nutrient minerals are easily identifiable and are considered essential for many biological functions. Nutrient minerals play key roles in metabolic processes such as muscle activity, endocrine functions, reproduction, skeletal strength, and overall growth and development. Even though most of the nutrient minerals in my system were beginning to fall within my normal reference ranges, some of the nutrients are still clearly in excess or deficiency. Some of these excesses are as a result of the treatments I was undergoing, and some of the deficiencies occurred as I eliminated certain foods from my diet as a result of pursuing various protocols. Again, the reference ranges for each individual will vary.

Let's take a closer look at the chart above. I'd like to give you some practical examples of what the excesses and deficiencies in these nutrient minerals can indicate as regards actual physical symptoms or chronic conditions that may be present.

The examples in this chapter have been drawn from my actual test results, and the interpretations provided with the generous assistance of Dr. William Crawford, of the Crawford Center, in Mobile, Alabama. A highly respected medical professional, Dr. Crawford is widely regarded as a definitive expert in the field of nutrient level and imbalance studies and treatment of debilitating or chronic conditions that may be present in a patient as a result. The following examples will give a general indication of the conditions that may result from an excess or deficiency of specific nutrients, or as a result of a group of nutrients out of balance in the body.

Again, these examples are for illustration only. Should you find that you have a similar excess or deficiency in one or more of these categories, it does not necessarily indicate that you have, or will contract, the described illness or chronic ailment. I cannot stress enough that "proper" nutrient levels are as individual as fingerprints, and you should work closely with your doctor or specialist when determining what your personal optimum levels should be.

For our first example, let's examine the copper levels present in my system at the time of this test. Notice the high level of copper indicated on my chart. Copper is one of the most important nutrient minerals, as it has an effect on so many systems and functions of the body, including the interference with production or retention of other essential nutrient minerals. Excess copper is stored in the liver, kidneys, and in some areas of the brain. Too much copper can result in abnormal tastes when eating. Food can taste strange, even unpleasant. Patients with an excess of copper in the system often have an increased craving for sweets. Unlike other foods, the taste of sweet edibles is not affected by an excess of copper. This may be why I find it difficult to give up the honey I use with tea, even though you've read how I began to follow the Zero Dairy, Zero Sugar nutritional program, and experienced health improvement when following the diet.

A chronic or long-term result of high copper levels is often weight gain, sometimes serious gain. How often have you heard overweight persons, even possibly yourself, admit that they cannot stay away from sweets, even though they know that these foods are making them fat? Sweet addiction may not be a "lack of will power" at all, as we've all been taught to think. It may be your body's way of telling you that you have too much copper in your system.

High copper concentration may also be the reason that overweight persons think that certain "healthy" foods taste terrible. Again, have you ever heard successful dieters attest to the fact that, although they once hated celery, broccoli, and cauliflower, they can't get enough of them now? That may not be such a crazy statement after all. When copper levels are reduced in the system, unsweetened foods begin to lose the strange taste they may have once had.

Excess copper in the system can also result in "age spots," small brown patches in the skin. If you are age forty or older, you may have begun to notice these spots appearing on your hands, forearms, forehead, or neck area, or you may have observed them on other older members of your family and friends. Sometimes this can be purely a result of the aging process. Although Chart 11-3 shows that the function of the thymus gland is directly affected by copper levels, the retention of copper can occur when the adrenal glands are operating below par. This often occurs as a part of aging, as the body loses desires it experienced in its prime. Interestingly, this may also account for a slowing of the aging process in persons involved with activities requiring higher adrenal gland activity. Athletes, soldiers, martial artists engaged in competition on a regular basis, police, or emergency personnel often find themselves in adrenaline-intensive situations. These are, for the most part, physically fit and healthy individuals.

Think of some of the most popular action heroes of today's films. Those who perform their own stunts and action scenes invariably look younger and more fit than their counterparts who prefer the use of a double, or stand-in. In fact, most of today's celluloid heroes are quite a bit older than you think! It is additionally interesting to note that once the above-mentioned groups of persons retire, however, they seem to age rather quickly. This may be due to the fact that they no longer find the need for increased adrenaline production as often as they did during their respective careers.

High copper can also be scientifically linked to depression and unexplained mood swings. This is shown to be particularly true of women just before their menstrual period. If you are a woman who experiences severe mood swings, or bouts of unexplained crying near the onset of your menstrual cycle, you may have a high level of copper in your system.

I found myself subject to frequent emotional extremes during my illness, especially after I was first diagnosed. Before the onset of my MS, I would have described myself as a tranquil extrovert. Hardly a contradiction in terms, this means that I was outgoing and friendly while maintaining an inner peace. Of course, I was not always peaceful during times of crisis or unpleasant circumstances, but few of us are. However, my emotional reaction during those incidents was appropriate to the situation. After my diagnosis, I would experience emotional highs, or lows, with less than normal provocation. Although some of my reactions can be attributed to an awareness of the gravity of my physical condition, an excess of copper in my system undoubtedly enhanced my responses.

Chronic high levels of copper may result in chronic depression, regardless of gender. This is due to the neurotransmitter imbalances in the brain caused by the condition. Neurotransmitters help to regulate many brain functions, including moods. High copper also interferes with other nutrient minerals, such as iron, zinc, and manganese. If you examine my chart, you will note that my levels of all three of these nutrient minerals are lower than is acceptable. Over time, as my copper levels decreased, these nutrient mineral levels were also restored to a normal balance.

Additionally, copper is antagonistic to iron, which means that the two minerals function in opposition to one another, maintaining a check-and-balance relationship. You will note that my iron level is below the acceptable reference range, while my copper level is high. The lack of production and storage of adequate iron is no doubt due to the excess levels of copper. Because copper is antagonistic to iron, a condition known as "iron deficiency anemia" can occur. We will discuss the implications of an imbalance in the ratio of copper to iron later in this chapter.

Next, note the level of zinc present in my system when this particular test was conducted. It reads just below the low end of the "normal" reference range. Dr. Crawford maintains that a zinc deficiency can be responsible for visual disturbances a patient may develop. Often, MS patients experience blurred or failing vision as their condition progresses. Zinc deficiency may be a major contributor to a number of optically related illnesses or conditions, including glaucoma, retinitis, and malnutrition blindness. In impoverished areas of the world, adequate nutrition is nearly impossible on a consistent basis. Zinc is obtained naturally from protein-rich foods, which are sorely lacking in the diet of these unfortunate people. Every day, thousands of children in these areas under the age of fourteen are losing their vision, permanently. Much of this may be due to the extreme deficiency of zinc in their systems.

Next, you will notice that the chromium level indicated on the chart is at the low end of the acceptable range. Chromium levels indicate your body's "glucose tolerance factor," the amount of dietary glucose obtained from carbohydrates or sugar that the body can efficiently metabolize. Hypoglycemics, persons who have a glucose deficiency commonly termed "low blood sugar," almost invariably have noticeable chromium deficiencies. Raising the chromium level in the system raises the blood sugar level, and increases the body's ability to metabolize carbohydrates and sugars efficiently. Because of their system's inability to metabolize carbohydrates and sugars effectively, persons who are afflicted with hypoglycemia need a higher amount of proteins than those persons with normal blood sugar levels.

Note also that the level of cobalt in my system is well above the acceptable range. Excess cobalt has been indirectly associated with anemia because cobalt is also antagonistic to iron and prevents the proper use of iron by your metabolism. Many persons who suffer from common forms of anemia are found to have excess cobalt in their systems, a condition referred to as "cobalt toxicity." If this excess is not corrected, certain blood deficiencies, such as anemia, can become chronic.

Chart 11-7 illustrates the levels of toxic minerals, or "heavy metals" present in my system. Their ability to interfere with normal metabolic functions has been scientifically proven. These elements are commonly found in the environment and are therefore present to a certain degree in any biological ecosystem. However, the presence of these metals indicates a definite cause for concern when system accumulation is excessive. Heavy metals have a tendency to accumulate in the body unless a treatment method such as chelation is utilized to cleanse the system and restore the levels to a normal range. Chelation helped to remove the mercury in my system and can be used to purge the body of other heavy metals as well. The tendency to accumulate heavy metals in the body is apparent in other life forms, particularly animals and fish. Mercury has been known to reach poisonous levels in some food fish as a result of pollution in their environment.

Chart 11-7: Hair Analysis—Toxic Mineral Range Test Results

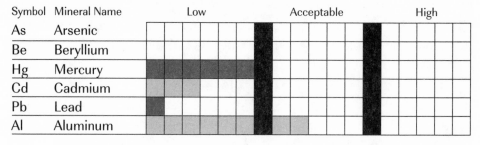

Symbol	Mineral Name	Low						Acceptable					High				
As	Arsenic																
Be	Beryllium																
Hg	Mercury																
Cd	Cadmium																
Pb	Lead																
Al	Aluminum																

Arsenic is a universally recognized poison, found naturally in some types of cactus and certain fruits, including grapes. Trace amounts of arsenic are not uncommon in very aged bottles of wine, for instance. The body will naturally build a resistance to arsenic, but an excess amount of this toxin can produce insanity, convulsions, paralysis, and death.

Although the effects of toxic metal presence and levels are not yet fully understood in all cases, it should be noted here that certain toxic metals in addition to arsenic, specifically lead and mercury, have been proven to be definite poisoners to which the body can only develop a certain amount of immunity. This chart indicates that in March 1999, the presence of almost all toxic metals was below the predetermined acceptable average levels, except for mercury and aluminum.

Before I began chelation therapy, most of these levels were off of the scale, proving, at least through my experience, that chelation has a definite benefit in removing mercury and other toxic heavy metals from the system. Through continuing use of supplements and careful adherence to my personal dietary requirements, the levels of these toxic metals eventually returned to the acceptable reference ranges.

Chart 11-8: These additional minerals are not as well known, nor are existing studies as extensive as those conducted on the nutrient and toxic minerals. Although they are considered possibly essential to bodily function, results regarding the correct amounts, proportions, and their relationship to other materials in the system are not definitive. Additional studies are still being conducted as to their value or detriment to the human system. Reflecting my test results of March 1999, this chart is shown simply to illustrate the thoroughness of the BCI analyses conducted for each individual patient.

Chart 11-8: Hair Analysis—Additional Mineral Range Test Results

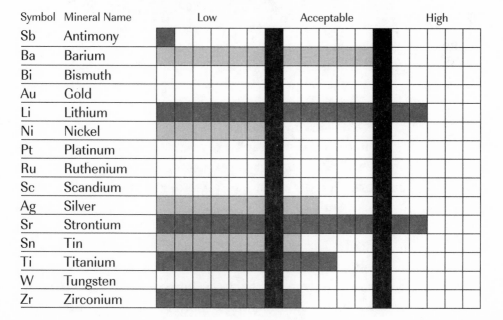

Symbol	Mineral Name	Low	Acceptable	High
Sb	Antimony			
Ba	Barium			
Bi	Bismuth			
Au	Gold			
Li	Lithium			
Ni	Nickel			
Pt	Platinum			
Ru	Ruthenium			
Sc	Scandium			
Ag	Silver			
Sr	Strontium			
Sn	Tin			
Ti	Titanium			
W	Tungsten			
Zr	Zirconium			

A ratio is the calculated comparison of a relationship between the presence of two minerals. Minerals are considered to be in relationship, or ratio, when both affect the same gland, organ, or system function. Ratios are calculated by dividing the first mineral level by the second mineral level. If the normal ratio between two minerals present in the human system is disturbed or out of alignment, significant studies show that essential biological functions can be adversely affected. Even at extremely low levels, the positive (synergistic) or negative (antagonistic) ratios of these minerals can affect the metabolic processes.

Chart 11-9 illustrates the mineral ratio balances and imbalances present in my system in March 1999.

Chart 11-9: Hair Analysis—Significant Mineral Ratio Results

Symbol	Mineral Name	Low	Acceptable	High
Ca/P	Calcium/Phosphorus			
Na/K	Sodium/Potassium			
Ca/K	Calcium/Potassium			
Zn/Cu	Zinc/Copper			
Na/Mg	Sodium/Magnesium			
Ca/Mg	Calcium/Magnesium			
Fe/Cu	Iron/Copper			

Let's take a moment to examine some of the ratios of these minerals present at the time these tests were conducted, and what they may indicate. Once again, these examples are for illustration only. Any interpretation of mineral ratios found in the system of the reader should be discussed with a physician or medical specialist before any method of treatment is instituted.

First, we'll examine my calcium/phosphorus ratio. You will note that it is extremely high, well beyond the acceptable reference range. Calcium and phosphorus have an opposite, or antagonistic, effect on the body's metabolism. Calcium acts as a metabolic sedative, slowing down the body's processing of raw materials. Phosphorus, on the other hand, stimulates the metabolism. When there is an excess of calcium in the system in relation to phosphorus, the calcium cancels the effect of the phosphorus, slowing the metabolism and causing reduced energy levels. Persons suffering from chronic fatigue are often found to have excessive calcium in their systems.

It will also be noted that my calcium/potassium ratio is extremely high. Calcium (Ca) and potassium (K) are also antagonistic to one another. Often, a calcium/potassium imbalance is found in patients with decreased thyroid activity, including persons suffering from a growth deficiency or obesity. Although decreased thyroid activity may be the cause of high calcium and lowered potassium in some individuals, the reverse may also be true: that an excess of calcium may inhibit the function of the thyroid gland and its processes. This ratio imbalance may manifest itself outwardly in other ways as well, including the appearance of dry skin or chronic constipation. A person experiencing either of these common conditions should not automatically assume a Ca/K imbalance, as several other factors are known to cause these common ailments, including change of diet and environmental intolerances or allergies.

The next ratio we should consider is the low zinc/copper ratio indicated on my chart. Copper is associated with the essential body enzyme histamine, and has the ability, when found in excess, to destroy this enzyme. Zinc, on the other hand, is essential for the storage of histamine. Patients found with a high copper/low zinc ratio are found to have low serum histamine. Low levels of this enzyme, when the condition becomes chronic, result in allergies and food intolerances in many persons. Conversely, when this imbalance is corrected and brought into normal range, patients find that the food, flower, or pet that caused them so much discomfort no longer has that adverse effect on their systems. Histamine is also essential to the production of the system antibodies that fight infection. This factor becomes particularly important when considering the viral origins of MS.

The sodium/magnesium ratio is also below the reference range considered acceptable. The function of the adrenal glands is directly related to this important ratio. Excess magnesium results in decreased adrenal cortical function, and may also contribute to the manifestation of dry skin, constipation, and chronic fatigue. When first diagnosed with MS, I found myself often becoming quickly fatigued without excess exertion.

This test illustrates that my iron/copper ratio was returning to the acceptable reference range. Copper is antagonistic to iron and contributes to iron deficiency anemia. Iron is essential to the development of many essential body systems, including brain growth and functionality. Many OB/GYN practitioners routinely prescribe daily iron supplements for pregnant or nursing mothers in an effort to prevent the lifetime side effects of an iron deficiency or iron/copper imbalance.

Part of the process in finding a cure for MS was identifying the cause of the virus. Due to the indicated condition of these ratios, and the additional high calcium/magnesium and low zinc/copper ratio present in previous tests, Dr. Crawford felt that the pattern might be indicative of the presence of the Epstein-Barr Virus (EBV) and recommended that I be tested for the disease as soon as possible.

After my test results were analyzed by Bio-Cypher Laboratories of Burbank, California, Dr. Crawford's suspicions were confirmed. The tests clearly indicated that the serology implied a previous EBV infection. We are now actively working to completely eliminate this virus from my system.

Many times, a patient suffering from MS will be initially diagnosed as having EBV. It may only be with more thorough or broader-spectrum testing conducted after treatments for EBV are ineffective that the patient will be re-diagnosed as actually having multiple sclerosis. In fact, in the early years of diagnosis, patients suffering from multiple sclerosis or EBV were often cross-diagnosed, or the diseases were combined and not considered dissimilar. Modern medicine clearly makes the distinction, however, and the treatment of each affliction is separate and specific.

In an effort to aid sufferers of EBV, I have included a listing of vitamin and mineral supplements found to be effective in the treatment of this illness in the next chapter, "Achieving Balance through Vitamin, Mineral, and Supplement Therapies." I additionally expand upon the noteworthy practices of Dr. Crawford and his work on imbalance correction through natural methods.

Many times, a patient suffering from MS will be initially diagnosed as having Epstein-Barr Virus. It may only be with more thorough or broader-spectrum testing conducted after treatments for Epstein-Barr Virus are ineffective that the patient will be re-diagnosed as actually having multiple sclerosis.

As I discussed in chapter 10, I have recently begun a new treatment aimed at correcting the excess of calcium in my system. I am taking calcium orotates, an oral calcium supplement, prescribed for me by Dr. Crawford. Although some highly respected practitioners would disagree, arguing that adding calcium to a system already overloaded was in essence "carrying coals to Newcastle" and certainly not normal procedure, the treatment is working. Successful on a twofold front, the regimen of 3000 mg. of calcium orotates per day (500 mg.–900 mg. is considered a "normal" prescription) resulted in my calcium levels lowering by about one-third in the period of time between the initial test and the chart reproduced above. Additionally, the ingestion of these oratates has resulted in a reduction of the serology levels (the amounts found in the bloodstream) for EBV, showing that this stubborn invader is steadily being pushed from my system. As the study of mineral ratios and their relation to optimum health or chronic conditions becomes more extensively detailed, it may soon become possible to correct a number of chronic illnesses or deficiencies by restoring mineral levels to normal ranges and ratios to one another.

Toxic mineral ratios at high levels do not always indicate that the patient will experience the clinical symptoms associated with those particular heavy minerals. However, research studies have proven that high concentrations or inappropriate ratios of these minerals can cause an antagonistic or adverse effect on various essential nutrient minerals, which, if not corrected, eventually begin to affect the function of the essential nutrient minerals in the body.

Chart 11-10 reflects my toxic mineral ratios during the same testing period of March 1999. I had already completed chelation at this time. Notice that the mercury ratios are below the reference range. Calcium ratios are again out of balance, as are the iron and lead ratios. Referring to Charts 11-6 and 11-7, you will note that my calcium, sulfur, and selenium levels are all disproportionately high when compared to the amount of lead in my system, accounting for these deficient or excessive ratios. Part of the reason for the low lead level reading at this time was the chelation therapy itself, which removed other metals from my system along with the excess mercury.

My iron levels measured within the acceptable reference range, but the low amounts of mercury in my system caused my iron/mercury ratio to chart as deficient. These results are another solid reason for performing a BCI analysis before beginning any therapy or treatment program. Determining your initial system composition assists you and your health care professional in planning therapies that address your particular excesses, deficiencies, or imbalances while maintaining the proper ratios of these elements to one another.

Chart 11-10: Hair Analysis—Toxic
Mineral Ratio Range Results

Symbol	Mineral Name	Low						Acceptable						High				
Ca/Pb	Calcium/Lead																	
Fe/Pb	Iron/Lead																	
Fe/Hg	Iron/Mercury																	
Se/Hg	Selenium/Mercury																	
Zn/Cd	Zinc/Cadmium																	
Zn/Hg	Zinc/Mercury																	
S/Hg	Sulfur/Mercury																	
S/Cd	Sulfur/Cadmium																	
S/Pb	Sulfur/Lead																	

I hope that the inclusion of these analyses charts has served to illustrate the importance of these tests. Knowing the score—possessing detailed knowledge of what exactly is occurring in your body—can be an invaluable weapon in the fight against illness. These tests can also become an important safeguard against future illness, as imbalances detected early can be corrected before further and more extensive damage occurs as a result of those imbalances.

Now that we have learned how the proper levels of minerals, metals, and elements present in the body can positively or negatively affect our metabolism and its optimum function, the next chapter will discuss how the addition of vitamin and mineral supplements can enhance, promote, and expedite the healing process in your system. I review each significant vitamin and mineral as it specifically relates to those afflicted with multiple sclerosis. I will show you which supplements have become a part of my daily routine and how they have contributed to the excellent state of health I enjoy today.

12
Achieving Balance through Vitamin, Mineral, and Supplement Therapies

We are beginning to learn that our bodies are much more than the shell we exist within which allows us to interact with the physical world around us. The human body is a finely tuned instrument. When in optimum operating condition, it is athletic, healthy, and vibrant. Out of balance, it becomes sluggish, uncoordinated, and suffers system breakdowns, which can be life threatening or even fatal.

One of the major turning points on my road to a cure was understanding the role that vitamins and minerals play in the health and proper nutrition of the system. In this chapter we will explore the vitamins and minerals that are most important to the MS patient, particularly vitamin C and the vitamin B group. We will also examine the role of nutritional and mineral supplements in restoring the system balance of the MS-afflicted, and the daily supplement and vitamin regimen I still adhere to today.

As we have learned from the chapter on BioCybernetics, determining the actual levels of vitamins, minerals, elements, and nutrients in your system is essential to your efforts to restore any imbalances that may be present. Besides a

BioCybernetics analysis, there are a number of other methods that you can use to determine your excess or deficiency in vital substances. Blood tests can determine the presence of certain vitamins that accumulate in the body, although some, like vitamin D, are not retained for long by the body, and therefore cannot be reliably measured by blood or urine testing. Probably two of the best ways to determine your vitamin levels is through symptom evaluation and dietary intake.

Because common symptoms can arise from a number of diverse and unrelated causes, I recommend that you evaluate your dietary intake as the most reliable way to determine whether or not you are ingesting the Dietary Reference Intake (DRI) for your personal needs. You may be familiar with these dietary requirements under their former name, the RDA, or Recommended Dietary Allowance. Currently, this table of daily nutrient intake is being revised in a joint cooperative venture between the governments of the United States and Canada. We will explore this topic in greater depth in chapter 15, "Life After Dairy: A Practical Guide to Alternate Eating," where we will examine the roles of calcium, magnesium, and phosphorus in the human diet, and chapter 16, "Making the Right Choices: Understanding the Role of Food in Creating a Nutrition Program that Works," where we will explore the principles of proper nutrition.

You are the person who knows best what you eat. You are also the person who will have to make the dietary adjustments necessary to replenish or replace those vitamins and nutrients that your body needs but does not have in adequate supply, either through the introduction of new foods or through supplementation. These two upcoming chapters will examine some dietary choices you can review, with their individual nutrient counts. For evaluations of food items with the individual nutrient counts we will discuss here, see "Making the Right Choices: A Nutrition Program that Works."

Science has made great strides toward understanding the composition of substances and life forms at the most basic level, the cell, and the chemicals that comprise each one. This field of study is known today as molecular biology. One of the most prominent figures in the world of molecular biology was the Nobel-Prize-winning chemist, the late Dr. Linus Pauling. Dr. Pauling's discoveries and the health recommendations that resulted were instrumental in my choices of nutrient supplementation in my fight against MS. Because his work was so crucial to my success, I have included this look at the life of Linus Carl Pauling, Ph.D., and how his research relates to the multiple sclerosis sufferer.

The Forest and the Trees— A Look at Linus Pauling

Dr. Pauling began his career as a chemical engineer, receiving his B.S. in 1922 from Oregon Agricultural College, later to become Oregon State University. Three years later he received his Ph.D. from the California Institute of Technology, where he would remain in a professorship for nearly four decades. His work concentrated mainly on the crystal structure of different minerals (Woodrow Wilson National Fellowship Foundation 1999). While at Cal Tech, Dr. Pauling began to examine the molecular structure of other substances and how the individual elements combined to form more complex structures. In late 1930, Dr. Pauling's study entitled "The Nature of the Chemical Bond" was first published in the *Journal of the American Chemical Society* (Oregon State University 1999). Nine years later, he expanded this article into a full-length book of the same name that remains one of the most referenced works in fields of chemical study. In 1935, he began to study what would become known as molecular biology. He examined hemoglobin in particular, and the effects that magnetism had on venal and arterial blood cells. This research led to further study of the building blocks of all living matter and the source of energy from food.

Although invited personally by his long-time friend Albert Einstein to become a member of the Emergency Committee of Atomic Scientists during the Second World War, Dr. Pauling declined to work on the Manhattan Project, being firmly opposed to war and all atomic weapons. In 1947, U.S. President Harry S. Truman awarded Dr. Pauling the Presidential Medal of Merit for his work on crystal structures, the nature of the chemical bond, and his efforts, with his wife, Ava Helen Miller Pauling, for world peace. Dr. Pauling's consistent efforts to end global hostilities earned him not only recognition, but also persecution. His book *No More War* sufficiently angered political zealots and powerful military manufacturers, making it impossible for him to obtain a passport for almost four years (Woodrow Wilson National Fellowship Foundation 1999). These nonscientific activities, though humanitarian, compromised his research and hindered his career.

In 1948, Dr. Pauling began research into the description of the DNA chain. His models were predicated on an alpha-helix structure, or single twisting chain. He was not permitted to attend a conference held in London in the spring of 1952, his passport application again denied despite a personal letter from Dr. Einstein accompanying his request. At that conference, the landmark photographs of DNA taken by Rosalind Franklin and associates at King's College in London were displayed (Woodrow Wilson National Fellowship Association 1999). Had Dr. Pauling been allowed to attend, he would have seen that DNA consisted of a double chain, a breakthrough conclusion reached by scientists James Watson and Francis Crick, who attended the conference and studied the pictures, later earning a Nobel Prize for their depiction of the double-helix structure of DNA.

His efforts on behalf of the nuclear test ban treaty earned him the Nobel Prize for Peace in 1962. Three years later, Dr. Pauling again redirected the focus of his research after responding to a letter from Irwin Stone, an outspoken advocate of the benefits of Vitamin C (Oregon State University 1999).

His studies would become the field of orthomolecular medicine and resulted in two major milestones: the publication of his landmark study *Vitamin C and the Common Cold* in 1970, and the advent of the Institute of Orthomolecular Medicine in 1973. There he worked with Arthur B. Robinson and Keene Dimick. This nonprofit health research organization was later to become known as the Linus Pauling Institute of Science and Medicine. In 1996, this highly regarded and internationally recognized research facility relocated to Oregon State University, and is known today as the Linus Pauling Institute.

Dr. Pauling's later work becomes especially significant to the MS patient, as it primarily focused on the effects of massive doses of Vitamin C on certain types of cancer and the clinical benefits of injections of vitamins in the B family on other chronic and life-threatening diseases, including MS. *Cancer and Vitamin C,* coauthored with Ewan Cameron, was published in 1979. *How to Live Longer and Feel Better* appeared in print in 1986, when Dr. Pauling was 85 years old. His thorough, commonsense approach to nutrition and the human body is highly regarded in the medical community, serving as the foundation for many popular diets and nutrition supplement regimens advocated by health professionals today. I highly recommend that you purchase and read this book. This information shared by Dr. Pauling, gained from a lifetime of research, is invaluable to both the MS patient and the healthy individual.

Dr. Linus Pauling left us in 1994, at 93 years of age. His legacy, the Linus Pauling Institute, continues his work in determining the role of food elements in maintaining human health and preventing and treating disease through research and education (Linus Pauling Institute 1999). Dr. Pauling's work was instrumental in the determination of adequate intake levels of essential vitamins and nutrients required to promote optimum human health. His research contributed to the U.S. government standard for vitamin and nutrient intake known as the RDA, and more recently, as the DRI. We will look at the DRI for essential vitamins and minerals in the next section.

Uncle Sam Wants You—To Eat
Your Vitamins and Minerals!

For over fifty years, scientists and nutrition experts have worked to produce a standard set of nutrient and vitamin levels necessary to maintain human health. Collectively known until 1997 as the RDA, these standards are currently undergoing major revisions. When complete they will be reissued as the DRI, or Dietary Reference Intake (USDA 1999). The new standards reflect the emerging changes in the evaluation of daily essential nutrient intakes, largely brought about by recent advances in scientific nutrition fields such as orthomolecular medicine, Linus Pauling's specialty.

These new standards should be used as a minimum nutritional guideline. I have already shown you through BioCybernetics analysis that each person is an individual, and the requirements for your optimum health will not be the same as those of your parents, your siblings, or your children. If, after testing, you find that your system is deficient in certain vitamins or minerals, you will need to supplement your intake of those substances. Your supplements should exceed the RDA or DRI for that mineral or vitamin until the deficiency has been corrected.

Chart 12-1 depicts the current RDA for vitamins and certain minerals, last compiled in 1989. To date, the DRI standards have not been publicly issued for all of these elements. I have included the DRI chart for vitamin D, calcium, magnesium, and phosphorus in chapter 15, "Life After Dairy: A Practical Guide to Alternate Eating."

Use this chart for reference. Remember, these are guidelines. Your individual dietary requirements will vary. If you are a 235-lb., 36-year-old male, your needs will be different from those of a 150-lb. male of the same age. Or, if you are a nursing mother of twins, you will require a different amount of nutrients than a mom who has only one breast-feeding child. There are many other factors that determine your ideal daily

Chart 12-1 USDA DRI—Dietary Reference Intake Guidelines

Recommended Levels in Milligrams (MG) unless Otherwise Specified

Age (Years)	Pr*	A	E	K	C	Th	Rb	Ni	B6	Fo	B$_{12}$	Fe	Z	Io	Se
Infants (All)															
0.0-0.5 yr.	13	375	3	5	30	.3	.4	5	.3	25	.3	6	5	40	10
0.5-1.0 yr.	14	375	4	10	35	.4	.5	6	.6	35	.5	10	5	50	15
Children (All)															
1 yr.-3 yr.	16	400	6	15	40	.7	.8	9	1.0	50	.7	10	10	70	20
4 yr.-6 yr.	24	500	7	20	45	.9	1.1	12	1.1	75	1.0	10	10	90	20
7 yr.-10 yr.	28	700	7	30	45	1.0	1.2	13	1.4	100	1.4	10	10	120	30
Males															
11-14	45	1000	10	45	50	1.3	1.5	17	1.7	150	2.0	12	15	150	40
15-18	59	1000	10	65	60	1.5	1.8	20	2.0	200	2.0	12	15	150	50
19-24	58	1000	10	70	60	1.5	1.7	19	2.0	200	2.0	10	15	150	70
25-50	63	1000	10	80	60	1.5	1.7	19	2.0	200	2.0	10	15	150	70
51+	63	1000	10	80	60	1.2	1.4	15	2.0	200	2.0	10	15	150	70
Females															
11-14	46	800	8	45	50	1.1	1.3	15	1.4	150	2.0	15	12	150	45
15-18	44	800	8	55	60	1.1	1.3	15	1.5	180	2.0	15	12	150	50
19-24	46	800	8	60	60	1.1	1.3	15	1.6	180	2.0	15	12	150	55
25-50	50	800	8	65	60	1.1	1.3	15	1.6	180	2.0	15	12	150	55
51+	50	800	8	65	60	1.0	1.2	13	1.6	180	2.0	10	12	150	55
Pregnant	60	800	10	65	70	1.5	1.6	17	2.2	400	2.2	30	15	175	65
Lactating															
1st 6 mos.	65	1300	12	65	95	1.6	1.8	20	2.1	280	2.6	15	19	200	75
2nd 6 mos.	62	1200	11	65	90	1.6	1.7	20	2.1	260	2.6	15	16	200	75

Table KEY * = Grams

Pr = Protein	Th = Thiamine	Fo = Folate	Io = Iodine
A = Vitamin A	Rb = Riboflavin	B12 = Vitamin B12	Se = Selenium
E = Vitamin E	Ni = Niacin	Fe = Iron	C = Vitamin C
B6 = Vitamin B6	Z = Zinc		

intake: blood conditions like diabetes or hypoglycemia, existing vitamin or nutrient deficiencies, or diseases such as MS. Later in this chapter we'll take a look at the vitamin and mineral supplement pack that I take daily. You will note that the amounts differ from those shown here as the correct daily intake for my age group. However, working with my BCI analyses, Dr. Weeks and Dr. Crawford, I know that the amounts in the daily nutrient package are right for me.

Now that we have the chart as an overview, let's break it down and take a look at the individual elements. Let's examine each vitamin or nutrient component, and discover what they are, where you can find them in natural foods, and how they benefit the body, particularly the body of a person afflicted with multiple sclerosis.

Vitamins and Minerals—The Raw Materials of Health

Think of your body, for the moment, as a construction site. The foods that you eat contain the raw materials your body construction site uses to produce the final product: health. Just as in an actual construction site, the amount of raw materials delivered to complete the project is crucial. Deliver too few materials, and the project is completed poorly, or not at all. Too many materials, and the project becomes costly, inefficient, and the job site a safety hazard.

We can think of the foods that we eat as our raw materials. Deliver too little wood to our job site, and the frame of our building is weak, poorly constructed, will not hold up under tough weather conditions, and will not stand the test of time. Deliver too little calcium, magnesium, and phosphorus to our bodies, and our frame, our bones, will be weak, possibly stunted in growth, easily injured during strenuous activities, and may develop osteoporosis later in life. If our job site does not have enough glass, our building will be dark, lightless. If our bodies do not get enough vitamin A, our eyes will not be able to see properly, and our world will grow dark. And, just as other raw materials are necessary for a sound, strong building, without the minerals and vitamins that we require, our body building will not be sturdy either.

Sometimes, depending on the project, certain materials are required more than others. A Southwestern style home will require more adobe, stone, and brick than would a classic Victorian farmhouse. A beach home will need more concrete and sturdy pylons for its foundation than would a lakeside cabin. The same is true for our bodies. The person who is MS-afflicted requires more of certain vitamins and minerals, and less of others, than does a "normal," healthy person. Although we will briefly touch upon all of the elements in the chart above, we will examine in more depth the vitamins and minerals that have been the most important in the treatment of my MS. Some of them have had RDA or DRI determinations made for them, some have not.

These are the vitamins and minerals that most helped me during the period of my affliction, many of which I still take on a daily basis. You may not need as many, or even the same ones as I did. Your own genetics, blood type, physical condition, age, and strength of the disease will dictate which elements you most and least need. This chapter should not be viewed as a vitamin and mineral handbook, by any means, and should not be used to substitute for testing or consultations with a health care professional. Just because Dr. Celeste may take 8,000 mg. per day of vitamin C (I do, by the way) does not mean that you should go out and buy the MegaBig 1000 count Mighty Pill collection.

It also doesn't mean that you need to start groaning about carrying dozens of pills around in a gym bag everywhere you go. Almost all of the substances we discuss here can be found in common food items. In chapters 15 and 16, I will show you how to find the foods that will give you the most of each of these important elements. You may need to take supplements, either daily or occasionally, but you do not need to become a slave to endless bottles of pills. As in all things, common sense is the key. Learn what vitamins and minerals are important to your system, and what foods supply those elements in sufficient quantity to meet your individual nutritional or health repair needs. Eat those foods, and use supplements for those nutrients that you either cannot supply through eating or need in excessive quantity.

For ease of reference, I have discussed the elements found in Chart 12-1 in alphabetical order. I have additionally included others that have been particularly important to me in my healing process. These do not yet have an RDA or DRI established. You will need to consult with your doctor and have testing performed to determine your specific needs.

Vitamin A is found in two forms: beta-carotene, known as provitamin A, and retinol, or preformed vitamin A. Vitamin A is a fat-soluble vitamin and is stored by your body. Because it is a stored vitamin, an excess, or toxicity, can occur. When taking vitamin A as a supplement, care must be taken not to overload your system. Some symptoms of vitamin A toxicity can include nausea and vomiting, diarrhea, and hair loss. Additionally, retinol as a supplement is not recommended for pregnant women, as it may cause complications in pregnancy and fetal difficulty. Vitamin A deficiency may manifest itself as night blindness, dry and brittle hair, or tooth and gum problems.

Retinol, or preformed vitamin A, is only found in foods from animal sources. Retinol from these sources is absorbed easily through digestion and is immediately utilized by the body. The best natural sources of retinol are animal and poultry livers, and oils made from fish liver, such as cod liver oil. This fact may be of special importance to vegans, who eschew all animal-produced foods.

Beta-carotene, or provitamin A, is found largely in foods from plant sources, although good amounts are also in cheeses and butter. This form of vitamin A must be converted by the body into a retinol-like form before it can be absorbed into the system and utilized. Yellow or dark green fruits and vegetables are the best sources of beta-carotene, like cantaloupe melons, apricots, carrots and broccoli. You can find other foods that are good sources of vitamin A in chapter 16.

Vitamin A is important to the MS-afflicted because it functions as an antioxidant, helping to keep your system free of toxins. It also protects and strengthens cell membranes, particularly mucous membranes, thereby helping increase resistance to respiratory infections and airborne viruses. It is essential to maintaining healthy vision. Many MS sufferers experience one of the most disabling and frightening symptoms of the disease: blurred, failing, or double vision. You will learn more about MS-induced blindness later in chapter 14, "Deadly Savior—Bee Venom Treatment."

The B family of vitamins is sometimes referred to as the B-complex series. Interrelated and working with one another, B vitamins contribute to the proper function of many of our essential life systems. Let's take a look at the ones that are the most important in MS recovery and continuing health.

Vitamin B_1, or thiamine, is a water-soluble vitamin. It is not stored by our bodies and is not considered to be toxic. However, because it works in conjunction with other members of the B family, too much B_1 can lead to an imbalance, thereby cutting down on the efficiency and ability of the rest of the complex to perform their separate functions. Thiamine deficiency can manifest as depression, memory loss, water retention, and muscle weakness.

The best food sources of thiamine are pork meats, animal organ meats, like liver, brewer's yeast, bran, whole grains, and enriched breads or flours. You can find other foods that are good sources of thiamine in chapter 16. Vitamin B_1 is considered to be an "unstable" or fragile vitamin; exposure to heat, air, and water during cooking can reduce the amount of B_1 in your foods. You may want to consider supplementation of this essential element to ensure that you are receiving an adequate daily supply.

Thiamine is particularly important to the MS patient because it maintains the central nervous system and strong muscle tissue. You remember from my personal story that some of the very first symptoms I experienced were muscle weakness in my step aerobics class and temporary paralysis on that disastrous Hawaiian hiking trip. Many patients with rapidly accelerating MS find themselves in a wheelchair before too long. Increased doses of daily thiamine help to fight muscle deterioration and maintain communication between the central nervous system and other areas of the body.

Vitamin B_2, also known as riboflavin, helps your body to form two important enzymes: flavin mononucleotide and flavin dinucleotide. The two enzymes work together to metabolize sugars, fats, and proteins. Vitamin B_2 is water-soluble. It is not stored by the body and therefore nontoxic. However, as with all of the B family, too much of one can lead to a deficiency or decreased efficiency of the others. Riboflavin deficiency can manifest in eye sensitivity to light, hair loss, and cold sores.

Animal organ meats, like liver, are again the best sources for riboflavin, as they are for almost all of the B family. Animal organ meats are also a terrific source of other important nutrients, such as calcium and phosphorus. B_2 can also be found in poultry, eggs, milk, cheeses, whole grains, enriched breads, dried beans, and leafy green vegetables. You can find other foods that are good sources of vitamin B_2 in chapters 15 and 16. One important additional fact to remember: riboflavin is light sensitive. Sunlight can destroy the riboflavin content in certain foods, like milk and cheese. It is best to purchase milk in cartons instead of plastic containers, although plastic may be more convenient and keep the milk fresh for a longer period of time. If you store your cheeses such as Parmesan or Romano in containers, keep them out of the sunlight.

Riboflavin is important to the MS-afflicted because it aids in the maintenance of cell membranes, especially mucous membranes. Like vitamin A, B_2 reinforces your resistance to respiratory infection and encourages clear vision. It also helps to strengthen and maintain cell respiration, the ability of your cells to pass oxygen and other gases through their walls. B_2

also is essential in food metabolism, allowing your body to maximize the value of each item that you eat, increasing your energy levels and the value of the vitamins and minerals in those foods.

Vitamin B_3 is also part of the B-complex group. Known commonly as niacin, it is water-soluble and not stored by the body. Although essentially nontoxic, niacin when taken in large doses can cause burning or itching skin or depression. When a niacin deficiency exists, symptoms can manifest as dermatitis, or skin rash, dementia, diarrhea, and nervousness without cause. Niacin deficiency can also be responsible for a disease known as pellagra, which includes all of the above symptoms.

Niacin, unlike other members of the B family, can be manufactured by your body. If there is no existing B-family deficiency, the amino acid tryptophan will produce niacin, although the amount of the amino acid needed to produce sufficient niacin is excessive. A much better source of B_3 is tuna fish and lean cuts of meat. Other good sources are basically the same as for the other members of the B-complex, described above, with the inclusion here of most nuts. See chapters 15 and 16 for additional niacin sources.

Niacin's body value is threefold. First, it maintains your nervous system health, a primary concern for the MS patient. Breakdown of nervous system response, resulting in an inability to move or coordinate your limbs, is a common symptom of progressing MS. Second, B_3 maintains and strengthens your blood circulation system. As movement becomes more limited, poor circulation can often be the result. Third, niacin aids in digestion and the metabolism of carbohydrates, fats, and proteins, increasing your energy levels and the nutrient value of foods.

Vitamin B_5 in the B-complex group is also known as pantothenic acid. The name comes from the Greek word "panthos," which means "everywhere." Pantothenic acid is found literally everywhere, in every living organism. B_5 is water-soluble and is not stored by the body, although it is an indigenous part of our own cells. It is a nontoxic vitamin, but excessive doses can cause other complications. Vitamin B_5 deficiency symptoms include fatigue, muscle cramps, stomach pains, and vomiting. Again, as the best natural source, animal organ meats come up the big winner, as do egg yolks, poultry, dark green vegetables, whole grains, and nuts. However, all food items of plant or animal origin do contain pantothenic acid, making it one of the easiest vitamins to obtain on an adequate daily basis.

Pantothenic acid in ample supply is vital to the MS-afflicted because the function of this important B vitamin is cell building and tissue generation. We will learn later in this chapter how certain components of our cells are damaged by MS. Vitamin B_5 is crucial in the battle against this damage, and is a powerful resource for rebuilding of damaged cells and production of new cells to replace those that have been destroyed by the disease. Also, B_5 aids in the metabolism of carbohydrates, fats, and proteins, as do others in the B family.

Vitamin B_6, scientifically referred to as pyridoxine, is another of the B-complex group so essential to daily health and vitality. B_6 is water-soluble and not stored in the body. Again, although nontoxic, massive doses can interfere with the function of others in the B family group. The symptoms of B_6 deficiency range from the mild to the severe, and include swollen ankles and fingers, skin rashes, nervous system disorders, low white blood cell count, and anemia.

Pyridoxine in the highest concentrations is found naturally in beef, liver, avocados, bananas, cantaloupe melons, leafy dark green vegetables, whole grains, and nuts. Other excellent sources are eggs, molasses, and brewer's yeast. You can compare the amounts of B_6 found in foods in chapter 16. Those of you on a high-protein diet will require more than the RDA recommended for your age and gender, as will smokers, women who use oral contraceptives or receive hormone replacement, and those with some types of heart disease. Your health care professional can help determine what amount is right for you.

Vitamin B_6 is essential to the MS patient for several reasons. In addition to aiding in the absorption of B_{12}, vitamin B_6 triggers the functioning of over sixty enzymes in the body. It is necessary for the production of insulin, adrenaline, and antibody white blood cells. It also aids in the metabolism of protein, which is why high-protein diets require greater dosages. MS can be impeded in its progress by the antibodies found in your white blood cells. Ingesting the proper amounts of B_6 will help your body produce the strong white blood cells so indispensable in the fight against diseases of all kinds.

Vitamin B_{12}, or cobalamin, is another water-soluble element that is not stored in the body and is therefore not considered to be toxic. One of the least-known vitamins of the B family, B_{12} is also one of the last true vitamins to have been discovered, identified by scientists after the Second World War. B_{12} is also the only vitamin that contains essential mineral elements. Cobalamin is necessary for the production of red blood cells, and metabolizes fatty acids, carbohydrates, and proteins. Deficiency may lead to pernicious anemia, menstrual difficulty, mental problems, and general listlessness.

The *only* food sources for B_{12} are products of animal origin. Cobalamin is not found naturally in vegetables or plants. Strict vegetarians will have to supplement this most important member of the B-complex group. Again, animal organ meats, such as beef liver and kidney, are the best natural sources of vitamin B_{12}. Dairy products are also high in cobalamin, as are eggs and poultry. You can compare food values in chapters 15 and 16.

Popularly known as the "wonder vitamin" because of its many purposes, cobalamin is truly the wonder vitamin for MS patients because B_{12} maintains and protects the "myelin sheath" that surrounds the cells of the central nervous system. Damage and lesions to this sheath are the hallmarks of multiple sclerosis and the cause of all of the mobility and coordination problems that subsequently arise. Therefore, it is imperative that you receive at a minimum the RDA of this vitamin. It is also essential that you receive amounts of B_6 and calcium sufficient to process the cobalamin, because your body cannot utilize this cornerstone of MS repair without them. Later in this chapter, we will discuss the myelin that surrounds our nerve cells and what role it plays in the progress or elimination of MS.

I take a supplement called Calcium 2-AEP each day. It comes in a pill form known as calcium orotates. I mention it here because the "orotate" portion of the substance name comes from the inclusion of orotic acid, or Vitamin B_{13}. This supplement aids in the absorption and utilization of B_{12}. Because the orotates are taken in conjunction with B_{12} and other B-family supplements, they draw upon my excess stores of calcium to meet the demands of the additional B_{12} ingested or injected, thereby depleting the excess and returning my system levels and ratios to the normal range. I discuss the orotate protocol in greater detail later in this chapter, including a look at the work of the eminent internist responsible for advances in the treatment of MS with this substance, Dr. Hans A. Nieper.

One of the protocols I have followed throughout the latter part of finding a cure is a regimen of B-complex compounds, calculated doses injected intravenously on a weekly basis. This protocol, along with the Calcium 2-AEP orotates, was prescribed for me by Dr. William Crawford. I continue to use these two important protocols today.

Vitamin BC, known as folic acid or folacin, is also a member of the B family. Folic acid is water-soluble and can be stored by the body. An extremely fragile vitamin, it is easily destroyed by light, heat, and air. Responsible for the metabolism of sugars and amino acids, folacin is essential in the manufacture of all cells and is required for cell reproduction and division. It is routinely prescribed for pregnant women as it maintains nervous system health and mental stability.

Even though it is a storable vitamin, it is estimated that over 90 percent of Americans have a folic acid deficiency. Severe cases can manifest as anemia, listlessness, memory loss, and insomnia. It is important to note here that massive doses of folic acid taken to correct a deficiency can mask the symptoms of pernicious anemia, a severe condition that can result from a B_{12} deficiency. It is important to have a blood test performed before taking large doses of any vitamin to replace a lack in your system. Your doctor or health care professional can help you with this procedure.

The MS patient must prevent a deficiency of Vitamin BC (folic acid) because it is so important to the maintenance and repair of the nervous system. Nerve transmitter damage is a consequence of progressing MS. An adequate supply of this vital element will help to strengthen your nervous system and possibly reverse the effects of the existing damage.

Folic acid or folacin takes its name from "foliage" as it is most often found in dark green leafy vegetables such as broccoli and spinach. Asparagus is an excellent source, as are carrots, egg yolks, most melons, avocados, brewer's yeast, and animal livers. Dried beans and peas also score highly. You can find other foods rich in folic acid in chapter 16.

The MS patient must prevent a deficiency of Vitamin BC because it is so important to the maintenance and repair of the nervous system. Nerve transmitter damage is a consequence of progressing MS. An adequate supply of this vital element will help to strengthen your nervous system and possibly reverse the effects of the existing damage.

Vitamin C is probably the best known of all of the vitamins. Scientifically referred to as ascorbic acid, vitamin C has been proven to promote the healing process and is prescribed for a number of ailments, including the common cold, and some forms of cancer. Dr. Linus Pauling did much important work on the subject. Ascorbic acid is a water-soluble vitamin that is not stored in the body and therefore not toxic.

Interestingly enough, most animals can internally produce their own supply of vitamin C, but humans and members of the ape family must rely on outside sources. Vitamin C aids in the production of collagen and red blood cells. Collagen has been found to slow the effects of aging on the human skin, so older readers should be certain to receive the minimum RDA for your age group and gender. Ascorbic acid also aids in the maintenance of healthy teeth, bones, and gums. Perhaps the most commonly known result of a severe vitamin C deficiency is a disease known as scurvy, but a lack of this element can also lead to a number of additional problems.

The good news for vegetarians is that the best sources of vitamin C are fresh fruits and vegetables. The best sources are citrus fruits like oranges and lemons, leafy green vegetables, tomatoes, melons, green peppers, Brussels sprouts, cabbages, and potatoes. Before you rush out for the Biggie French Fry, remember this: Vitamin C is extremely oxygen sensitive and can be destroyed by light, heat, air, and certain forms of cooking. I highly recommend that you purchase a food and nutrition guide that will help you choose the best sources to include in your daily diet. You can learn more about food and nutrition guides in chapters 15 and 16.

Because vitamin C is so essential to healthy living, the MS patient should be certain to receive a sufficient amount in the daily diet. Usually, an aware and conversant doctor will prescribe daily doses that are far above the minimum RDA to maximize the healing properties it contains and promotes. Dr. Weeks has prescribed a daily supplemental dosage between 6,000 and 8,000 milligrams, in addition to the vitamin C I receive from the foods that I eat. Your doctor may decide that you do not need that much, or possibly that you may need more. As with all other nutrient supplements, many other factors determine your needs, like height, weight, age and gender, and your medical history. Your doctor will help you determine your optimum intake.

Chromium is a mineral I have utilized in my progress toward a cure. There is currently no RDA established for chromium, and studies as to its complete function and effectiveness are ongoing. Chromium is a metal and can be stored by the body. Although there are several different forms of chromium, only chromium-III is utilized by the body. Certain kinds of this metal can be cancer causing, particularly chromium-VI, found in metal plating and used in welding shops. A BioCybernetics analysis will reveal the level of chromium in your system and help you to plot an increase or decrease in dosage. Chromium aids in the utilization of glucose and may help to bind insulin to insulin receptors, thereby being of great benefit to persons suffering from Type 2 diabetes. You can learn more about Type 2 diabetes in chapter 13.

The best available natural sources of chromium-III are beef liver, American cheese, brewer's yeast, and wheat germ. Other good sources include other animal meats and fats, fish, fresh fruit, whole grains, carrots, potatoes, spinach, alfalfa, brown sugar, and molasses (Sawyer et al. 1994). Because the Food and Drug Administration does not yet regulate the quality of chromium supplements, you should choose carefully when considering a supplier.

Exercise caution when hearing claims of benefits, and read the labels of supplements before you buy, taking specific note of what else the supplement may contain. Although there is ongoing research on the benefit of chromium, or chromium-picolinate compound, in the treatment of obesity, there is, as yet, no scientifically proven result. The same is presently true of claims that chromium or chromium-picolinate aids in body building without the combinations of proper diet and exercise.

I currently take 200 mcg. (micromilligrams) of chromium daily, because my BioCybernetics analysis showed that my levels of this element were below the normal range. These levels have increased in subsequent testing, indicating that my body is storing a portion of the intake. Because chromium as a dietary aid is a relatively new study, I would not advise that you begin daily supplementation unless recommended by your physician or specialist. The long-term toxic effects of excess chromium have not yet been adequately determined.

Vitamin E, or tocopherol, is considered to be one of the most important antioxidant vitamins. It is fat-soluble and therefore stored in the body, but only for a short period of time. It can also be toxic when taken in high doses. Tocopherol is composed of eight parts, each named for the corresponding first eight letters of the Greek alphabet: alpha, beta, kappa, delta, epsilon, gamma, hydra, and lambda. Alpha-tocopherol is considered the most potent form.

Vitamin E has several important functions. It aids in the production of red blood cells, supplies oxygen through the circulation of blood, helps to maintain healthy muscle and tissue, protects vitamin A and essential fatty acids from oxidation, and regenerates skin cells. It is also thought to strengthen the immune system and promote the body's healing process. Because this vitamin is so plentiful in foods, vitamin E deficiency is relatively rare. However, those who consume excessive alcohol should be aware that a vitamin E deficiency can contribute to cirrhosis of the liver, a condition promoted and exacerbated by the frequent excess consumption of alcoholic beverages. Vitamin E is found in so many common foods that you are certain of ingesting at least some of the RDA each time that you eat. The highest concentrations, however, are found in oils, soybeans, wheat germ, seeds, whole grains, and eggs. Leafy green vegetables also have good amounts per serving. You can find comparisons of the vitamin E content of foods in chapter 16.

The benefits to the MS patient of doses of vitamin E are far-reaching, the most important being its ability to boost the immune system and maintain healthy muscles and tissues. When nervous system damage occurs, muscles have a tendency to grow weak and even atrophy from disuse. Vitamin E will help keep your muscles and connecting tissues strong and healthy while you fight the disease.

The next group of nutrients is also part of my daily supplement intake. I will touch on them only briefly here. With the exception of lecithin, a BioCybernetics analysis will show you what the levels of each of these are in your system. There are several web sites on the Internet where you can learn about these supplements, or you can request a product description catalog from a reliable natural vitamin and nutrient supplier. I will give you several good sources in the resources section.

The benefits to the MS patient of doses of vitamin E are far-reaching, the most important being its ability to boost the immune system and maintain healthy muscles and tissues. Vitamin E will help keep your muscles and connecting tissues strong and healthy while you fight the disease.

Choline is a phosphytidal supplemental vitamin that maintains the integrity of cell membranes, particularly liver cell membranes. Additionally, choline regulates the distribution of fats and other nutrients, and can aid in the detoxification of the system. Choline supplements can be obtained in natural or synthetic form. I recommend that you use the natural versions, as the synthetic forms can be difficult for some persons to digest and may produce adverse reactions.

Lecithin is a food emulsifier consisting of components called phospholipids. Lecithin supplements are produced from soybeans. Originally developed after the Second World War specifically to aid in food processing, lecithin today is used for a variety of nutritional purposes. Most importantly, lecithin is used as a base material for the production and purification of phospholipids, the building blocks of cell membranes.

Virusine is the product name of a special amino acid compound formula clinically proven to be effective against the common cold and certain viral infections. MS patients are more susceptible to viruses, as are other autoimmune disease sufferers. Virusine is commercially available in supplement form from any number of larger vitamin and nutrient distributors. Again, I will give you several sources in the resources section.

Selenium is an essential trace mineral that cannot be manufactured by the body. It can be stored and become toxic in prolonged excessive doses. It is considered to be a powerful antioxidant, between fifty to one hundred times more potent than an equal dosage of Vitamin E. Selenium also aids in good vision, liver function, and cardiovascular health. Selenium is found in the greatest concentrations in servings of tuna fish, broccoli, tomatoes, onions, whole wheat grain, bran, and wheat germ. I take 150 mcg. of selenium per day, but your individual needs will probably vary.

Zinc is another mineral found in the human system. It plays an important part in over eighty enzyme functions and is also vital in maintaining proper ratio balances between many other important minerals, as we have learned in chapter 11. Zinc deficiency can manifest in a number of symptoms, including slow healing, blurred or impaired vision and other senses, sexual dysfunction, and growth retardation in children.

One of the most crucial functions of zinc as regards the MS sufferer is its support of the immune system and the integrity of cell membranes. You can find zinc in the highest amounts in animal meats, oysters, other shellfish, eggs, brewer's yeast, and whole grains. For a detailed explanation regarding the importance of zinc in several body mineral ratios, see chapter 11. A comparison of foods and their zinc content can be found in chapter 16.

The use of these supplements with the Calcium 2-AEP orotates and a product called Progesterone Cream in the treatment of multiple sclerosis is growing in credibility and practice in orthodox medicine today, due largely to the work of the late Dr. Hans A. Nieper. This final section will examine the career of Dr. Nieper and his pioneering work in the treatment of multiple sclerosis through natural, or biologic, medicine.

Naturally Inclined—Dr. Hans A. Nieper and Multiple Sclerosis

The late Dr. Hans A. Nieper believed that "toxic treatments do more harm than good in the long run. The best physician is your own body. We must strengthen, not weaken, its defenses." Those afflicted with a number of debilitating and life-threatening diseases today, particularly MS, owe a debt of gratitude to the brilliant researcher and internist Hans A. Nieper, M.D., Ph.D. Born in Hannover, Germany, in 1928, the son of a neurologist, Dr. Nieper originally began his career as an internist, specializing in cancer therapy and the treatment of heart disease through "biologic" or natural substance medicine. Through his own scientific research and clinical practice, Dr. Nieper's focus began to turn to the treatment of multiple sclerosis.

Dr. Nieper theorized that the best weapon available against invading diseases of the body was a natural defense. He was firmly of the opinion that to treat cancer, heart disease, and, later, multiple sclerosis with a number of man-made medicines was simply a stopgap against the progression of these ailments and did not help the body to repair the damage done by the affliction. He began to study the natural transporting capabilities of mineral carriers in the form of aspertates and orotates, and to investigate the causes and effects of MS through clinical treatment of his own patients.

Dr. Nieper began to treat MS sufferers in the mid 1960's, a specialty he continued for over twenty years. At the time of the writing of his landmark study, *The Treatment of Multiple Sclerosis* (1990), Dr. Nieper had treated over 1,300 patients in various stages of MS. He was one of the few physicians, if not the only one, specializing in MS at the time, and his patients came to him from all over the world. In fact, by his own estimation, almost 80 percent of his patients came from North America. He attributed this fact to joyful recommendation from successfully treated sufferers who had benefited from his methods.

In fact, this in-depth study was the major force behind my decision to pursue Dr. Nieper's protocol and one of the first documents that I explored shortly after my initial diagnosis. Originally published in the *Townsend Letter for Doctors* in November 1990, it is now, along with Dr. Nieper's complete library of publications and studies, part of the A. Keith Brewer Science Library in Wisconsin. If you have not read this important study, I strongly suggest that you do so, to familiarize yourself with the nature of MS and why it can be successfully treated with Dr. Nieper's methods. A complete copy of this article is available on the Internet, courtesy of *Explore! Publications*. (Their web site address is included in the Bibliography.)

To understand the revolutionary approach that Dr. Nieper pursued in the treatment of multiple sclerosis, you will first need to understand the nature of the damage MS inflicts upon the body. I will briefly review the effects of the disease so the MS patient can understand the significance that Calcium 2-AEP and progesterone cream play in successful treatment.

Even if we possess no formal medical knowledge, most of us know that all of our voluntary bodily functions are controlled by the brain, which sends signals, or neurological impulses, to our body parts through the central nervous system. The nerve fiber that carries these impulses to our muscles and other systems is called the central axon. The central axon is insulated by a multilayered sheath of 5–30 layers. This sheath greatly resembles a large tobacco leaf, wrapped around the central axon somewhat like a tobacco leaf is wrapped around a fine cigar. The layers of the sheath are known as myelin, or collectively, as the myelin sheath. Myelin is produced by a unique type of cell called an oligodendrocyte. The entire group of cells is known as the oligodendria.

The cells that make up the myelin layer are structurally identical to other body cells. This means that they have the same basic characteristics and properties, including the ability to pass substances, gases, and electrical impulses through their membranes. The human nervous system functions according to the laws of physics and the principles of electricity. Nerve fibers contain an electric charge of specific polarity. The cells in the myelin sheath have an opposite electrical polarity. Together, they act in the same manner as an electrical condenser does, converting gravitational field energy to the electrical energy essential for the function of the central axon. Those of you who have a background in electronics, electrical engineering, or similar fields will understand this principle easily. In layman's terms, these opposite polarities achieve a balanced flow, which allows the system to operate efficiently and correctly without "shorting out."

In order for the myelin, and the central axon, to retain their proper polarity, the electrical charge has to bind to the cell membrane. As in all of our cell functions, specific substances are necessary for this process to occur. Substances that bind electrical charges to the cell membranes are known as neurotransmitters. Aspartic acid salts, or aspartates, are a textbook example of a neurotransmitter and are found on the inside of the outer cell membrane. Another critical neurotransmitter is an amino acid compound known as AEP, which we will examine next.

This main essential compound is made up of colamin phosphate, scientifically termed 2-amino-ethanol-phosphate, or mercifully, 2-AEP for short. Without enough AEP in each cell, binding of the electrical charge cannot occur, or occurs inefficiently. The cells in MS patients have become defective and do not produce the AEP necessary to promote electrical binding. Not only the myelin sheath cells, but the porosity of all the cells of the MS-afflicted is affected in this way.

Because the membrane system does not function properly, the cells of MS patients, and other autoimmune disease sufferers, cannot properly defend against viral invaders, thereby making them extremely susceptible to initial infection and subsequent spread of disease. The AEP deficiency results in the malfunction of the body's antibody system, triggering eventual complete destruction of the myelin sheath through a progression known as demyelinization.

The beginning of this destruction is felt as the tingling and numbness experienced in the extremities of most early MS patients. As the demyelinization progresses, the impulses from the brain reach the parts of our body along increasingly faulty connections, or bad wiring. Finally, just as with a frayed electrical cord or damaged cable, the signal can no longer reach the intended target, essentially "shorting out" and rendering the body paralyzed in that area. At the extreme end of demyelinization, involuntary impulses like breathing and heartbeat are affected, producing an often fatal result.

Dr. Nieper points out that at this time, scientists do not know why the loss of AEP in the cell membrane results in reduced or halted electrical binding, only that it definitely occurs as a result. They are also just beginning to determine what causes the AEP production to drop. Research has shown that genetic and hereditary factors may play a part in determining who is at the greatest risk. This may be true in my case, as my father was diagnosed with MS while in the United States Navy.

High levels of aluminum in the system may also play a major part in the inhibition of AEP production, although definitive research as to how aluminum does this is not yet available. Again, this is another powerful reason to undergo a BioCybernetics analysis, as soon as possible. Not all human bodies collect aluminum, so you cannot automatically assume that because you have MS, your aluminum levels are too high or your aluminum ratios are out of balance. Until you do have an analysis, you may want to take note of two of the ways that the average person is exposed to aluminum on a regular basis: deodorants and beverages.

Some deodorants contain a compound known as aluminum hydroxide. Read your deodorant label carefully to see if it contains this substance. Not all of them do, especially those made from natural substances. Even though we all know that good personal hygiene is important, you may want to switch to a personal care product that does not contain aluminum hydroxide.

One of the single most convenient and popular beverages available to Western society today is soda. Most brands of soda are available in aluminum cans. Although there are standards for the manufacture of cans in place, certain carbonated beverages, particularly colas, contain certain corrosive properties. Spilled on the paint of your car, for instance, they will ruin the finish. Fruit juices are also sold commercially in cans, particularly the "nectar" juices like apricot, mango, and peach. These are not always produced in the United States and may not have the same standards for food and can safety. In fact, there have been times when I have purchased a cold can of nectar-type juice from a deli or quick mart, and I can taste the aluminum from the can. Aluminum has a distinctively metallic taste. If this happens to you, throw the juice out! If you can taste the aluminum, it's a pretty good bet there is more than the usual trace amount contaminating the juice.

Both of these beverage types are available in glass and plastic bottles. Everybody should drink some juice on a regular basis, unless you have a prohibiting or monitored medical condition such as diabetes. If you must drink soda, and I think you should avoid it in excess, try switching to glass or plastic containers. Plastic is best, as it has a plastic cap as well, but the small aluminum top of a glass bottle is still a better choice than an entire aluminum can. Switching the container type for your beverages is certainly a simple and painless way to remove a source of possible toxic substances from your environment.

Dr. Nieper understood that the body possesses specific built-in repair mechanisms that correct and eliminate damages done, if those systems are properly in place and functioning efficiently. Along with the maintenance of the electrical bond to the cellular membrane, AEP is important to the repair of the central nervous system. A vital catalyst necessary for the production of AEP in the cells is calcium. That is the primary reason that AEP is combined with calcium in the Calcium 2-AEP supplement.

However, the proper absorption and utilization of calcium cannot occur unless other vitamin and mineral nutrients are also supplied in adequate proportions, specifically magnesium, phosphorus, and vitamins D and the B family. Without proper levels of these substances, calcium absorption and utilization are diminished, thereby reducing the amount of AEP produced by the cells, leading to the conditions described above.

Because of this scientifically proven correlation and Dr. Nieper's successful protocol combinations, Dr. Crawford additionally prescribes a compound called Magnesium-Potassium AEP orotates, or phosetamin, which I take daily in conjunction with the Calcium 2-AEP. Dr. Nieper also routinely prescribed these two supplements in combination as a result of the synthesis, at his request, of colaminphosphate salts by the world-renowned and internationally recognized chemist, the late Dr. Franz Koehler.

Dr. Koehler found that the combination of these two compounds produces a sealing substance in the outer cell membranes, preventing the penetration of the cells by harmful substances and viral infections. The addition of the orotates to these salts, which I explained earlier, allows the sealing substance to be produced along the inner cell membrane, which is the function of the orotate part of the compound, or vitamin B_{13}.

Although now as I am almost completely rid of MS, I take these supplements orally, these compounds are ideally received in intravenous form in the beginning stages of treatment. Both Dr. Nieper's and Dr. Crawford's research and experience with MS patients has shown that intravenous injection, either as a series of injections into an implanted catheter or as a controlled drip through an IV, is the only way to build a sufficient concentration of the colamin phosphate on the cell membrane, thereby allowing the insulation and repair systems to begin to function properly. Dr. Nieper recommends that this protocol continue for a period of not less than four years, with periods as long as seven years proving ideal in more virulent cases.

Dr. Nieper's research also explored other elements necessary for the production of AEP and maintenance of the myelin sheath, including certain types of steroids, specifically the group known as adrenal cortex steroids. Although it is currently popular, controversial, and in some states illegal to include steroids in body building or athletic performance regimens, steroids are also naturally produced by the human body. These naturally produced steroids are essential to the function of the repair mechanisms for the myelin sheath. Not only must they be present for repairs to occur, they must also contain a sufficient degree of electrical excitement. This is achieved through the energy conversion processes occurring in the cell membrane. In MS patients, the membrane is faulty, thereby reducing the electrical stimulus available to the adrenal cortex steroids.

It is not my purpose in this book to either explore or argue the steroid supplement question, except to say that, according to Dr. Nieper and other scientific researchers, the commonly prescribed steroid ACTH, or adrenocorticotropic hormone, is far from beneficial to MS patients. ACTH does produce a temporary improvement in the symptoms of MS sufferers, but it ultimately taxes the already overstressed adrenal cortex system. A good analogy would be driving your car when low on motor oil. You can get away with it for a period of time, although you will definitely cause wear and internal harm to your engine. If you continue to drive without the correct amount of motor oil, sooner or later you will stress your engine to the point of no return and it will break down permanently. ACTH, when used by the MS patient over a prolonged period, causes a steady deterioration of the adrenal cortex leading to the eventual collapse of the entire system and irreparable permanent disability. Dr. Nieper discontinued the use of ACTH in the late 1970's and refused to use it for any of his patients after that period because of the long-term damage it has been proven to cause.

If your doctor is currently prescribing ACTH for your condition, contact him or her immediately. Put the book down, go to the telephone, and tell your doctor that you do not wish to take ACTH one more day! Prednisone and Triamcinolon, also marketed as Volon, are Dr. Nieper's recommended alternatives, the latter especially in cases of the inflammation of the optical nerves that sometimes accompanies MS. If your medical situation requires that you do continue with ACTH temporarily, it is vital that you also include the required foods in your diet that supply the adrenal cortex system, foods high in vitamin D_2 and vitamin A, beta-carotene. It is also essential that you take additional high supplemental doses of vitamin C and probably between 50 mg. and 200 mg. of selenium daily. Note that my daily supplement package at the close of this chapter includes all of these components. Even though I do not take ACTH, these compounds are essential to adrenal cortex health and optimum function and should be included in the daily supplement regimen of all MS patients.

The work of Dr. Nieper extended far beyond the treatment of multiple sclerosis, and I have only briefly touched upon his protocols as regards this disease. I recommend that you familiarize yourself with the complete versions of his studies on MS as part of your own research. Additionally, I highly recommend the Crawford Center in Mobile, Alabama, as an excellent treatment facility, which practices the Nieper protocols in MS treatment. Without Dr. Crawford and his continuing care, I am certain that I would not be in the superb condition I am today. You can find contact information for the Crawford Center in the resources section.

Dr. Hans Nieper left us in 1998, after only seventy years on Earth; however, MS, cancer, and heart patients all over the world enjoy quality lives today because of this learned man. The work that he started will continue with his trusted colleagues, but he will be missed. I regret that I never had the opportunity to meet with him personally. His discoveries have allowed me to finally rid my body of MS. I would've liked to thank him.

The last special substance that I use and that we will discuss here is progesterone cream. This is a topical ointment containing the female sex hormone progesterone, produced naturally in the human body by a group of cells known as the Schwann cells, located in the peripheral nerves, which synthesize it from the naturally occurring compound pregnenolone. Schwann cells also produce myelin in the peripheral nerves, as do the oligodendria in the central nervous system. Progesterone is a neurosteroid, similar to the steroids, which interact with the AEP in the oligodendria to produce myelination. Studies have shown that progesterone may not always function strictly as a sex hormone and may indeed have completely separate functions in other areas of the body, including the myelinization of cells.

Progesterone cream and its parent substance, pregnenolone, when topically applied to the areas of damaged nerves where demyelinization has occurred, has been clinically proven to increase the concentration of these substances in the blood to between five to ten times the amounts present in the untreated areas. This results in increased production by the Schwann cells and the formation of new nerve fibers, strengthening the process of myelinization, the production of healthy levels of myelin in the peripheral nerve sheathing cells. To date, there have been no conclusive studies proving that pregnenolone or progesterone cream has any positive effect on myelin production in the central nervous system, as the elements contributing to the functions of the central and peripheral nervous systems are, although related, entirely different in aspect.

One disturbing fact that may hold special significance for European and U.S. readers is that certain chemical substances inhibit the conversion of pregnenolone into progesterone and severely decrease the thickness of newly formed myelin sheath cells. One such substance is RU-486, the "home abortion" drug. RU-486 terminates a pregnancy by blocking the action of progesterone. RU-486 is widely used in Europe, especially in France. If you have been diagnosed with MS, I strongly urge you to seriously consider the alternatives to RU-486. It is not my intention to address the legal or moral issues of abortion, which have no bearing on the subject of multiple sclerosis. I do advise against using any substance that decreases the levels or inhibits production of myelin in your system.

I apply progesterone cream to my forearms and legs, and have seen a definite improvement in my mobility and muscle tone. Although I believe that all patients would benefit from the use of this topical protocol, I may see an increased benefit because I am a woman, and progesterone is a female hormonal substance. Consult with your doctor, or investigate the subject further on your own. A topical progesterone cream that can be applied to the face and neck is now under development. This cream may prove to be beneficial in the restoration of proper function of the eye and face muscles, which is important to MS patients as facial muscle slackness can often be a symptom of the progression of this disease. If your doctor is unfamiliar with topical progesterone cream, I invite you to contact me. You will find my information in the resources section.

Review the last section of this chapter carefully. Because of my busy schedule, I don't always meet my personal RDA and DRI of vitamins and minerals through the foods that I eat. Therefore, a personal supplementation plan has been developed especially for me through my work with Drs. Crawford and Weeks. The chart will give you an idea of the substances that you might find beneficial in your own healing regimen.

Supplemental Benefits—My Personal Daily Regimen

The final section of this chapter is for reference only. The chart that follows details the composition of the supplemental nutrient pack I take twice daily. The dosages listed here are specific to my condition, determined through periodic BCI, blood, and other laboratory tests, and close consultation with Drs. Crawford and Weeks. My progress is closely monitored, and I consult with each doctor on a regular basis. Adjustments have been made to the substances and dosages in the past, and will be made again as my system returns to normal levels and the last of the MS fades.

Again, I stress that you do not rush to begin taking the same supplements in the same dosages because I do, even if I am virtually cured of my affliction. Your system and body needs are *different*. You may require all, some, or none of these substances, or need others that are not listed here at all. The dosages right for you will depend on factors such as gender, age, ethnicity, physical condition, and additional medications you are taking or protocols you are following. This is not a "fly by the seat of your pants" operation. This is your *health*. Some of these substances are toxic when taken in too great a dosage, and all of them can interfere with the function of the others if taken in incorrect proportions or combinations. Ask your doctor. And, if your doctor thinks that vitamins and nutrition are not all that important, then get a new doctor! Your life may depend on it.

Chart 12-2 on page 257 illustrates the Nutritional Supplement Package I currently take twice daily.

As my journey to wellness progressed, you will recall that I instituted a number of major dietary changes. Drs. Matthew Van Benshoten and Joseph McSweyne had experienced success when treating autoimmune patients with a zero dairy and zero sugar diet. I strictly followed this protocol for over a year, and I found the difference in my health extremely noticeable. A number of blood and allergy tests that I have had performed on my MS patients showed one interesting correlation: nearly all tested immunoglobulin-G radioallergosorbant test (IgG RAST) positive for cow's milk allergy.

In the next chapter, we will examine the role of dairy in nutrition. Is it a necessary part of our dietary intake, a vital

Chart 12-2 Twice Daily Nutritional Supplement Package Prescribed for Dr. Celeste Pepe

All Measurements in Units of Measurements as Noted

Nutrient	Dosage	%DV	Nutrient	Dosage	%DV
Vitamin A	7500 IU	150	Alpha-Lipoic Acid	5 mg	*
Vitamin B6	10 mg	500	Borage Seed	75 mg	*
Vitamin B12	15 mcg	250	Boron	1.5 mg	*
Vitamin C	250 mcg	417	Broccoli +	25 mg	*
Vitamin D3	200 IU	50	Cabbage +	25 mg	*
Vitamin E	150 IU	500	Citrus Bioflavonoids	12.5 mg	*
Vitamin K1	20 mcg	25	Curcumin	25 mg	*
Biotin	150 mcg	50	Evening Primrose Oil	75 mg	*
Calcium	500 mg	50	Inositol	1.25 mg	*
Chromium	100 mcg	83	Isoflavones	12.5 mg	*
Copper	1 mg	50	Leucoanthocyanin	5 mg	*
Folic Acid	300mcg	75	Lutein	1 mg	*
Iodine	37.5 mcg	25	Lycopene	.5 mg	*
Iron	5 mg	28	Quercetin	25 mg	*
Magnesium	250 mg	63	Vanadium	10 mcg	*
Manganese	1.8 mg	90	Silicon	5 mg	*
Niacin	20 mg	100			
Pantothenic Acid	15 mg	150	**KEY**		
Riboflavin	1.7 mcg	100	I U = International Units		
Selenium	50 mcg	71	Mg = Milligrams		
Thiamine	1.5 mcg	100	Mcg = Micromilligrams		
Zinc	7.5 mg	50	* = No RDA or DRI established		

source of essential nutrients? Or, are dairy products detrimental to our health, the hidden cause of a number of ailments, as some physicians and nutritionists claim that they are? Let's examine both sides in "Dangerous Dairy," the next chapter.

13

Dangerous Dairy

How do you convince people that something that they have been taught all of their lives was a good thing could actually be harming them? How do you get them to believe that everything that they may have been told from the time they were very young, by people that they trusted the most, may be completely wrong?

Those were the questions I asked myself while constructing this chapter. Although you have learned from my personal story that I made several significant dietary changes during the course of my search for a cure for MS, those were *my* choices. Reading about what one person has done does not necessarily mean that you, the reader, will put any stock in the notions yourself. Therein lay the problem. I wished to present the information in this chapter in such a way as to allow the reader to follow the logic behind the decisions, without discounting what may seem to be an extreme choice. Finally, I decided on a devil's advocate approach. It is my intention to present as many sides to this controversial argument as can be substantiated by scientific results. I will not be discussing conspiracy theories or the effect of political pressure on public advertising campaigns or government studies. That is not at all my intention here.

Explore the information in this chapter carefully. I warn you: most of the concepts contained here will no doubt fly in the face of everything that you have been led to believe regarding one of the staples of the average American and European diet: dairy products. Are dairy products harmful to your health? Or, are they one of the great benefits of this bountiful planet and a necessary component to our diet and nutrition? Let's explore the topic together, and then you can decide for yourself the truth behind "dangerous dairy."

Elsie: Maligned or Malignant?

No matter where you have spent most of your life, most of us have grown up with the familiar, gentle face of Elsie the Cow, beaming benevolently at us from the Borden's can or carton. Her kind, smiling countenance radiated trust, assuring us that the contents of the container were nutritious and tasty. How could they possibly hurt you?

How many of us have come through the door after school to a plate of Mom's cookies and a big glass of fresh milk? Didn't our parents, teachers, and coaches take us out for ice cream as a special treat? And what about Heidi? No way could the kindly old grandfather ever be making poison cheese up on that mountain! How on earth could something as supposedly nutritious as dairy products be harmful? Who would ever believe that? The truth is that dairy products can indeed be harmful, in certain cases. Let's take a look at some of the evidence on both sides of the issue, and see where dairy products fit, if at all, into our diets.

"Kids, Drink Your Milk!" Good or Bad Advice?

This familiar command seems an ideal place to start exploring the role of dairy products in the human diet. Arguments rage on both sides as to whether or not dairy calcium is essential, or harmful, for the human infant.

The late Dr. Frank Aram Oski, former Director of Pediatrics at Johns Hopkins University School of Medicine, contended that cow's milk could be severely damaging to infants. His well-known book, *Don't Drink Your Milk*, the latest edition of which was published in 1992, contains much documented evidence regarding the health damage that can be caused by dairy products. Dr. Oski and other like-minded professionals advocate feeding with mother's breast milk for an extended period of time, stating that breast milk contains all of the nutrients necessary for a solid foundation for human growth. Dr. Oski further believed that the mental capacity of an infant could be reduced by feeding cow's milk and that this reduction in intelligence would be lifelong if cow's milk was a major staple of a baby's diet. His recommendation was that cow's milk, and all dairy products, should be completely eliminated from the diet of infants or young children, and that new mothers who are breast-feeding children should eschew all consumption of dairy products in order to avoid the passing of dairy elements along to the infant through the mother's milk.

Although Dr. Oski was known as a leader in his field and a well-respected member of the pediatric medical community, recent studies suggest that his mandate to eliminate dairy is incorrect and may be damaging to children who are denied dairy products. Several important studies have recently been completed that support the contention that the elements found in dairy products, most notably dairy calcium, phosphorus, and vitamin D_2, are essential for the health and development of infants and young children. Reduction or elimination of dairy can seriously increase the risk of debilitating childhood ailments.

The American Medical Association (AMA) is recognized as one of the leading authorities on current medical information and practice. The AMA published a June 15, 1999 report carried by *Reuters Health News* entitled "Low Calcium Raises Kids' Lead Poisoning Risk." Citing a study by Dr. John H. Bogden and associates at the New Jersey University of Medicine and Dentistry, and the New Jersey Medical School, the report, originally published in the June 1999 issue of the *Environmental Health Perspectives Journal*, states that "increased calcium intake can be a key factor in protecting young children from lead contamination."

The study, involving 314 inner-city children living in Newark, New Jersey was conducted in that area as the incidences of pediatric lead poisoning were among the highest in the United States. Researchers found that 31 percent of the 1- to 3-year-olds studied had a daily calcium intake well below the government recommended minimum of 500 mgs./day, and 59 percent of the 4- to 8-year-olds consumed less than the 800 mgs./day recommended for their group. Dietary calcium helps to prevent the gastrointestinal absorption of lead and other harmful minerals, including some that are listed in the heavy metals group (see chapter 11). The study also points out that "diets that are high in calcium-containing foods (i.e. dairy products) are also rich in other nutrients essential to bodily growth and function." Dr. Bogden and his colleagues believe that the public should be educated as to the importance of calcium-rich diets in the protection against pediatric lead poisoning. They consider the best natural sources of dietary calcium for young children to be found in dairy products.

The importance of dairy calcium in the diets of infants and young children is also supported by the results of a study addressed in the August 19, 1999 issue of the *New England Journal of Medicine*. In this issue, an editorial entitled "Rickets Today—Children Still Need Milk and Sunshine," by Dr. Nicholas Bishop of the University of Sheffield, England, correlates studies that support the original research done in 1919 and 1921 regarding the importance of vitamin D and dairy calcium in the development and maintenance of skeletal heath.

Vitamin D_3 is produced in the human skin by the action of sunlight, and vitamin D_2 is obtained through food consumption. Each has equal biologic potency. Processed by first the liver and then the kidneys, vitamin D_2 "acts through specific receptors to increase calcium absorption in the intestine and, with the parathyroid hormone, mobilizes calcium from bone to maintain serum calcium concentrations." (Bishop 1999). Calcium deficiency can lead to a number of complications, especially in children and young adults during the years of skeletal growth. A common complication, especially in certain geographic areas or cultural societies, is the manifestation of a condition known as rickets.

Although rickets is an ancient disease afflicting countless children throughout the centuries, even with the advances of modern science it still remains a major health problem, not only in the underdeveloped countries of the world, but also with the immigration of people from these locations to developed countries such as the UK and the United States. Rickets usually begins to manifest in children at eighteen months of age or more, although cases in premature infants is not uncommon.

Rickets produces poor or delayed motor development and attendant skills, short stature, and bowed legs or knock knees, where the limbs are turned toward each other as opposed to the parallel limbs of healthy children. Whether due to cultural differences or language barriers in the cases of immigrants, these children are largely kept indoors, fully clothed, and experience prolonged breast-feeding without vitamin D supplementation. An additional consequence of rickets and dietary calcium deficiency in young children is an increased risk of pneumonia, the primary cause of morbidity and mortality in children aged under five years old, worldwide.

Cases of both nutritional rickets and pneumonia are common in developing countries such as Ethiopia. A study was conducted over a five-year period at the Ethio-Swedish Children's Hospital in Addis Ababa, Ethiopia involving 1000 children. The study showed that the cases of children with pneumonia who also had rickets were thirteen times as high (210 cases out of 500 admissions) as the group of control children who received adequate dietary dairy calcium where pneumonia but no evidence of rickets was present (20 out of 500 admissions). Adjustments were made for contributing factors such as family size, birth order, and crowded living quarters. The children who developed both pneumonia and rickets were raised by prolonged months of exclusive breast-feeding with no vitamin or calcium supplementation. The study also exhibited that inadequate calcium in the mothers of these children produced bony pelvic deformities, which increased incidents of obstructed labor, stillborn births, and death during childbirth (Muhe et al. 1997, 349:1801–1804).

Therefore, it is evident that vitamin D deficiency and inadequate dietary calcium contribute to an increased risk of contracting both pneumonia and rickets in children under five years of age. Efforts to prevent these deficiencies by calcium supplementation may result in a significant reduction of the risk of morbidity and mortality in children from these causes. The standard treatment for rickets is vitamin D. Deficiency of this vitamin is not the only cause, however. Rickets can develop in premature babies who have outgrown their daily dietary intake of calcium and phosphate that is found in mother's milk alone. These babies should be given more calcium and phosphate, not vitamin D (Bishop 1999, 341:602–604).

Another independent study was conducted using Nigerian children as subjects (Thatcher et al. 1999, 341:563–568). Although these children got more than adequate amounts of sunlight, allowing for sufficient production of vitamin D_3, these children still developed rickets. This study concentrated on the treatment and cure of rickets after the disease was present. The research charted three groups of children, all with rickets. One group was given the standard treatment of vitamin D supplementation alone. The second group was treated with an addition of dietary calcium, and a third group was given both supplements. The results showed that the children in the second and third groups evidenced a greater increase of serum calcium (calcium levels in the blood) than did those in the first group. The researchers thereby concluded that rickets could be reversed and even cured by supplementing the calcium lacking in the diet of these children, which largely consists of maize porridge, which is low in calcium and high in fiber. Dietary calcium comes from dairy products, which are not readily available and are eaten only occasionally as a result. In order to prevent rickets, pneumonia or other like complications or diseases in infants and children, the study concludes that dairy calcium is essential.

Therefore, in these cases in particular, the contention of Dr. Oski and others that the extended breast-feeding of children is sufficient with no additional supplementation, can indeed be harmful to infants and young children, placing them at greater risk for these diseases. Additional studies have shown that some genetic factors in certain children may enable them to resist the effects of rickets and other calcium-deficient diseases while consuming a diet low in calcium (Ames et al. 1999, 14:740–746). However, it may be wise to include dairy calcium as an integral part of a baby's or young child's diet where these resistance factors are not present.

It appears that perhaps dairy products have unfairly been given a bad reputation, at least as regards the benefits to infants and young children. What about older children, young adults, and mature individuals? Let's take a look at the evidence in these cases as presented in recent scientific studies.

From Birth to Kindergarten: How Important Is Dairy?

Does the need for dairy products diminish as we grow older? Or, do we begin to develop allergic reactions to milk and other dairy products as we begin to grow and change? There is a contention in the medical community that cow's milk can contribute to the onset of Type 1 diabetes.

What is the connection, if any, between Type 1 diabetes and the consumption of dairy products? To understand how this may be possible, we need first to examine the nature of diabetes. Diabetes mellitus, the medical term for this illness, affects nearly 16 million Americans and is one of this nation's leading causes of premature death. The word "diabetes" comes from the Greek word for siphon, which describes the excessive thirst and frequent need to urinate experienced by the afflicted. "Mellitus," the Greek word for "honey," refers to the urine of the diabetic. It is filled with sugar and consequently sweet. Type 1 diabetics are insulin dependent, and therefore this form of the disease is abbreviated in the medical community as IDDM, for insulin dependent diabetes mellitus. Type 1 diabetes was initially found to strike young children, and so was originally termed "juvenile onset diabetes." That term is no longer in use, as further scientific research has found that this form of the illness will also strike young adults. Although adults can contract IDDM even into their thirties, the majority of cases are diagnosed in persons who are less than twenty years of age. Type 1 diabetes accounts for about five to ten percent of the total diabetic population.

People suffering from IDDM are insulin dependent. That means that they must take injections of insulin each day in order for their systems to properly utilize glucose, the body fuel that we produce and use from digesting carbohydrates. Without insulin, the diabetic cannot process glucose and move it into the body cells to be used as fuel. Therefore, the glucose continues to build up in the blood, creating a condition known as hyperglycemia. If the condition becomes extreme, the patient will experience insulin shock, and even death if emergency treatment is not rendered immediately.

In spite of the fact that anyone can contract this form of the disease, it seems to be most common among Caucasians. Research is currently being conducted to determine how much of a role genetics plays in the risk for this disease. Although several genetic factors may contribute to the risk of contraction, scientists have not as yet located a single gene, or group of genes that undeniably cause the disease.

IDDM, though not classified as an autoimmune condition, is similar in nature. This means that the body mistakes its own defense mechanism as harmful and destroys the cells that attack the virus, mistaking them for invading germs. The cells that process insulin from glucose in foods are created in the pancreas and are known as "beta cells," or islet cells, as they are actually formed in the part of the pancreas known as the Islets of Langerhans. The body of a diabetic sees these cells as invaders, and attacks them, rendering it impossible to produce insulin.

Interestingly, research is beginning to show that diabetes can manifest itself after the body has experienced a viral infection, much like MS can develop after a childhood virus. The viruses that affect a prediabetic most often are German measles, polio, and mumps. These viruses contain proteins that appear to be very similar to the proteins found in the insulin-producing beta calls. The body begins to attack the cells along with the viral germs, destroying insulin-producing ability and causing diabetes (Diabetes.com Health Library 1999).

Here is where the possible connection to cow's milk comes into play. Cow's milk contains a protein, bovine serum albumin, which is very similar to a molecule found in the beta cells in the human body. The child's body may therefore mistake its own beta cells for invading proteins and begin to destroy them, producing a diabetic condition.

Controversy has raged over this diagnosis for years. Studies that appear to support and disprove the theory are both in evidence. An ecological correlation study conducted in 1991 at the Aker Diabetes Research Center in Oslo, Norway, analyzed data from twelve developed countries, including the United States and Great Britain. Children who consumed cow's milk and later contracted IDDM showed a measurable correlation. These results supported the theory that cow's milk may contain a triggering element in the development of IDDM in children (Dahl-Jorgensen, Joner, and Hanssen 1991, 14:1801–13).

It is important to note here that the studies cited in this chapter refer to antibodies. The general picture of an immune system antibody is a white blood cell designed to fight infection. That image is correct, but it is not complete. The immune system produces several different kinds of antibodies. Not all of them are located in the bloodstream. Some are manufactured in the internal organs and programmed to attack specific foreign substances. When these studies refer to cow's milk antibodies, or diabetes antibodies, the reference denotes antibodies that are manufactured to react to the specific substances relevant to diabetes.

Two recent studies have also indicated that some elements found in cow's milk baby formula may have a similar triggering effect. The first, conducted in 1997 by the National Public Health Institute of Finland, produced interesting results (Vaarala et al. 1998, 47:131–135). Children were studied from birth to the first nine months of life and divided into three groups: children who received a cow's milk (CM) formula, those who were exclusively breast-fed, and those who received a hydrolyze casein (HC) formula (Hydrolysis is a processing method used in food, enzyme, and chemical production. In lay terms, additional water molecules are added to the original substance to be converted. Chemicals, substances, enzymes, and foods that utilize the addition of water molecules in this way are referred to as "hydrolyzed."). The mothers of the breast-fed children were not given dietary restrictions.

A test known as IgG, or immunoglobulin-G antibody test, was performed on the blood hemoglobin of each of the subjects at six and nine months of age. The test was performed to detect the presence of antibodies specifically targeted to bovine insulin, which was present in both the CM and HC formulas. These antibodies bind with the bovine insulin and feed upon it, destroying the insulin cell. The scientists postulated that if the children were developing antibodies to this bovine insulin, the antibodies might confuse human insulin with the bovine insulin and begin to destroy the human insulin-producing cells as well, thereby creating a low insulin, or diabetic, condition.

Children fed the cow's milk formula (CM) showed a greater incidence of antibody production than those who were fed the HC formula or those who were breast-fed. At nine months of age, the percentages for CM children dropped slightly, while the HC children increased slightly. The breast-fed children largely remained unchanged. The conclusion drawn was that there is a correlation between the exposure to bovine insulin and the development of antibodies to human insulin, which may later trigger IDDM, when infants are fed cow's milk formula. The study did not include children who were given whole or partially skimmed fluid cow's milk to drink.

The second study that supports the theory that cow's milk may trigger IDDM in those children already at genetic risk for the disease was completed in 1999, in Finland. Some of the same scientists from the first study also participated in this new research. Again, children were studied from birth, but this study followed them through age eighteen months. The subjects were divided into four groups: those given cow's milk formula in the first twelve weeks of life, children who were exclusively breast-fed for that same period or longer, children who had already tested positive for Type 1 or other diabetic antibodies, and healthy children who were given a varied diet. The diets of the mothers of the breast-fed children were not restricted.

This study showed that the children who were given a CM formula in the very beginning stages of life had a greater incidence of IgG-detected antibodies bonding to the bovine insulin found in the formula than those who were not fed the CM formula so early. Levels of IgG-detected bonding decreased in all groups at twelve and eighteen months, except for the children who had already developed diabetic antibodies prior to the testing period. These children showed increased bonding. The conclusion drawn was that CM formula is an environmental trigger to bovine insulin immunization in infancy, which may later be diverted into immunization to human insulin, thus increasing the risk for the development of IDDM in children who are already genetically predisposed toward the condition (Vaarala et al. 1999, 48:1389-1394).

In contrast, other studies indicate that there is little or no correlation between dairy products and the increased risk of IDDM. Scientists at the University of Rome studied children from nine regions of Italy ranging in age from birth to fourteen years. These children were breast-fed and additionally consumed fluid cow's milk and a variety of cheeses. The correlation between fluid milk consumption and the incidence of IDDM was lower than the 1991 Norwegian study, but still enough to indicate significance as regards fluid cow's milk acting as a trigger mechanism. Consumption of cheeses showed no correlation whatsoever as regards IDDM, and the study is careful to point out that in these regions, especially Sardinia, consumption of cow's milk cannot be judged the sole contributing factor to IDDM manifestation (Fava, Leslie, and Pozilli 1994, 17:1488–1490).

A further study in Bonn, Germany reevaluated earlier findings that cow's milk protein was definitely linked to IDDM. Over seven hundred infants were studied. They were divided into six groups, ranging from those who were exclusively breast-fed for at least four weeks to those who were given an extensively hydrolyzed cow's milk formula for that period and then were given fluid cow's milk. The study showed that the breast-fed children, those breast-fed plus fed extensively hydrolyzed CM formula, and those fed the extensively hydrolyzed CM formula then fluid milk showed a slow rise in antibody production, and the children fed exclusively fluid cow's milk showed two high peaks of antibody production (Keller et al. 1996, 155:331–337).

Those infants given fluid cow's milk after breast-feeding during the first three months of life showed a higher tendency to develop antibodies than the children in the same group who were introduced to fluid cow's milk at a later date. Other groups showed no significant change in antibody production. The conclusion drawn was that the age at which cow's milk is introduced increases or decreases the risk factor. The later the fluid cow's milk is introduced to the child, the lesser the risk of developing IDDM tendencies.

Finally, claims have been made by physicians that the unhealthy elements in cow's milk and dairy products can be adversely passed along to both the fetus and the breast-feeding newborn, sometimes causing irreparable harm. Research conducted in a cooperative effort between scientists from the Medizinische Fakultat der Humboldt-Universitat, the Department of Obstetrics at the University Hospital Rudolf Virchow, and the Department of Gynecology and Obstetrics at the Benjamin Franklin Hospital, Free University, all located in Berlin, Germany, studied the possible benefit or detriment to newborn infants in families at risk for food allergies if the mother avoided milk, dairy products, and eggs during pregnancy and nursing.

The expectant mothers were divided into three groups: those who were told to restrict their diet in the last trimester (three months) of pregnancy and through the first three months of breast-feeding, completely avoiding milk, dairy products, and eggs; those who began the dietary restrictions at the time of delivery and through the first three months of breast-feeding; and those who were given no restrictions during either pregnancy or the nursing period. There were no further restrictions placed on any of the groups.

The children were tested for specific sensitivity to milk and eggs at six and twelve months of age. The researchers found that there was no significant difference among the three groups studied. Therefore, the study concluded that the scientists were unable to demonstrate that there was any significant preventative effect to be had by the mother of an infant avoiding eggs and dairy, either in the final stages of pregnancy, when the fetus absorbs more elements directly from the mother's system than at any other time in development, or during the crucial first three months of life, when exclusive breast-feeding is the optimum nourishment supply for a newborn human (Herrmann et al. 1996, 155:770–777).

So, what is the best answer? Are dairy products, specifically fluid cow's milk, beneficial or harmful to infants and young children? I believe the correct viewpoint lies somewhere in the middle. Infants given any foreign substance at too early a stage in their life have a tendency to develop an immunity or allergic reaction, regardless of the nature of the substance. The infant immune system is just beginning to function and may not have developed the refinement necessary to distinguish between harmful and beneficial elements. An older child's system is better equipped to handle new and different foods.

Mothers of newborns should be encouraged to breast-feed exclusively in the first months of life, gradually introducing other foods into the infant's diet. By all indications, cow's milk formula may not be as beneficial as once thought, although millions of infants consume it each day around the world. Fluid cow's milk seems to be a better choice than processed cow's milk formulas as toddlers begin to explore the vast variety of foods available. In my experience as a nutritionist, this would be logical, as processing of any natural food almost always alters or reduces the benefits found in the natural form.

What about older children, young and mature adults, and the elderly? Do dairy products retain their usefulness in health, or do the benefits fall into a limited window of life, a time when dairy is healthy, and afterwards harmful? Let's examine the scientific studies, which address these questions next.

Building Strong Bones, Benefits for a Lifetime: Where Does Dairy Fit?

Osteoporosis is a disease characterized by loss of bone mass, reduced bone strength, and increasing risk of fractures.

Eighty percent of all diagnosed cases are women, particularly Caucasian and Asian women, who have been shown to statistically be at twice the risk for the disease. Osteoporosis is known as the "silent disease," as many who are afflicted do not know of the worsening condition of their skeletal health until they are into their sixties. Your bone mass density and skeletal structure are normally determined by the time you have reached thirty to thirty-five years of age. Therefore, calcium plays an essential role in skeletal growth and health early in life. Arguably one of the best sources of natural calcium and the combination nutrients vitamin D and phosphorus necessary to fully utilize it is found in cow's milk and dairy products.

How early in life is a calcium and vitamin D sufficient diet important to building the satisfactory bone mass and skeletal strength necessary to carry your body through the rest of your life? Although a significant portion of doctors were against the consumption of dairy products during the mid 1980's–1990's, the community was still widely divided on the issue. As further research was completed, scientists began to discover that dairy products were perhaps undeserving of their bad reputation.

A 1996 article in *Pediatric Nursing* quoted the National Institute of Health Consensus Development Conference, which focused on, among other medical matters, osteoporosis and the risk of fractures later in life (Gallo 1996, 22:369–374,422). The conclusion of the conference was that "recommendations for optimal calcium intake encourage the increased intake of calcium." Regardless of the source, the position was that adequate calcium was necessary to proper skeletal health.

Scientists in Geneva, Switzerland researched the effects of a calcium-enriched diet on girls ranging from seven to nine years old. The study was a double-blind, randomized, placebo-controlled trial. Half of the young subjects were given two food products containing 850 mg. of calcium per day for one year. The other half were given a placebo (a pill with no value) supplement, containing no calcium. After the testing period, bone mass, bone density, and skeletal strength were measured. The subjects who received the calcium-rich diet showed a greater increase in all three categories than did the placebo group, although not all parts of the skeleton showed noticeable differences. The conclusion drawn was that calcium-enriched foods significantly increased bone mass in girls who were prepubertal, girls who had not yet entered the menses cycle (Bonjour et al. 1997, 99:1287–1294).

In 1999, researchers at the Department of Foods and Nutrition and Health at Purdue University in Lafayette, Indiana completed a study that proved conclusively that the consumption of fluid cow's milk benefited the skeletal health and growth of bone mass necessary to build healthy bones that would last a lifetime (Teagarden et al. 1999, 69:1014–1017). Young girls and women ranging in age from early childhood to thirty-one years of age were studied for a food frequency level. Subjects were charted for milk consumption in three categories: those who consumed milk or milk products seldom or never; those who drank milk sometimes; and those who had milk with almost every meal during their early childhood to twelve years of age, and through adolescence, twelve to nineteen years of age. Results clearly showed that higher milk intake during adolescence is associated with greater total body, spine, and radial bone mineral measurement during the period of development of peak bone mass.

Science has proven with these recent studies that vitamin D and calcium are vital to healthy skeletal growth and strength. Long-term studies, especially, showed a distinct benefit gained in the area of skeletal health from regular cow's milk consumption through childhood, adolescent, and adult years. Therefore, we can conclude that adequate dietary calcium and vitamin D intake are crucial throughout the developmental stages of life, particularly for females. Some questions remain, however.

How important is dietary calcium intake later in life? What about the benefit or detriment found in other components of cow's milk, namely saturated fat? Do the elements of cow's milk and dairy products considered undesirable or possibly harmful create significant risks or adverse effects to outweigh obtaining the proven benefits of dietary calcium from this source? Let's examine those questions next.

Dairy for Life: Friend, or Foe?

Women, as a general rule, have a bone mass measuring ten to twenty-five percent less than a man of similar proportions, making them more susceptible to the ravages of osteoporosis. Once a woman has reached the stage of life known as post-menopausal, after her menses cycle has come to a close, she begins to lose bone mass, sometimes rapidly. As bone mass decreases, the risk of osteoporosis and fracture increases. Can this process be reversed or minimized through the use of calcium and vitamin D supplementation? Research is beginning to indicate that they may, indeed, be helpful.

The U.S. Department of Agriculture's Human Nutrition Research Center on Aging studied postmenopausal women for the effects of calcium and vitamin D supplementation on critical long bone mass and spinal bone mass loss (Dawson-Hughes 1996). Calcium supplementation only modestly reduced the long bone mass loss, but had little or no effect on slowing the loss of bone mass in the spine. It was further noted that supplementation of calcium and vitamin D in combination aided the effects of the calcium-only supplements. Additionally, in those women studied who had a dairy calcium-replete diet, supplements of calcium and vitamin D in combination did help to reduce bone loss and decrease fracture risk.

The USDA study was conducted in late 1995 and published in 1996. Two years later, a three-year study conducted on both men and women over the age of 65 was completed at Johns Hopkins University School of Hygiene and Public Health in Baltimore, Maryland. This research was conducted to determine the impact of combined calcium and vitamin D supplementation on nonvertebral (not involving the spine) fracture incidents. The study charted the progress and fracture incident rate of 389 men and women divided into two main groups—those receiving 500 mg. of calcium and 700 IU of vitamin D daily, and those who received a placebo (no value) supplement.

The group that received the real supplements was found to have moderate bone mass loss and significantly decreased incidents of fractures as compared to the placebo group. The benefits to both genders, male and female, were apparent. The study concludes that daily supplementation with calcium and vitamin D in combination did in fact slow the process of bone mass loss and reduce the risk of debilitating and disfiguring fractures (O'Brien 1998).

It is obvious that calcium and vitamin D are essential nutrients for the human body, aiding in growth, development, and long-term skeletal health. Subjects in the studies who included dairy products as a regular part of their diet received a greater benefit from additional non-dairy calcium and vitamin D supplements, even later in life. Evidence supports the conclusion that dairy calcium is more effectively utilized by the human system than non-dairy supplements because of the concentrations of additional elements in the dairy product. Vitamin D, magnesium, and phosphorus are all necessary to the efficient processing of the calcium. But, what about the other "unwanted" elements in dairy products? For years, diet gurus and some nutritionists have been outspoken about the dangers of the unwanted saturated fats in whole milk, advocating instead the consumption of skim or reduced-fat-percentage products. Are they correct?

Researchers who conducted the landmark Framingham Heart Study do not think so. In fact, this twenty-year study of the dietary habits of 832 men between the ages of forty-five and sixty-five showed quite the reverse. The study conclusively showed that the higher the consumption of certain types of fat in the subject's diet, the lower the risk of the most common type of stroke (Gilman et al. 1997).

Let's look at the evidence. Stroke is one of the leading killers of adult men and a significant cause of death in women in the United States today. Although men are at a higher risk as a gender, women do carry a measurable risk as well. Strokes can occur without warning and cause paralysis, loss of memory, heart and brain damage, and death. The most common type is ischemic stoke. Ischemic stroke is caused by a blockage of a blood vessel in the brain or in the neck. Eighty percent of all strokes are of the ischemic type, and more than half of these are fatal.

The Framingham Study scientists found that increased intake of total dietary fat, especially certain types of fat, was directly correlated to a decreased risk of developing ischemic stroke. The effects of the intake of three types of fat were analyzed: saturated fat, found in meat and dairy products; monounsaturated fat, found in canola, nut, and olive oils; and polyunsaturated fat, found in fish and vegetable oils. These three fats provide the most concentrated source of energy fuel for our bodies.

The researchers determined that for every three percent increase in total saturated and monounsaturated dietary fat intake in the men studied, there was a fifteen percent decrease in the risk of ischemic stroke. Polyunsaturated fat, although applauded by most nutritionists, did not have the same association, and provided no appreciable benefit in the reduction of risk. Dr. Matthew W. Gillman and his colleagues concluded: "Our data suggests that fat intake does not increase the risk of stroke . . . fat intake was strongly inversely associated with ischemic stroke incidence. . . " (Gilman et al. 1997).

Dr. Gillman's group also wisely cautions that the study warrants other follow-up research, and recommends specifically testing other groups, for instance, an extended study of female subjects comparative to the males in the Framingham study, or subjects of both genders varying in age, before massive public dietary recommendations are made based on this one study, no matter how comprehensive and long term it certainly had been. In conclusion, they summarize their findings this way: "Nonetheless, the results of this study raise the possibility that restriction of fat intake (referring to saturated and monounsaturated fats) among residents of Western societies, as recommended by the U.S. Cholesterol Education Program and others, does not decrease—and could increase—overall risk of ischemic stroke" (Gilman 1997). The work of Dr. Gillman and his colleagues was supported by the National Heart, Lung and Blood Institute, Harvard Medical School, and the Harvard Pilgrim Health Care Foundation.

Does the Framingham study indicate that all males would be healthier with a diet that liberally includes fat-laden fast food burgers and milk shakes? Not necessarily. Remember, not everything is good for everybody! Before incorporating drastic increases of fat into your diet, I insist you read and understand chapter 16. Your genetic, ethnic, and blood types also determine how your body will utilize one substance for its maximum benefits and derive little or no benefit from another. However, the facts are worth considering, as they clearly contradict those things that we have been recently taught to accept about the foods we eat.

Although non-dairy source supplements can be taken to adjust deficiencies, recent scientific evidence proves that nothing can substitute for a lifetime of consumption of adequate amounts of these vital elements to human health: calcium, vitamin D, and phosphorus. These elements occur naturally in dairy products, in proportions ideal for efficient utilization by the human body. Without lifelong inclusion of these products, or their equivalents as part of total dietary intake, supplements alone will not repair deficiency damage, stop the loss of bone mass from that most important component of the skeleton, the spine, or reduce the risk of stroke. Last, dairy foods are rich in other essential nutrients. In addition to calcium, vitamin D, and phosphorus, dairy products contain riboflavin, protein, and magnesium, all vital to optimum human health.

After review of all of this research, plus dozens of other studies that I have not cited here, several facts become apparent. First: calcium, vitamin D, and phosphorus are essential nutrients for the growth, development, and health of the human skeletal system. Second: certain kinds of dietary fats, particularly the saturated fats found in dairy products and animal meats, and monounsaturated fats found in canola, nut, and olive oils are important to maintain the health of vital organs such as the heart and brain, preventing crippling or fatal strokes, especially in males. Third: the most natural sources for these nutrients in ideal proportions are cow's milk and dairy products. This conclusion is particularly supported by the studies conducted on bone mass and skeletal growth, which indicate that consumption of dairy products over a lifetime results in the maximum utilization of the calcium inherent in these foods.

But what about the evidence that supports the connection between diabetes in children and milk products? What about persons suffering from various autoimmune diseases? What about the people who cannot digest milk, or its main component, lactose? What are the consequences to persons who are found to have overly high levels of calcium already in their systems? What role do allergies play in the consumption of dairy products? How do these conditions affect their overall skeletal health? Are they fated to a lifetime of adverse health conditions simply because their bodies cannot tolerate these substances? Let's examine the importance of milk and dairy allergies in the next section.

Does Milk Really Do a Body Good?
Lactose Intolerance and Dairy Diseases

Why is it that some of us can drink milk all our lives, stuff ourselves on ice cream, melted cheese sandwiches, and manicotti, while others among us can't even eat a cup of cottage cheese without searing heartburn? Why do some children thrive on milk and others experience behavioral problems or serious illness? The answer is twofold: inability to process the sugar in cow's milk and dairy products called lactose, and hidden milk allergies. What is "dairy sensitivity" or, to use today's popular term, "lactose intolerance"? Who suffers from it? Can it be prevented, or cured? What role does dairy play in aggravating or alleviating the condition?

Lactose intolerance, also referred to as lactose maldigestion, is the inability to digest the natural disaccharide (complex) sugar found in cow's milk and other dairy products. This sugar breaks down during digestion into two monosaccharide (simple) sugars: glucose and galactose. Lactose is digested by the action of an enzyme, beta-galactosidase, produced in the human small intestine, and referred to as lactase. Newborn babies produce lactase to digest similar sugars found in mother's breast milk. As children develop and different solid foods are added to their diet, the body's need for lactase decreases. The production of the enzyme therefore usually declines.

Scientists believe that lactose intolerance may be genetically linked. People in certain areas of the world, or with certain genetic histories, continue to produce lactase throughout adulthood, particularly Caucasians of Scandinavian, Nordic, or Germanic descent. Other Caucasians not of these origins do continue to produce lactase beyond childhood, as do some other ethnic groups. Correlating this fact with our review of osteoporosis, this may be why all Caucasians are so at risk for the disease. Perhaps their bodies require a lifelong supply of calcium, particularly dairy calcium, as lactase would not need to be produced if calcium were only to be derived from other, non-dairy sources.

Prospective studies have begun to show that the decrease of lactase production may be related to the reduced consumption of products containing milk sugars, such as milk, although data at this point are not conclusive. Other diseases or life events may cause the small intestine to stop producing lactase. Major surgery, radiation, or treatment with broad-spectrum antibiotics can cause the condition, and it has been known to occur as the aftereffect of gastroenteritis, an inflammation of the intestinal tract. Actually, any condition that produces trauma to the intestines can result in either a temporary or permanent loss of lactase production.

An estimated 30 percent of all adults in the United States suffer from lactose maldigestion or intolerance. How do you know if you are lactose intolerant? The symptoms include bloating, stomach pain, heartburn, flatulence, and diarrhea, although these common signs of human imbalance can be caused by other factors or diseases. Some people may have a lactase deficiency and show no symptoms, as factors such as body weight and age may influence how much dairy a person must consume before symptoms do manifest. Many physicians dogmatically counsel their lactose intolerant patients to avoid dairy products, thereby possibly setting these patients up for a calcium/vitamin D deficiency unless appropriate supplements are prescribed.

Studies show that these lactose intolerant patients are able to consume limited amounts of fluid milk, and a variety of other dairy foods before symptoms manifest. A clinical trial conducted in 1998 at the Minneapolis Veterans Affairs Medical Center examined lactose maldigestion and digestion when the diet was supplemented with dairy products. Sixty-two women participated in this double-blind, randomized study. Thirty-one of the women were healthy, and the other half had previously been diagnosed as lactose intolerant. Symptoms were charted on a weekly basis. The subjects received measured quantities of cow's milk, cheese, and yogurt daily, equal to the consumption of 1500 mg. of calcium. The results showed that although the lactose-intolerant women experienced significantly increased episodes of flatus (passing wind), the symptoms of bloating, painful gas, and diarrhea did not occur (Suarez et al. 1998, 68:1118–1122). The healthy group showed no significant ill effects. The results indicate that even persons with actual lactose intolerance can consume dairy products in enough quantity to receive adequate dietary dairy calcium intake without serious detriment to their health.

A review of similar studies in Germany also correlated the data from several tests involving lactose intolerance (de Vrese, Sieber, and Stransky 1998, 128:1393–1400). The combined data indicated that most lactose intolerant patients were able to ingest on average small amounts (about one cup) of milk daily without ill effects. They were also able to consume hard and semi-hard cheeses (Parmesan, Romano, Swiss, cheddar, etc.), and most soft cheeses (mozzarella, brie, cream cheese, etc.). Hard and semi-hard cheeses do not contain lactose, and soft cheeses average only about ten percent lactose content. These products are a very important source of dietary calcium and other nutrients, and probably should not be eliminated from the diet unless absolutely indicated.

Lactose intolerance tests have been conducted with children. Scientists at the David Grant U.S. Air Force Medical Center tested the digestion of dietary dairy calcium by comparing the effects of consuming standard cow's milk and products containing live bacteria such as acidophilus milk and unfermented milk that had been inoculated with live yogurt bacteria (Montes et al. 1995, 78:1657–1664). Nine out of ten subjects who showed symptoms when fed standard milk experienced a reduction in symptoms when fed acidophilus milk, and five out of six experienced reduced symptoms when fed milk injected with live yogurt cultures.

Other, similar tests conducted over the last ten years have illustrated clearly that lactose intolerant persons—children and adults—experienced a three- to fourfold reduction in symptoms when fed yogurt that was nonpasteurized and contained a substantial amount of beta-galactase enzymes, released into the intestine by the digestion of the yogurt. The beta-galactase, or lactase enzyme, then began to aid in the digestion of the yogurt. Therefore, it may be inferred that the tendency to lactose intolerance in some persons may be significantly reduced when those persons consume dairy products containing digestive enzymes. These individuals would be able to ingest the required amounts of daily dietary calcium by choosing those dairy products that contained these helpful enzymes and avoiding those products that did not contain them.

Dairy products have also been implicated in cases of inflammatory bowel disease (IBD), also known as Crohn's Disease. A study involving Caucasian, non-Jewish subjects from Northern Europe was conducted by the Mayo Clinic (Newcomer and McGill 1983, 58:339–341). A deficiency in the lactase enzyme was found in only five of the eighty IBD patients studied. However, when the five IBD patients with the lactase deficiency had milk, although not other dairy products, removed from their diets, three of the five experienced reduced symptoms of IBD. Since so few of the IBD patients studied had lactase deficiency, the researchers concluded that lactase deficiency was "an uncommon cause of irritable bowel syndrome." (American Whole Health 1999).

A recent review of studies done on Crohn's Disease patients and their ability to tolerate diary products summarized that the prevalence of lactose malabsorption was significantly greater in those patients who were diagnosed with Crohn's in the small intestine as opposed to those with Crohn's in the large intestine or the colon, or who had developed ulcerative colitis (Mishkin 1997, 65:564-567). The studies reviewed additionally determined that other factors may be contributing to lactose intolerance in small-bowel Crohn's patients, such as the presence of bacterial overgrowth or small-intestine food transit time due to the presence of the Crohn's condition.

Patients who were diagnosed with Crohn's but did not fit into the categories above appeared to have the most prevalent incidents of lactose intolerance due to the genetics or ethnicity of each patient. In all cases, patients were able to tolerate a daily glass of milk without complications, and doctors were cautioned against dogmatically counseling similar patients to strict avoidance of dairy products without further careful study and determination of the needs of each patient on an individual basis. In no cases were the presence of dairy products in the diet found to have caused IBD.

Dairy products have additionally often been accused as being the cause of attacks in asthma sufferers. An Australian clinical trial completed in 1998 showed this hypothesis to be unfounded. Doctors and scientists from the Monash Medical School and the Alfred Hospital in Melbourne, Australia conducted a randomized, cross-over, double-blind, placebo-controlled trial involving twenty adult men and women with asthma (Woods 1998, 101:45-50). None of the subjects showed a positive skin prick test reaction to cow's milk. The subjects were fed either a single-dose drink equivalent to 300 ml. (about a cup and a half) of cow's milk or a placebo liquid on alternating days. Tests to measure changes in respiratory rhythm and peak expiratory flow were charted at the same interval on both the days that the subjects were given the actual drink and on the false dosage (placebo) days.

The results in the test measurements were compared between active challenge days and placebo challenge days. Nine patients showed changes in different categories. Three subjects showed changes in testing levels on active challenge days, two showed changes on placebo days, and four on both active and placebo days. The latter two categories indicated that patient perception as to their "dairy sensitivity" might be a factor in reaction differences. Of the patients who exhibited changes on active days, two showed changed levels only in one test, and, after retesting, showed no asthmatic reaction in either type of test. The conclusion drawn was that it is unlikely that dairy products have any specific effect on the bronchoconstriction (loss of breath) in most patients with asthma.

Last, on the subject of diseases allegedly caused by dairy products, let's look at one of the fastest-growing killers of adult women today: breast cancer. Worldwide, breast cancer takes the lives of an estimated 300,000 or more women annually. Tens of thousands more are permanently disfigured, physically or psychologically. The cost of surgical procedures, medications, and aftercare is staggering, and the damage to patients, families, and marriages is even more devastating.

Geographically and ethnically, the risk of breast cancer differs around the world. Women in Northern Europe are at the greatest risk for the disease, followed by those from North America, southern Africa, and tropical South America. Conversely, women in India, central Asia, the Middle East, and Northern Africa are well below the world average for fatalities. Again, as we have seen in the cases of diabetes and lactose intolerance, genetics and ethnic background may be important factors in determining the risk of contracting breast cancer. Research is presently in progress, but no conclusive results that confirm or disprove the hypothesis have yet been obtained.

Because proper dietary calcium and vitamin D are so important to skeletal health, especially in women, a recent extensive study regarding dairy products and breast cancer becomes doubly important. Researchers at the National Public Health Institute in Helsinki, Finland studied the relationship between the intake of dairy products and the risk of breast cancer (Knekt et al. 1996, 73:687-691).

The dietary history, habitual diet, and consumption of milk and other dairy products by 4,697 women were charted over a 25-year period. After adjustments in data were calculated for potential confounding factors such as age, body mass index, smoking, childbirth, occupation, and geographic area, the results exhibited clearly that a significant inverse gradient between milk intake and incidence of breast cancer was observed. In layman's terms, this means that the results, gathered over a study spanning a quarter century, showed that, specifically, the *more* cow's milk consumed by the subjects over the course of their lives and the study period, the *less* breast cancer cases were observed. Adjustments for other factors, types of food, and nutrients (carbohydrates, proteins, fats, vitamins, and other trace elements) still showed no significant alteration of the results. Also interestingly, this inverse ratio with other dairy products besides fluid cow's milk was not significant. Overall, out of the nearly 5000 women studied, only 88 cases of breast cancer were diagnosed.

The conclusion drawn after all of the data had been analyzed suggests that there is actually a protective effect gained from the drinking of cow's milk that overwhelms the associations between different other factors and the risk of breast cancer in women.

That's really something to think about. As a woman, breast cancer is certainly a concern that has crossed my mind, as it probably has for most other women in our society. Anything that can reduce the risk of contracting this killer is worth considering, especially if the evidence points to a natural substance.

As a doctor of nutrition, I would encourage everyone to be carefully tested for the presence of hidden food allergies, particularly milk allergies, at as early an age as is practical. I urge you to have these vital tests performed before embarking on a drastic change in your dairy intake.

As a doctor of nutrition, I would encourage everyone to be carefully tested for the presence of hidden food allergies, particularly milk allergies, at as early an age as is practical. If you are reading this chapter and have never been tested for dairy sensitivity or hidden milk allergy, I urge you to have these vital tests performed before embarking on a drastic change in your dairy intake. This next section will examine the role of hidden milk allergies, and the effect that they have on health and the susceptibility of milk allergic persons to other, more serious diseases.

Milk and Medicine: Examining Dairy Allergies

Allergies come in all types—pollen, fabrics, foods, pets—and a human being can develop an allergic reaction to almost any substance. Most allergic reactions are readily apparent. Sneezing, wheezing, watery eyes, runny nose, itching, hives, and vomiting are all symptoms of allergic reaction. As we will learn in chapter 14, allergic reaction to some substances, such as bee venom, can cause serious and potentially fatal reactions.

Allergies occur when your body is overly sensitive to a foreign substance, whether consumed as food or found in the environment. No research to date has yet pinpointed the single cause of any one form of allergy, or the absolute cause of the development of sensitivity. Scientists have, however, developed an excellent and specific testing system for identifying and isolating those elements to which the allergic person reacts. There are two main types of allergy testing used today. The IgE, or immunoglobulin-E test, is used to identify the cause of an exhibiting allergy, such as reactions to dog hair, chocolate, eggs, or fruit juice. This test is widely used successfully by allergists in determining the offending substances and effectively treating their patients with dietary changes or prescription medicines that eliminate or control the symptoms.

Another even more detailed test for allergy also detects nonpresenting, or "hidden," allergies. These allergies are found most often with food. The technical name for the test is the immunoglobulin-G radioallergosorbant test, or IgG RAST method. The IgG RAST examines white blood cells and tests their reactions to various food substances, and elements found in those substances, like proteins, sugars, and enzymes. The IgG RAST is valuable as it is able to detect allergic reaction on a cellular level. Patients with hidden allergies may not manifest the outward symptoms I've mentioned above. Symptoms of hidden allergy may be intestinal bleeding, migraine headaches, loss of energy, weight loss without deliberate dieting, susceptibility to minor illnesses such as coughs and colds due to lowered resistance, and an increased risk for the development of other, more serious illnesses such as Type 1 diabetes.

Cow's milk proteins rank as one of the three most common causes of hidden food allergies. Allergy to cow's milk seems to develop at an early age, although older children and adults have also been known to test positively. Allergic reaction to bovine serum albumin is most common, and adverse reactions to the four types of casein, another protein found in cow's milk, have also been frequently observed. Casein is present after milk has been mildly acidified. It is a multipurpose protein, used for a variety of food and non-food purposes, from supplements to the manufacture of buttons and other small plastic objects.

Conversely, those afflicted with chronic or some autoimmune diseases may develop hidden food allergies as a *result* of the particular disease. As IgG RAST becomes more widely used, results will be able to show whether the milk allergy is responsible for the development of other ailments, or, if the allergy to milk is developed as a result of the ailment contracted.

One interesting fact that lends weight to this hypothesis, at least in my professional experience, is that I have tested dozens of MS suffers over the last five years for hidden food allergies, and all of them have tested positively for some form of milk allergic reaction. Yet, I have already shown MS is a viral infection, so we know that it is virtually impossible for the disease to have been caused by the intake of dairy products. We can also eliminate contaminants or foreign agents in the milk. The odds of all MS sufferers having drunk sufficient quantities of the same contaminated batch, or for the various regulatory agencies of the separate governments of all of the countries with MS patients to have collectively missed this mysterious toxin are beyond astronomical. In fact, it's a ludicrous idea. Therefore, the answer cannot be that milk allergies cause MS.

However, it would be interesting to see the results of a study in the reverse. I have not noted which specific milk proteins cause an allergic reaction in MS patients, nor have I had the opportunity to test MS patients for milk allergy when they are initially diagnosed for MS, or begin to present MS-type symptoms. Perhaps studies will be conducted on this interesting hypothesis in the future.

Now that we have explored the importance of hidden allergies, let's examine the solutions, if any, to the problem of cow's milk allergy, and the supply of substitute sources to replace the elements found in dairy products.

You need to understand the importance of having an IgG RAST performed. If you have recently had such a test, then the information that I am about to share with you next will be particularly valuable. If you have never had this test performed, or have not had one within the last year, I strongly urge you to schedule testing without delay, especially if you are suffering from MS. Even if you are not an MS or autoimmune disease sufferer, you should still have the test conducted.

Parents should have their children tested, even those only a few months old. Even if a child comes back negative for all reactions, it may be wise to have them periodically retested throughout their adolescence, when normal milk consumption is statistically proven to be highest. The test is simple, and relatively painless. Blood is drawn and sent to a laboratory for analysis. Your family doctor probably already uses a laboratory that performs IgE and IgG testing. I have included contact information on the one that I use for my patients in the resources section.

The results will prove to be invaluable in your progress toward optimum health. If you test completely negatively, you can concentrate on supplying your body with its optimum level of dietary calcium, vitamin D, and phosphorus by a daily intake of all dairy products. If your results indicate some or all positive indications, you will need to make major changes to your diet. You will need to eliminate some foods that you have eaten, and probably highly relished, all or most of your life. And, you will need to introduce either greater quantities of what may be already familiar foods, or perhaps include some new and different foods, vitamins, and nutritional supplements as part of your total diet.

Maintaining a nutritional balance is of the utmost importance. I stress this point throughout this book. Without this balance, your body cannot process the fuel you give to it, manufacture the substances it needs from that fuel, and maintain your optimal health. Keep your body out of balance long enough, and you will not be able to ward off any number of assailants, from infections to crippling viruses like multiple sclerosis, EBV, diabetes, and cancer. You will gain or lose tremendous amounts of weight, lose energy, and have parts of your body, from your spine to your reproductive organs, begin to malfunction and deteriorate from the lack of the substances that they require for survival.

A word to "healthy" readers as well: no matter how strong you may be physically, or how little illness you have ever experienced in your life, you would do well to remember our analogy from chapter 12. You can only run your car for so long without oil. Sooner or later, the engine will break down. Although you may feel perfectly healthy, you should still consider testing. You may prevent serious consequences later.

How do we maintain that healthy balance once a milk allergy has been detected in our blood? There are several ways in which to accomplish this task. First: not all dairy may need to be eliminated from your total diet. You may simply have to avoid pasteurized cow's milk and products made from it. Second: if you have a casein allergy, you can obtain non-pasteurized milk, acidophilus milk, and casein-free products. Be certain to read the label of any new product or food that you eat before you try it. Regulations on casein content in foods vary, and what may be casein-free to the FDA or other regulatory agency may still be too much casein for you. You will find a chart with some good substitute milk and ice cream choices in chapter 15, along with a comparison of the relative amounts of substitute you will need to drink in order to obtain the same level of nutrient intake.

You may not have to eliminate all cheeses, for instance. Hard and semi-hard cheeses may be perfectly acceptable parts of your diet, and, as they are important sources of calcium and other essential nutrients, you should not eliminate them if you do not need to. Yogurt with live cultures is also an excellent source of dietary calcium and contains very little lactose. Even some soft cheeses may be okay for you to eat. Consult with your physician or nutritionist, who will be familiar with you, or your child's case. They will help you to determine the optimum nutrient intake you need to achieve daily in order to maintain your best health, and which dairy products you should avoid. If you do need to eliminate cheese, again, you will also find a chart located in chapter 15 with some excellent items that you could choose to help you obtain the same nutrients you lost when dairy was eliminated.

Additionally, there are many vegetables that contain natural calcium, such as broccoli. Vitamin D_3 is manufactured by the action of sunlight on your skin, so you can increase the amounts you receive with some daily periods of outdoor exercise, or sunbathing. Vitamin D_2 is also important, however, and it is *not* enough for you to eat some salads and lie out in a lawn chair to receive an adequate supply. Phosphorus is also crucial to the efficient utilization of calcium. You will need to obtain a supplement form of these two essential elements. We will discuss which supplements are best, and which vegetables and other foods provide the most benefit in chapter 15. I have provided a chart for you to compare milk and other dairy foods to substitute foods that will give you the same nutrient levels there as well. You can find a list of some good places to purchase nutritional supplements in the resources section.

Finally, a word for parents who may be concerned about feeding their children a diet of vitamin pills instead of food. Consider a study conducted by researchers at the University of North Carolina Division of Orthopaedics (Madsen and Henderson 1997, 33:209–212). Fifty-eight children of both sexes between the ages of five and sixteen who were previously diagnosed with a positive IgG RAST for milk allergy were studied for low calcium-intake levels. The ethnic or economic backgrounds of the children were not noted in the review. Vitamin D and phosphorus levels were not tested.

The subjects were given nutritional counseling sessions and those who were found to have low calcium intake (53 percent) were advised to add calcium supplements and other calcium-containing foods to their diets. The remainder of the patients were already supplementing their diet or substituting appropriately valuable foods. The 31 subjects in the low calcium-intake group were reevaluated nearly two years later for changes to intake levels. Calcium intake had been increased in each child on the average of 360mg./day (about the same as is found in 12 oz. of milk), and supplements were now being used by 52 percent of the group.

Even though these were positive changes, 48 percent of the children still failed to meet the RDA for their corresponding size, gender, and age level. The researchers noted that the families of the patients who failed to meet their RDA after the follow-up period simply were not placing enough importance on, or diligently overseeing, the calcium intake of their children. The scientists concluded that although supplementation and alternate non-dairy food choices would adjust dietary calcium to the proper levels, where it could be maintained with the institution of habitual dietary habits, they felt that families should be educated as to the importance of maintaining these dietary intake levels.

The decision to eliminate dairy products from my diet was difficult because I missed so many of my favorite foods. I knew the importance of the step for me, however, and made my choice based upon the evidence from my personal test results. After a period of going without dairy, I felt healthier than I had in some time, and some of my MS symptoms disappeared or decreased. I began to replace my lost dairy with other equally delicious and satisfying foods that provided some of the nutrients that I would no longer be receiving through dairy. I have detailed these substitute choices in chapter 15. Although you may always miss some of your old dairy favorites, you can find lots of other tasty items to put into their place, and the benefits to eliminating dairy for you will far outweigh the regret you may feel now.

The decision to eliminate dairy products from my diet was difficult because I missed so many of my favorite foods. After a period of going without dairy, I felt healthier than I had in some time, and some of my MS symptoms disappeared or decreased. In fact, it probably would have been more dangerous for me to keep dairy in my diet.

Eliminating dairy, although difficult, was certainly not the most dangerous treatment method that I explored on my road to a cure for multiple sclerosis. In fact, it probably would have been more dangerous for me to keep dairy in my diet. Strange as some healing modules may initially seem, as a doctor, my instincts tell me to keep an open mind. Although I was familiar with, and had studied many natural herbal remedies and several ancient medical practices, I found I was still in for some surprises. The most dangerous part of my healing journey was still to come.

14

Deadly Savior—Bee Venom Treatment

Perhaps the most controversial, and certainly the most dangerous of all of the treatments I experienced in my search for a cure for MS was Bee Venom Treatment, or BVT: the systematic injection of the poisonous venom of the common black and yellow honeybee, *Apis mellifera*.

This healing module is definitely *not* for the uninitiated or the faint of heart. Painful and possibly deadly, the treatment can achieve almost miraculous results. In this chapter I will explain this fascinating and little known treatment option, and why it may be beneficial for the MS-afflicted. I will examine the history and treatment protocols of BVT, and present interviews with Dr. Theodore Cherbuliez of the American Apitherapy Society (AAS) and Mrs. Pat Wagner, "The Bee Lady of Waldorf."

Apitherapy, which takes its name from the Greek word *apis*, or "bee," has been recommended from ancient times as a preventative and curative for a number of ailments. Apitherapy is defined as the use of bees, honey, propolis, and other products of the hive for healing and medicinal purposes. Hippocrates, the great Hellenic Greek physician, advocated apitherapy in *Hippocratus Corpus*, which was written around the year 400 B.C.

Hippocrates was known as the "Father of Medicine" for his revolutionary approach to treating and healing the human condition. Hippocrates viewed medicine and the causes of ailments not to be of divine retribution nor supernatural intervention, but rather that they: " . . . arise from causes . . . namely, those things which enter and quit the body. . . . And each has its own peculiar nature and power, and none is of an ambiguous nature, or irremediable. And the most of them are curable by the same means as those by which any other thing is food to one, and injurious to another." (1981, 14–1)

Hippocrates encouraged the physicians of his day to treat the ailments with natural healing remedies:

"Thus, then, the physician should understand and distinguish the season of each, so that at one time he may attend to the nourishment and increase, and at another to abstraction and diminution. And in this disease as in all others, he must strive not to feed the disease, but endeavor to wear it out by administering whatever is most opposed to each disease, and not that which favors and is allied to it.

"For by that which is allied to it, it gains vigor and increase, but it wears out and disappears under the use of that which is opposed to it. But whoever is acquainted with such a change in men, and can render a man humid and dry, hot and cold by regimen, could also cure this disease, if he recognizes the proper season for administering his remedies, without minding purifications, spells, and all other illiberal practices of a like kind" (1981, 2:139–183).

Hippocrates is considered to be one of the first recorded naturopaths. He advocated the use of natural substances in the treatment of a number of ailments. He believed that all illness was as a result of imbalances in the body, which could be corrected with diet and natural substance supplementation. Many of the healing protocols he prescribed, like apitherapy, are still in use around the world today. The Bible also tells us of the benefits of honey as a major part of the diet. John the Baptist existed in the wilderness on a diet consisting mainly of locusts (a kind of fig) and wild bee honey (Matthew 3:4; Mark 1:6). Chinese medicine, ancient and modern, also prescribes apitherapy as a curative for disease.

If apitherapy has been advocated and practiced for nearly two and one half millennia, why then are its protocols not more widely recognized as treatment options? There are several answers to this question. First, apitherapy *is* widely practiced outside of the United States. Other countries throughout the world are conversant with its methods and benefits, and apitherapists are considered to be fully accredited healers. American medicine during the last half century has developed a distinct tendency toward elitist snobbery. Members of the medical community often discount, dismiss, or unfairly denigrate as "folk medicine" natural remedies or traditional healing arts in favor of "modern" treatments: manufactured medications and usually expensive professional care.

Some of these "wonder drugs," like penicillin and the Salk vaccine, have advanced the cause of medicine and saved millions of lives. Others, like Betaseron and ACTH, are advocated as "breakthrough" treatments, but are in reality expensive disease management tools, offering no real healing to the patient. My personal opinion on the reason behind this attitude shift would take some time to express and is not really relevant to the subject at hand. Suffice it to say that modern medicine has become big business, and the patient does not always benefit because of it.

Some of the practice of apitherapy is accepted and utilized in this country, though few recognize the treatments as part of this healing art. Many naturopaths, nutritionists, and health food professionals advocate honey, propolis, and royal jelly as excellent natural sources of vitamins, antioxidants, and nutrition. However, other apitherapy protocols, like BVT, are virtually unknown. Why?

In the case of BVT, one reason is probably the unpleasantness of the treatment. Regardless of the duration of the discomfort or the amount of swelling that may or may not occur, this is not a pleasant remedy. Bee stings *do* hurt. As each person's individual tolerance for pain varies, the amount of discomfort will also vary. Some patients find BVT merely a mild discomfort, like getting a tattoo or a mild sunburn, while others experience far more pain.

Another explanation may be simple fear. All of our lives we have been taught, by our parents, teachers, scoutmasters, and camp counselors as well as by painful personal experience that bees should be left alone. Bees are not pets to be handled, they are stinging insects to be avoided or pain and possible serious reactions to the sting will almost certainly be the consequence. The idea of deliberately placing a bee onto any portion of your body and encouraging it to sting you causes most people to shake their heads and back away. If you are afflicted with MS, however, you probably live with pain every day. The relative discomfort of a small bee sting pales in comparison to the pain endured by those afflicted with this crippling disease, and anything that brings relief or offers improvement in your condition is worth considering.

BVT offers much more than relief or improvement for the MS patient. When used properly, BVT can arrest and has been proven to actually reverse MS in some cases. You already know that when I experienced the therapy myself, the numbness that had been present in my left leg for over four years was cured. It has never returned. BVT is an important, natural healing modality. In this next section, I will introduce you to an individual who is recognized as one of the leading authorities in the United States on BVT and its use in the treatment of MS patients: Mrs. Pat Wagner. Executive board member of the American Apiary Society (AAS) and herself an MS patient, this certified apitherapist was instrumental in my decision to try BVT on my condition.

Pat Wagner: "The Bee Lady of Waldorf"

One of the most unique individuals active in alternative medicine today is Mrs. Pat Wagner, the "Bee Lady of Waldorf." (The title bestowed upon her by appreciative physicians and patients refers to her home in Waldorf, Maryland.) One of the most prominent voices raised in praise of the effectiveness of BVT, Mrs. Wagner has appeared on television news programs, has been the subject of several televised documentaries, and has been interviewed by several major newspapers and magazines. Author of the self-help book *How Well Are You Willing To Bee?* (1994), Pat has successfully assisted over ten thousand patients in BVT therapy, with amazing results.

I have included this full-length August 1999 interview with Pat Wagner because of her practical expertise and firsthand experience with BVT. My questions appear in italics, her answers below each one in regular text. I want you to pay particular attention to the horrifying litany of prescription drugs she was given as her condition steadily worsened and her physical condition when she began BVT. Let's find out what she has to say about apitherapy, bees, and the benefits of BVT:

For the benefit of my readers who may not as yet have read your book, How Well Are You Willing To Bee? *could you tell us when and where you were diagnosed with multiple sclerosis? How old were you when the diagnosis was made?*

I was initially diagnosed with multiple sclerosis in the spring of 1970, at Georgetown University Hospital in Washington, D.C. I was nineteen years old at the time.

What prompted you to seek medical assistance? What symptoms were you experiencing at the time?

My foot had fallen asleep for three weeks and there was some numbness in my limbs, along with a slight stumbling when I walked.

Were you additionally diagnosed with other illnesses at that time?

Yes, I was. Scars of tuberculosis were found on one of my lungs. Because the medication ACTH can activate TB and cause a reoccurrence, I had to take a drug called INH to prevent any activation of the TB whenever I was taking ACTH. This would happen two to three times per year, usually when I was in the hospital.

My dad was diagnosed while in military service as having MS. Is any other blood relative in your family afflicted with MS or another debilitating disease?

No, no one else in my family has been afflicted with a major or chronic disease.

What medications were prescribed for you by your doctor?

I was given ACTH and Prednisone for the neurological flare-ups; Meprobamate, Dexedrine, and Dantrium for muscle spasms; Dalmane, Valium, and Halcyon as sleep aids; Ditropan to combat bladder incontinence and Lomotil for bowel incontinence; and the antibiotics erythromycin and penicillin, as well as Keflex for urinary tract infection. I was also prescribed Seconal for my increasing anxiety attacks; Timoptic eye drops for iritis; and Tylenol #3, Indomethacin, Percocet, Vicodin, Fiorinol, Soma, and morphine for the pain.

Were these medications changed throughout the progress of the disease?

Basically they remained unchanged except to fill the prescriptions with the generic drug equivalent when possible for cost savings. I was only prescribed morphine once, during a period of hospitalization. My entire body, from my toes to my eye muscles and the muscle surrounding my brain, had begun contracting uncontrollably.

When did you realize that the prescribed course of healing wasn't working?

In 1991. A doctor treating me prescribed 80 milligrams of Prednisone (tapered down as usual). He immediately gave the same thing again and there was no change in my condition.

What was your physical condition at that time?

I was numb in my arms, hands, partially in my face, and especially from the waist down. My bones felt like they were made of ice. I had no bowel or bladder control. I couldn't wiggle any of my toes or move my feet, roll over or sit up by myself, or hear out of my right ear. I slept about eighteen hours a day and trembled when I tried to put food or drink to my mouth, let alone a toothbrush. My vision had deteriorated so badly that I couldn't see clearly enough to tell if the person in front of me was male or female, black or white, wearing glasses or bearded. I couldn't even see my own reflection in the mirror. I couldn't remember even the simplest things, and I seemed to be angered easily and often.

What event, information, or person prompted you to explore BVT and apitherapy as alternative healing modules?

I was originally introduced to bee stings (BVT) alone, but later learned about the use of all the products of the hive, which is the practice of apitherapy. As for learning about bee stings, it came about through the suggestion of a friend of my mother's. He was a beekeeper and had just learned from the bee inspector about the use of honeybees for many ailments, including one person who had MS and was trying bee stings. My mother called and asked me if I wanted to try bee stings.

That friend of my mother, the bee inspector, and his wife came to my home a few evenings later. I was given my first sting on the outside of my left knee. Twenty minutes after that sting, my entire left leg was no longer bone cold. I then got stung once on the back of each shoulder and once on the upper part of each buttock. The next day, I was totally free of the bone coldness except for some that remained in my hands and feet.

When did you begin BVT in earnest?

I began bee venom treatment on March 24, 1992.

Did you eliminate all medications at that time and rely solely upon the curative properties of BVT, or did you continue with some medications while undergoing BVT?

I continued with the medications until I realized that the venom from the honeybees was taking care of many of my problems. I then weaned myself off of my medications, with this exception: I now, on an "as needed" basis, take 5 mg. of Valium. I also occasionally, on the same basis, take 5 mgs. of Dexedrine. These are prescribed for me by my doctor as per my request.

Why did you continue with the Valium and the Dexedrine?

I continued using Valium at those times when I felt I needed good rest. I then asked my doctor to prescribe Dexedrine to be used one-half to one hour after taking the Valium. My doctor stated that the Valium would relax my muscles and I could move about more easily without tiring by taking the Dexedrine. Both medications are now seldom used.

In your book, you attribute the application of BVT as "the sole cause of my turnabout with the ravages of multiple sclerosis." Why?

I attribute my turnabout with the course of my MS to honeybees and BVT because of the things—like warming my bones—BVT restored that no medications I was given had been able to do. The medications caused additional symptomatic problems in addition to my MS, like constipation and erratic sleep, among other things. I realized that I would be better off not further complicating an already complicated disease. When the bee venom cleared up my "fuzzy thinking," my mental clarity, it was much more apparent to me that the medical world did not hold the answer to my illness.

You've described several symptoms you've experienced. Which of those are now eradicated by your use of BVT and apitherapy?

All of the symptoms I was experiencing before beginning BVT are now gone, with the exception of some imbalance due to weakness in my right leg, which was the part of my body most affected by the MS. When I experience long days that go into the night, I will often feel additional weakness in my leg the next day. Also, my vision is not yet 20/20 and I sometimes have urinary urgency, mostly due to sipping water when I don't get the chance to stop and just drink a whole glass at one time.

Let's change the topic for the moment, and talk a little about diet and nutrition. What prompted you to eliminate dairy and "white foods" such as white bread and white sugar from your diet?

I began realizing that I was having bowel problems, especially after ingesting dairy products. I decided to try eliminating them from my diet. I saw a big change in my digestion. I also learned through the American Apitherapy Society (AAS) that eliminating white bread and white sugar might be beneficial. At the time, I was using very large amounts of sugar. When I changed from sugar to honey, I found that my energy and emotional levels became much more normal, as opposed to the roller coaster ride that I had been on by using sugar . . . especially to the extent that I had been using it.

Did anyone prescribe these or additional dietary changes for you, and when did you make the changes?

Dr. Bradford S. Weeks, who was then president of the AAS, didn't prescribe them but suggested that I might benefit by trying them. I changed my diet after I began BVT.

Have you been tested for the presence of MS or other conditions since you have begun BVT and apitherapy?

When I first started BVT, I was given an MRI. It showed the presence of a lot of plaque, the lesions attributed to MS, in my brain.

Have you been additionally tested? If so, how recent was your last test, and would you share the results with my readers?

My second MRI was done in 1993. A year after starting BVT, I asked my doctor, Stuart Goodman, M.D., of Southern Maryland Hospital Center, for a second MRI. The results showed that the existing plaque had diminished and there were no new flares.

Do you think if you stopped practicing BVT, your symptoms of MS would return?

Yes, to some extent. I have tried going without using BVT for periods of time and some of my symptoms did reoccur. When I went back to BVT, the symptoms disappeared. As time passes, I find that I can now go for longer periods of time without using BVT before any symptoms are evidenced.

Let's explore the practice of BVT itself more thoroughly. At the time of your book's revised publication in 1997, you stated that you had administered BVT to nearly seven thousand persons. Would it be safe to say that you have treated at least ten thousand people by this time?

Since I am not a doctor, I haven't "treated" anyone. However, I have shared my knowledge of BVT and apitherapy with perhaps 12,000 people by now.

Do you practice as an apitherapist full time?

Yes, I do. In fact, I'm on call twenty-four hours a day, seven days a week!

Does the administration of apitherapy require licensing?

No licensing is required for the practice of apitherapy. However, the American Apitherapy Society is offering certification in apitherapy through their knowledge review course. This course is open to both medical professionals and laypersons. I have completed several apitherapy training courses and am myself a certified apitherapist.

How do you determine where to apply BVT for each patient?

BVT practitioners use many of the anatomical and nervous system charts utilized by acupuncturists. Where applicable, we plan treatment following those nerve medians and pressure points. When dealing with cases of arthritis or patients experiencing numbness in their extremities or other body parts, the affected area is stung directly.

I know that during the course of my own therapy, I increased my collected venom injections to the equivalent of twenty stings per session. Is this normal for all BVT patients, or does the amount of venom needed at each session vary?

The amount of venom needed for each patient will vary depending upon the severity of their medical condition or the extent of the existing damage. Some patients are prescribed as many as thirty stings per session, the equivalent of one-half cc of venom.

Is there anyone who should not *consider BVT?*

Yes. Anyone who is on a beta blocker. They should have their doctor prescribe another medication that is not a beta blocker in its place. If a person were to go into anaphylactic shock, epinephrine would not work while a beta blocker medication is being used by that person.

After the administration of BVT, does the patient experience a "euphoria," a feeling of "being high," or are increased energy levels the usual result, or a combination of both?

Often, "euphoria" is experienced shortly after administration of the stings. Increased energy levels are usually noticed, especially in those who have a low energy level in general.

Initially, how do you determine that the swelling arising from a test sting is beneficial purging or an allergic reaction?

First, two stings are required for testing. I usually don't see swelling with the first stings mainly because I give them near the spine or on the main trunk of the body, where swelling is less likely to occur. A swelling reaction (which is an allergic reaction) to BVT usually comes later in the course of giving stings. To me, swelling shows that your body is accepting BVT and that your adrenal glands are basically in good working order. I have been told that swelling is a good indication that your body will respond well to BVT.

In your book, you refer to "fluid changes" in the body occurring during the initial stages of BVT. Are these changes specific to MS patients, or are they a universal reaction to the stings?

They are universal. The fluid changes are usually caused by a change in your histamine levels. That change is what causes the itching. When it is severe and the palms of your hands turn red, it is a good idea to take a Benadryl Kapseal. This over-the-counter medication is usually needed only once during the course of BVT, usually in the beginning sessions. Other fluid changes can happen with sinuses, blood, etc. These are beneficial as will be noted by the person being stung.

The elements in bee venom stimulate adrenal function. Viewing BVT as a "hot start" for your system immune and repair functions, do you feel that this practice is "managing" the disease, or do you feel that the use of BVT can actually reverse MS and cure it?

BVT gives your system a "jump start." It helps "manage" your immune and repair systems, and thus the disease. I do believe that BVT alone can cure, especially when used in the early stages of a disease, particularly MS. Since MS is basically an inflammation of the nervous system, and BVT provides a strong anti-inflammatory substance, a patient can get rid of the inflammation causing many of the symptoms of MS. I do know of such cases. In the later stages, after plaque and scarring has occurred, all of the apitherapy protocols, and sometimes additional healing methods will most likely be needed, depending on the severity of the illness.

Finally, for the benefit of my readers, please tell us a little about the American Apitherapy Society (AAS). What is your connection with the organization?

The AAS is a nonprofit organization, which receives no outside funding. Its main purpose is to gather, organize, and disseminate information regarding honeybees and apitherapy to the medical community and the public at large. I am currently serving as an executive board member of the AAS.

Mrs. Pat Wagner is a vital, down-to-earth, regular person. To me, she is just another example of how God can use an afflicted person to bring great good and beneficial changes to the world, and turn the darkest of situations into something wonderful. I would like to take a moment here to sincerely thank Pat for all of her time and kind assistance she has rendered that has proved invaluable in the completion of this chapter.

Let's take a closer look at this unusual, but admittedly effective alternative medical practice. BVT is the application of honeybees to the human skin to produce a bee sting. The venom contained in the sting contains certain elements that render it useful in stimulating the body's own curative powers. When practiced correctly, bee venom treatment can produce nearly miraculous results.

Which Bees Are Best? Understanding the Difference in Species

What sorts of bees are used in apitherapy? Are all honeybees the same? There are several different kinds of honeybees, from our familiar black and yellow friends buzzing cheerfully about in our flower gardens to honey producers native to almost all parts of the world. There are the infamous "killer bees," supposedly unstoppable and moving farther into the North American continent each year.

Let's take a moment to discuss these "killer" bees, *Apis mellifera L. scutellata (Lepetelier)*. The Africanized honeybee

(AHB) is closely related to the common European Honeybee (EHB). According to research conducted by the U.S. and California State Departments of Agriculture, Texas A&M University (1999), and the University of California Riverside Entomology Department (1999), AHB's are smaller in size than our common bumblebee. They are extremely similar in appearance to the EHB, and nearly impossible to distinguish with the naked eye. Scientists make the distinction through capture, dissection, and microscopic analysis.

These are *not* the bees used in apitherapy or BVT. Then, why should they be important to this discussion? The answer to that question should quickly become apparent. I mention the AHB to emphasize a very important point: when considering either BVT or the full range of apitherapy, it is vital to know the source of your bees! Choose a reliable and recognized apiary, or bee supplier, especially when considering keeping and raising your own home colony of bees.

Africanized bees are the result of crossbreeding between wild African bees and the EHB. They were originally introduced during the 1950's to Brazil. The thought was that the high-honey-producing Africanized bee would be more easily acclimated to the environment, yielding more honey than the low-production South American (SA) bee, or the EHB, which did not fare well in the hot and humid South American climate. The "experiment" was indeed successful, raising Brazil from twenty-seventh in world honey production to fourth. However, serious consequences began to develop. The AHB proved far more difficult to domesticate than its SA counterpart. Honeybees have been bred for gentleness and calm interaction with their human guardians, the beekeepers. Although all bees will defend their hive if threatened, AHB colonies will perceive a threat at a far greater range, and with much fiercer intensity.

Their reputation as "killers" does not originate from the venom contained in their sting. AHB venom and honeybee venom contain exactly the same elements. As the AHB is smaller than the honeybee, it in fact carries *less* venom in its individual sting. The danger lies in the *number* of stings received by the victim. Most of us have been stung by at least one honeybee at some time in our lives. The AHB attacks in far greater numbers. Animals, livestock, and people have succumbed to the venom after receiving at times upwards of a hundred stings within a minute or two.

Africanized bees have been gradually moving northward. First encountered in Texas in 1990, AHB's have now been reported in Arizona, New Mexico, California, Nevada, Puerto Rico, and the Virgin Islands (USDA). Presently, more than 110 Texas counties have been quarantined against the AHB. Beekeepers may transport the colonies, but not outside of the quarantined zones. This is done to prevent the assisted spread of the AHB. If AHB populations become numerous, they will drive out or kill the gentler honeybee as they search for new territories. This could be disastrous economically, for both the beekeeping industry and the farmer, as AHB's do not pollinate nearly as many flowers or vegetable plants as their gentler cousin.

If you would like to learn more about the Africanized honeybee, I suggest that you contact the U.S. Department of Agriculture, or visit the web sites of the universities cited here. You will find their web addresses in the Bibliography. They all provide useful information about the AHB species and its progression into the United States.

Bee Venom: Deadly Poison or Nature's Medicine Chest?

Exactly what is contained in bee venom that makes it so useful? Let's take a look at the major components of the venom—its toxicology. Honeybee venom contains at least eighteen identifiable active substances (Rothfeld 1999). For ease of understanding, I have listed the eleven most substantial elements in Chart 14-1 with the area of the human system affected by each element.

Chart 14-1 Elements of Bee Venom

Element	Function/Effects
Melittin	Anti-Inflammatory (Hydrocortisol)
Adolapin	Anti-Inflammatory (Cyclooxygenase) Analgesic
Apamin	C3 Complement Potassium Blocker Nerve Transmission Enhancer
Compound X	Inflammatory Venom Response
Hyaluronidase	Tissue Softener
Phospholipase A2	Facilitates Substance Flow
Histamine	
Mast Cell Degranulating Protein (MCDP)	
Dopamine	Neurotransmitters
Norepinephrine	Increases Motor Activity
Seratonin	Affects Emotional Centers

Eight of these eleven components are the most relevant to BVT. Let's examine each and learn why they are beneficial to the human system.

Mellitin is one of the most powerful anti-inflammatory substances known to science. It is a hundred times more powerful than hydrocortisol. Mellitin stimulates the pituitary gland to naturally release the hormone ACTH, which causes the adrenal glands to produce cortisol, our own powerful natural healing substance, thereby activating the body's healing response system. (Another excellent source of cortisol is vitamin C.)

Adolapin is a powerful anti-inflammatory agent, and combines with mellitin to produce the pain experienced by the sting. Adolapin also possesses analgesic properties, which temper the reaction produced by the mellitin.

Apamin blocks calcium plus dependent potassium and enhances long-term synaptic (or nerve signal) transmissions.

Hyaluronidase acts upon hyaluronic acid, the substance that coats the walls of our cells. Hyaluronic acid acts like a glue, connecting the cells together. Hyaluronidase eats away at this glue, making it easier for healing substances to flow at the cellular level into the damaged area and for waste material and toxic substances to be removed.

Mast Cell Degranulating Peptide (MCDP) causes the release of histamines, which create the signs of sting injury such as swelling, itching, burning, and redness. Additionally, and this is important: MCDP is one of the most powerful naturally occurring seizure-inducing agents. The danger in receiving an overdose of this substance is another reason why the proper application of BVT is so crucial to the patient's safety.

Dopamine, norepinephrine, and seratonin are neurotransmitters. (We discussed the significance of neurotransmitters in chapter 12.) These stimulate and facilitate the signals and activities of the nervous system. They create the "flush" or "fire" feeling that spreads when injected or stung. Dopamine is particularly significant in that it is found to be deficient in those suffering from Parkinson's disease and persons experiencing deep psychosis requiring treatment with neuroleptic drugs. Its lack has also been noted as a primary factor in cases of major depressive states.

Almost all of these substances can be utilized positively by the human system. Why, then, do the stories of anaphylactic shock and allergic reactions persist? Because a bee by any other name can be deadly! Studies have shown that the bulk of allergic reactions occur as a result of yellow jacket and wasp stings. *Apis mellifera* venom does not normally cross-react within the human body. In fact, less than five percent of all reported allergic reactions occur as a result of a sting by the common honeybee (Rothfeld 1999).

However, allergic reaction to the common honeybee can occur if the amount of venom is great enough. This is exactly the reason that a patient considering BVT as a means of treatment should always have proper emergency treatment remedies immediately available, and engage in this healing module under the supervision of an apitherapist, a physician, or nurse familiar with the practice of BVT. After proper training by an experienced apitherapist, a patient can self-perform the therapy, but it is wisest to have another person familiar with the shock kit standing by to administer emergency procedures and contact the police or EMT services if necessary.

We've heard from Mrs. Pat Wagner regarding her practical experiences with apitherapy and the effects it has had on her personal battle with MS. Now, let's get the opinion of one of the foremost medical experts and advocates of apitherapy as a means of treatment: Theodore Cherbuliez, M.D., current president of the AAS. I contacted him in September 1999 to include a medical perspective on this protocol. A charming and most distinguished gentleman, he graciously assented to the interview and its inclusion here.

Dr. Cherbuliez is the author of the highly respected treatise "Bee Venom Therapy and Safety" (1997) and other noted works on the subject of apitherapy and BVT as legitimate treatments and healing options. Dr. Cherbuliez presently occupies the office of president for both the American Apitherapy Society (AAS) and Apimondia, the International Federation of Beekeepers Associations, headquartered in Rome, Italy. My questions are shown in italics, and Dr. Cherbuliez' answers appear in regular text below each one.

Could you tell me how you became involved with the practice of apitherapy?

Through Charles Mraz, a Vermont beekeeper. Mr. Mraz died recently at the age of ninety-four on September 6, 1999. Some fifteen years ago he did a demonstration of Bee Venom Therapy (BVT). I had known from way back that bee stings were good for arthritis, but had not paid this fact much attention. I had also noted, just in passing, that pain in both my shoulders had disappeared since I kept bees, which I had already been keeping for about ten years at that time.

Mr. Mraz suffered rheumatic disease at the age of twenty-five and he had successfully treated himself with bee stings. From then on, he treated anyone that came to him. Over the years, he acquired a worldwide reputation. He can justly be called the "Father of BVT" in the United States. He never charged any money for his treatments. Many physicians called him "the best rheumatologist in New England." I remained in quite close contact with him until he passed away.

As a medical doctor, is your specialty apitherapy, or is your practice focused in another direction?

My specialty is psychiatry, with particular emphasis on family treatment. I give apitherapy consultations on Saturday mornings.

Do you use apitherapy regularly in practice to treat your patients?

I do not mix the two practices. If a person I see as a psychiatrist wishes an apitherapy consultation, this will be offered separately for a Saturday morning.

For what illnesses do you recommend BVT as a treatment?

BVT is not an approved treatment in the United States. I consider it an experimental approach and do not recommend it. However, I do state that I have experience in the subject and can speak about the circumstances where BVT has been used successfully. I also can address the known limitations of this approach so that people consulting with me can make informed decisions. The majority of the people I see come to me with their minds already made up to go ahead with the procedure. For some of them, this is the last approach, while for others, they believe in it, but lack experience and need technical guidance.

What is your opinion as to the effectiveness of BVT as a means of treatment for MS? Could apitherapy be termed a "cure" for the disease, or a means to "manage" the symptoms and retard or halt progression of the disease?

We have no cure for the disease. Some people with MS experience such major improvement after undergoing BVT that they are nearly symptom-free and can lead a normal life. In my experience, however, even major improvement keeps the MS in the background, and not very far. A usual way of assessing the effect of BVT in MS is to look at the various manifestations of the condition in each individual.

Some have "good reputation," that is, they statistically respond well to the therapy. Fatigue as a symptom is the best example: it is quite frequently reported and often patients experience a rapid decrease of this as they enter therapy. Sometimes it seems that the progression of the illness has stopped altogether, at least for some period of time, which can span over years. Examples of regression of the deterioration are also not rare.

In your article "Bee Venom and Safety" *you provide much valuable and detailed information regarding the safe way to practice BVT. Would you briefly review the reactions that one might expect from a BVT sting?*

What seems important to me here is not what one can expect from one sting, but rather from a course of bee stings. My protocol directs me to offer to new patients one test and two stings. I propose and they dispose. It is, however, quite rare that a patient declines the second sting after having asked for the first. Practically every sting evokes pain, swelling, reddening, and itching to some degree. Pain, the most unwelcome event, is mostly of short duration. It infrequently exceeds one minute. The unusual reactions deserve special mention: I will mention here first deep pain in the joints, mostly in small joints, finger and wrist, and second, the formation of a bloody bubble on the site of the sting. It is interpreted as a strong reaction of the person to the venom, and suggests small doses, at least at the beginning. These two reactions are rare and can be observed at the beginning of treatment. Next comes the reaction that often comes in the second or third week of treatment. It typically takes the form of a gastrointestinal disturbance, occasionally with diarrhea and vomiting. Quite unpleasant, but usually followed by a clear improvement of the symptoms, hence its name "the healing crisis." An exaggeration, as this is only an improvement, not a cure.

In your expert opinion, what are the dangers, in percentage, of a patient experiencing anaphylactic shock when practicing BVT?

Anaphylaxis is an extreme form of allergy. The statistics I have give figures running against popular belief. About seven people in 1000 are allergic to honeybee venom, and of these seven a very small portion will have anaphylactic response. A very loose estimation suggests that the chances are of the order of 1 to 1,000,000.

Are you aware of any fatalities resulting from anaphylaxis after engaging in a BVT session?

Whatever the exact figure, we do not have, so far, any instance of death following a therapeutic sting.

In addition, what other adverse reactions can be triggered by BVT? Please note whether these reactions are common or rare.

There are a number of them. We have sometimes allergic reactions, developing slowly, for example some ten to thirty minutes after stinging and progressing slowly. These reactions can take many forms: a metallic taste in the mouth is the one that alarms people the most when not informed about its harmlessness. Transitory rashes, fever, abdominal cramps, and headaches are rare. The last three may herald a favorable change in the patient's condition.

I have seen, also rarely, a malaise that can last a whole day, somewhat similar to the healing crisis, but less marked. It has no explanation and, the malaise gone, treatment resumes, first at a lower dose than before, and then back to the previous level. A local reaction that may alarm people, comes as a large swelling, usually at an extremity, larger than ten centimeters. It can last several days and is not painful. It is easily confused with cellulitis. Its mechanism seems to be a trouble in the lymphatic return system. The proper approach is mechanical: the limb, leg, or arm must be elevated. One can wear a holding stocking if one has to walk.

You recommend that a patient have an anaphylactic shock kit, or Ana Kit, or Epi Pen immediately available during BVT. Would you explain what is contained in these emergency antidote kits? Do they require special skills to administer?

Absolutely. In fact I recommend, and do myself, that the kit be immediately available, close at hand, and not in a drawer. Once a month I open it, look at the instructions, and follow them out as if I were to use it. I don't want to have to read it when I need it! The kit contains a solution of epinephrine. When injected it provokes very quickly a constriction of the vessels, thereby counteracting the brusque vasodilation that is part of the anaphylactic reaction. No other skills are needed than those acquired by careful reading of the instructions of the kit.

Even if a patient does not have so severe a reaction, some discomfort will occur. What other methods can a patient pursue to ease this discomfort and reduce the swelling caused by the stings?

There are several types of discomfort. The first, pain, can be substantially decreased by cooling the skin at the sting site. A small metallic can, kept in the freezer, does a good job. Applied for ten to twenty seconds immediately before the sting and the person stung hardly notices the event until the skin naturally warms up. Do not cool after the sting is in place, as it would stop the pumping action of the sting apparatus. Itching can be handled with antihistaminics or with the commercially available cream called *Preparation H.* Scratching usually keeps the itching going and is not recommended. The swelling, other than the one discussed above, is no real problem. Reassurance is the best thing.

NSAIDs, non-steroid anti-inflammatory drugs, have been reported to cause an adverse reaction, nullify the effects of BVT, and reduce sting immunity. In a recent article entitled "Understanding Prescription Drugs" Dorothy L. Smith reports that over-the-counter medications such as Motrin, Ibuprofin, Tylenol, and Naproxen, and NSAIDs, such as Fenoprofen, Ketoprofen, Sulindac, Peroxicam, Suprofen, and Tolmetin, can reverse the immunity to bee stings and increase the risk of anaphylaxis. What is your opinion on this issue?

Whether these are allergic reactions is debated. The reality of their happening is not. They take indeed the form of allergic reactions. I have no knowledge that they reverse the immunity. The disturbances do not reoccur when the NSAID is discontinued.

As regards the previous question, have you ever personally had a patient with whom this was the case? If so, what medication caused the reaction, and what illness or condition were they taking the NSAID to treat?

None personally, but they are frequently described as antidotes. I have been told of cases involving MS and arthritis patients.

An opposing viewpoint on the effect of NSAIDs on "lost immunity" is presented by Dr. Ross A. Hauser of Caring Medical and Rehabilitation Services in his article "Regarding NSAIDs and Anaphylaxis" (1996). He believes that it is far more likely that these adverse reactions were to the medications themselves, and have little or no impact on BVT or exposure to bee venom. Do you agree or disagree, and why?

Even though the evidence is only anecdotal and has not been the object of a scientific investigation as it should and will be, I have read enough of these stories linking NSAIDs and venom to accept the high likelihood of a relationship between them.

The statement has been made, from several sources, that BVT can be practiced by the patient alone, without the necessity of a physician or medical professional in attendance. Do you agree or disagree?

One fact is that, at least in the United States, the number of physicians willing to supervise BVT is so low that it is just not possible. As the next best solution, I always recommend a consultation with someone well versed in BVT before starting such treatment. But even this is utopian, and my advice is not always followed.

Mellitin found in bee venom stimulates the production of cortisol. Please explain why cortisol is so important.

Cortisol, as representative of corticosteroids, influences the metabolisms of fat, proteins, and carbohydrates. It also assists the organism at resisting noxious stimuli and environmental changes: it is essential to well-being. Furthermore, cortisol has major anti-inflammatory properties.

Please share with us some information on the bee venom/apitoxin study presently being conducted in Brussels, Belgium. What does this study hope to prove or disprove, and how will it affect the practice of BVT?

As there were no recent studies on the relationship, or differences between fresh bee venom and the processed extract (which is sometimes also called bee venom but will be identified here as apitoxin), the AAS proposed to do a chromatographic study of the two products.

The study was conducted at the Université Catholique de Louvain in Brussels, Belgium. Even though the chemical analysis of the compounds is not completed, the differences are already marked. One hypothesis about this difference is that it reflects the activity of the enzymes, occurring naturally in the venom, but becoming activated in the apitoxin. To this first step, we plan to add clinical studies of their therapeutic activity, so as to know their respective indications. The latter are already partially explored.

I want my readers to have access to the best sources of information for all of the therapies that I have undergone in the course of my successful treatment. With that in mind, let's talk a moment about the American Apitherapy Society. As the president of this organization, would you explain its general purpose?

The AAS is a nonprofit membership organization established for the purpose of advancing the investigation of apitherapy, which is the healing use of all of the products of the hive. The AAS accomplishes this first by collecting information on apitherapy and maintaining a library containing printed information, raw data, audiovisual materials, and a database; and second, by informing the medical profession and the general public in matters relating to apitherapy, through the publishing of a periodic newsletter and conducting workshops.

Why would you recommend that people considering BVT contact the AAS? How can the AAS help them?

The AAS is a major source of assistance and regularly updated information about apitherapy in the United States. This help comes as printed information, personal contacts with AAS members practicing some form of apitherapy, and the opportunity to attend workshops and related courses.

Please talk about the "Apitherapy Knowledge Review Course" offered by the AAS. Should those persons considering apitherapy be interested in attending a course such as this one, or is it more applicable to those wishing to become apitherapists?

The AAS will organize for the third year an apitherapy course that will have two levels of knowledge. These courses have recently been renamed the "Charles Mraz Apitherapy Courses" (CMAC) in honor of this learned man, who died on September 6, 1999. They will take place in Salisbury, Maryland, in conjunction with the meetings of the Eastern Apicultural Society. Details will be printed in *Bee Informed*, the journal of the AAS. Anyone interested in apitherapy can take the courses.

Apimondia is the International Federation of Beekeepers Associations. It has seven permanent Commissions. One of them is the Apitherapy Commission, and you are currently its president. Apimondia lists member associations, including the AAS, from several countries across the globe. Could you tell us about Apimondia and its purpose?

Here is a quote from our statutes: "Apimondia is meant to promote apicultural scientific, technical and economic development in all countries and the fraternal cooperation of beekeepers associations and of individual beekeepers the world over. It also aims at putting into practice every initiative that can contribute efficiently to improving beekeeping practice and to rendering the products obtained from this activity profitable."

This federation is one hundred two years old and has some fifty member beekeeper associations. Currently its major contributions are the activities of its seven permanent Commissions and the organization, which holds a congress every other year. Apimondia's statutes are presently being revised with the intention of adapting this respectable institution to the globalized world of today.

There are several Apimondia member associations from European block countries, as well as Japan and Egypt. Is the practice of apitherapy more widely accepted in these locations than in the U.S.? Why or why not?

Apitherapy is far more widely accepted elsewhere. In the U.S., we are still in the dark ages concerning apitherapy. It is not only an unrecognized group of treatments, but is often the object of much fear, particularly regarding BVT. Apitherapy has a long way to go to be put on the scientific map, and this is one of the main missions of the Apitherapy Commission of Apimondia.

The Far East, China in particular, has some eighteen centuries of apitherapy tradition, further assisted by combining it with acupuncture to become Apiacupuncture. Eastern Europe,

Romania, and Russia have more than one hundred years of experience and been active in research and development.

What do you see as the future of apitherapy and BVT as regards the treatment or cure of multiple sclerosis?

For many, apitherapy with emphasis on BVT is their last chance, having exhausted the offering of official medicine. Observation has shown that BVT often results in improvement, sometimes dramatic, occasionally arresting or significantly slowing down the process of deterioration that makes MS into a dreaded illness.

One last question: Is there anyone for whom you would absolutely not recommend BVT, and if so, why?

I never recommend apitherapy, as I have devoted my interest, my passion, to thoroughly investigating it. Furthermore, as a physician, I am keenly aware of its medico-legal status, and therefore, even if inclined to do so, would not recommend it. Apitherapy, and in particular BVT should not be given to whoever does not want it. I would also be extremely careful with acute, unstable conditions of any kind.

I'd like to take this opportunity to openly thank Dr. Cherbuilez for his assistance, the enormous amount of time he donated to this interview, and his sincere desire to assist me in educating all persons, but particularly MS patients, on the benefit of BVT. I strongly encourage all that are interested in apitherapy to explore the work of the American Apitherapy Society and of Apimondia, and to visit their informative Internet web sites. Contact information for Dr. Theodore Cherbuilez and these organizations is included in the resources section.

Now that we've heard from one of the world's leading experts on the subject of apitherapy and BVT in particular, let's take a closer look at one of the risks of BVT, anaphylactic shock. As you have learned through his interview, Dr.

Cherbuilez considers it a very real danger, and although he has performed the procedure hundreds of times, he never ceases to review the emergency procedures that can save lives. His statement that he did not want to have to read up on the emergency measures when he needed them is very sound advice. We will examine anaphylactic shock and the emergency safety procedures in this next section.

Understanding Anaphylactic Shock

BVT is definitely not a "fly by the seat of your pants" operation. There are unquestionably inherent dangers in this type of treatment. Chart 14-2 on page 321 will be helpful to all patients considering BVT as a healing option. You may want to photocopy this chart and keep it handy for reference.

What should you do if you or someone who is undergoing BVT begins to experience these symptoms? Chart 14-3 on page 322 details the emergency steps you should take. I advise to you to make a copy of these emergency procedures and keep it posted near your treatment area, along with your emergency antidote kit.

If you do not know CPR, or cardiopulmonary resuscitation, I strongly suggest you learn. Even if you never decide to pursue BVT, CPR is a valuable, necessary, and lifesaving skill. From the victim of a serious accident to a child falling into a pool, CPR saves lives. You can easily learn this technique from any number of sources. Classes are usually free, have a nominal charge, or request a donation. Your local fire and rescue squads will have information on where you can take a CPR class. Or, you can contact the American Red Cross for further information.

Now that we are familiar with the dangers of anaphylactic shock, let's examine the emergency antidote kit that you should always have on hand, regardless of the length of time that you may have been practicing BVT or your expertise in applying the treatment. Sometimes known as an Allergy Kit, and marketed

Chart 14-2 Symptoms of Anaphylactic Shock

Symptom	Details
Unusual Skin Color	Pale or clammy in appearance or touch
Variable Pulse Rate	Heartbeat alternately races and slows with no activity changes
Confusion	Inability to remember decisions, facts, events, or persons
Dizziness	Inability to stand, bend over, extreme lightheadedness
Nausea or Vomiting	Found in combination with these other symptoms and also accompanied often by diarrhea
Muscle Cramps	Muscles reacting as if after a strenuous workout
Weakness	Lack of basic strength
Wheezing, Labored Breathing	Can be combined with coughing excessively or sneezing
Hives or Rash	Red blotches or pustules appearing on the skin accompanied by itching or burning sensations
Swelling of the face or throat	Similar in appearance to mumps
Fever	Temperature rises and falls, or "spikes" irregularly. Often accompanied by chills, a false feeling of intense cold
Anxiety or Paranoia	Intense feelings of dread or threat from no valid cause
Low Blood Pressure	Drastic variation or drop from normal pressure for the patient
Shock	Pupils wide and dilated, do not react to light. Patient heartbeat irregular and thready. Inability to recognize surroundings, persons, or respond to simple questions. Muscles rigid or completely lax, convulsions possible
Unconsciousness	Complete inability to respond. Breathing becomes shallow, aphasia can occur. Patient totally unaware of surroundings

most widely under the brand names Ana-Kit or Epi Pen, your emergency antidote kit should contain the following:

- **Epinephrine:** Preloaded syringe containing the correct average dosage.
- **Sterile Cotton Swabs and Alcohol Wipes:** For cleaning the area of skin prior to injection of the Epinephrine.
- **Antihistamine Tablets:** To counter minor allergic reactions such as burning or itching.

Chart 14-3 Anaphylactic Shock: Emergency Procedures

1. IMMEDIATELY administer the antidote kit, which contains epinephrine, a controlled prescription substance.
2. IF SYMPTOMS ARE NOT SEVERE, transport the patient to the nearest hospital or regular physician if available.
3. IF SYMPTOMS ARE SEVERE, immediately call 911 Emergency and request an ambulance! Be certain to tell the emergency dispatcher that ANAPHYLACTIC SHOCK is suspected.
4. While waiting for the ambulance, treat the patient for shock!
    A. Lay the patient on the floor or other flat surface where they cannot convulse and fall.
    B. Cover with a medium-weight blanket if indoors, heavy blanket if outdoors.
    C. Place a pillow, rolled coat, or blanket under the knees of the victim to maintain a slight elevation.
    D. Dim lights or create shade for the victim.
    E. Have a safe object handy to insert horizontally between the victim's teeth (like a horse's bit) should convulsions occur. A hard rubber dog bone is ideal, about 6"-8" long. It is safe, and will not break the victim's teeth. It is also easy for you to insert and remove, and cannot be accidentally swallowed.
    F. Perform CPR if necessary.
5. Be SURE to bring to the hospital:
    A. The antidote kit you have used.
    B. The bottle of collected venom you are injecting, or the jar of bees used in treatment.
    C. Any dead bees used in treatment.
    D. List of known patient allergies.

- **Tourniquet:** To tighten around the limb containing the stings to prevent the spread of the venom. Of course, if you are treating your neck or genital area, I do not recommend that you apply the tourniquet!
- **Instructions:** How to use the kit, should you be unable or unavailable to do so.

Always check the expiration date of each medication, and replace those which have expired, even if they appear to be "good." Once you have administered the kit, to yourself or to another patient, *seek medical treatment immediately!* Further lifesaving procedures may be necessary in a hospital environment.

Another useful point to remember, which could become crucial, is to keep your personal information current with your local pharmacy and your physician. As you've learned from reading my personal story, one of the most chilling moments I've ever experienced came when I read the letter of recall from Rite Aid Corporation, the pharmacy who had been supplying me with the Epi Pen. I would never have become aware of the potential danger had my address and telephone number been out of date with the local pharmacy or my doctors. It seems a small point, to be sure, but God is often in the details, and, in an emergency situation, Death could be there also.

As a doctor, I feel that I have a professional and moral obligation to include the following information in this chapter. The danger of anaphylactic shock is very real. I have shown you the complications that can arise from this condition, including death. In the health interest of my readers, I have reproduced the letter I received from the Rite Aid Corporation June 3, 1998 at the end of this chapter. Those of you who have an Epi Pen Kit should carefully check your kit immediately against the lot numbers contained in the letter. If you find that your kit is among those listed as defective, immediately return it to the Rite Aid Pharmacy, or other retail establishment from which you purchased it for a replacement.

Remember: you are dealing with controlled prescription substances, which can cause serious harm or death if used improperly. Defective kits can fail to reverse the effects of a severe allergic reaction, and irreversible harm or fatality can occur before alternate medical treatments can be rendered. I cannot stress enough the importance of vigilance and attention to detail when it comes to these, and all medications, whether prescribed or over-the-counter. Your very health, or the health of your patient, hangs in the balance. Please read this letter carefully. Remember, if you have an Epi Pen or Epi Pen Jr., please go and check the lot number. It could save your life!

Now that you know more about BVT, and have been introduced to apitherapy, you may decide to consider this entirely legitimate healing protocol. Although no one can guarantee the success of any healing therapy, the numbers of persons who have utilized BVT successfully is most encouraging, especially those patients afflicted with MS. Several commercial beekeepers, such as Ferris Apiaries, have Internet web sites, which allow you to order bees and products online and have them shipped directly to your location. Contact information for Ferris Apiaries is provided in the resources section.

We have learned that the ancient practices of BVT and apitherapy do indeed have merit and validity in today's world. I still undergo BVT periodically and would recommend it to any MS patient unless specifically prohibited by your doctor. I do strongly believe that diligent application of BVT and the use of other apitherapy products can aid in ridding the body of this deadly virus and are very positive and productive steps on the road to a cure.

In conclusion, we have learned that the ancient practices of BVT and apitherapy do indeed have merit and validity in today's world. I still undergo BVT periodically and would recommend it to any MS patient unless specifically prohibited by your doctor. The small pain and discomfort felt by the sting of this valuable and beneficial creature cannot possibly compare with the pain of a lifetime, and it would certainly be a shame if this method of treatment were not at least considered by the MS patient.

Although I find BVT and apitherapy to both be extremely beneficial to my present state of excellent health, for me they are a portion of the larger picture. I do not think that BVT is a cure for MS in and of itself. I do, however, strongly believe that diligent application of BVT and the use of other apitherapy products can aid in ridding the body of this deadly virus and are very positive and productive steps on the road to a cure.

The next chapter will examine another important step on my journey to wellness: chiropractic medicine, and how new knowledge and techniques can add up to health, vitality, and a return to a normal life.

RiteAid Corporation   June 3, 1998

Dear Epi Pen User:

The manufacturers of Epi Pen and Epi Pen Jr. have voluntarily instituted a program to withdraw specific defective lots and replace them with new product.

The reason for this withdrawal is that specific lot numbers, distributed between July 1997 and April 1998 may contain a sub-potent dose of epinephrine, which may be ineffective in a medical emergency.

If you received a prescription to EpiPen or EpiPen Jr. during this time, please check the product lot number. If it is one of the following lots please contact your Rite Aid Pharmacist to receive replacement merchandise.

Affected Lots: 7SX208, 7SX209, 7SX216, 7SX217, 7SX194, 7RX204, 7RX223, 7SR247, 7SR265, 7SR286, 7SR292, 7SR293, 7SR317, 7SR318, 7SR321, 7SR342, 7SR355, 7SR356, 7SR358, 7SR370, 7SR371, 7SR378, 7JR242, 7JR243, 7JR289, 7JR290, 7JR323, 7JR362, 7JR374, 7JR375, 8SR004, 8SR077, 8SR078, 7C6214, 7C6279, 7C8277, 7C8381, 7F7221, 7F7262, 7F7380, 7C5238, 7C5376, 7F8391, 7F8220, 7F8263, and 7CA382.

Once again, if your EpiPen or EpiPen Jr. is labeled with one of the above lot numbers it is important for you to contact your Rite Aid Pharmacist to receive a replacement pen.

Should you have any questions, please contact our toll-free drug information line at 1-800-RITE AID.

Thank you.
Your Pharmacist

Section III:
Controlling Your Destiny—Beating MS

15

Life after Dairy: A Practical Guide to Alternate Eating

Now that you have determined to make changes in your eating habits, you will need to implement those changes by adding new and beneficial foods to your diet. Here and in chapter 16 we will explore some interesting choices you might want to consider. In the next chapter we will discuss the nutritional benefits of selected or commonly eaten foods, and how to determine and develop a nutritional program that is right for your metabolic and blood type.

This chapter will deal primarily with menu choices for three classes of people: those who have no dairy restrictions, those who are dairy sensitive or lactose intolerant, and those who have tested IgG positive for cow's milk allergy. I will be listing foods that provide the best sources of dietary calcium, magnesium, and phosphorus for each type of person. Each chart will contain data on the concentration of target minerals, serving size, and preparation method for each food item so that you can choose and combine them to achieve your daily RDA of these essential nutrients.

I have not included the calorie counts on these foods in the charts. As we will explore more fully in chapter 16, calorie counting is not *all* important in maintaining a healthy, balanced system. How your body uses the calories that you eat is so much *more* important. This does not in any way imply that I endorse consuming ten thousand calories a day! I do, however, stress that each person has an *individual* calorie count that is right for them.

For the purposes of this chapter, I have included only the counts for calcium, magnesium, and phosphorus, as those are the nutrients we are trying to replace when dairy, or full dairy, is no longer a viable option. Some of these same foods will be listed again in chapter 16, along with some others. Each chart can be printed for handy reference to customize and plan your optimal diet, depending on your needs.

The information contained in the charts that you will find here, and in the next chapter, are the result of countless hours of research and legwork. I have utilized information gathered from a number of sources in the charts found here and in chapter 16, including the United States Department of Agriculture (USDA 1999), the USDA Food and Nutrition Service, popular fast food chains, and well-known food and candy manufacturers. I have researched almost one thousand separate foods in the process of completing these two chapters, and have included the ones that either provide the best sources of dietary nutrients, or that are commonly consumed by the average American so that you can get a real idea of what you are eating and examine those foods that you may wish to reconsider, increase your intake of, or eliminate.

I have also relied upon the data published in two of the most valuable books that I have found on the subject of the nutritional components of foods, *The Complete Book of Food Counts* (Netzer 1997a), and *The Complete Book of Vitamin and Mineral Counts* (Netzer 1997b). Both of these excellent reference works by nutritional expert Corinne T. Netzer contain exhaustively researched and invaluable data. I highly recommend that you obtain both of these books and keep them with you for reference as you try new foods, whether shopping for food items or while cooking. They are invaluable in planning a healthy diet for yourself and your family, which meets your personal Recommended Dietary Allowance (RDA).

In the beginning, changing your diet can be a big step. It's not easy to break old habits of any kind, and eating habits are arguably the hardest, especially the older you are. You become so accustomed to familiar foods. They are comforting in their sameness, like old friends. Or, they become part of your daily routine, like those morning trips to your favorite deli or donut shop, your favorite lunch places, your stop at the snack machine in the afternoon. The thought of giving all of those up is uncomfortable, unpleasant, and uninspiring, and a big part of the reason why most "diets" fail. Food is so much more than just sustenance. It's a time for social interaction, sensory pleasures, and emotional pleasures as well. A beer at the ballpark, chocolate when you're blue, chicken soup when you're feeling low, holiday cakes and cookies. It's hard to give them up.

Surprisingly, you may find that you may not have to! Well, not all of them, anyway. Let's face it: some of them, regardless of your dairy restrictions, really should go. Every single one of us eats something that we have no business putting into our mouths. Most of the time we know it, too.

I'm really not going to deal with "right" or "wrong" food choices here. This chapter will tell you which choices helped *me* on the road to a cure for MS and give you the information necessary to decide for yourselves. I may never get the opportunity to meet most of you, and reliable doctors do not prescribe for patients that they have never even seen. Read the information in this chapter carefully, and use the charts to plan meals that give you the most benefit, no matter which dietary category fits you best.

Before we examine our dietary choices, let's look at the U.S. Government's chart for the minimum RDA of the nutrients we receive from dairy products, specifically calcium, magnesium, and phosphorus. Remember, this is the national guideline. Your individual requirement may vary according to your metabolism, blood type, and physical state of health. As with any other procedure or healing module I explore in this book, I urge you to consult your family physician or nutritional specialist before instituting any radical changes in your food intake. They will help you plan a diet that fully supplies the nutrient levels that you personally require for optimum health.

Chart 15-1 illustrates the USDA's RDA Guidelines as published for 1999. The USDA, in cooperation with the government of Canada, has been in the process of revising the 1989 standard for RDA. The new allowances, known as DRI, Dietary Reference Intakes, will soon be available for all vitamins and nutrients formerly listed in the RDA, replacing that standard. The DRI reproduced here was released in 1997.

Chart 15-1 USDA DRI—Dietary Reference Intake Guidelines

All Recommended Levels in Milligrams (MG) and IU Units

Age (Years)	Vitamin D	Calcium	Magnesium	Phosphorus
Infants(All)				
0.0-0.5 yr.	5 IU	210mg.	100mg.	30 mg.
0.5-1.0 yr.	5	270	275	75
Children(All)				
1 yr.-3 yr.	5	500	460	80
4 yr.-8 yr.	5	800	500	130
Males				
9-13	5	1300	1250	240
14-18	5	1300	1250	410
19-30	5	1000	700	400
31-50	5	1000	700	420
51-70	10	1200	700	420
71+	10	1200	700	420
Females				
9-13	5	1300	1250	240
14-18	5	1300	1250	360
19-30	5	100	700	310
31-50	5	100	700	320
51-70	10	1200	700	320
71+	10	1200	700	320
Pregnant	*	*	*	+40
Lactating	*	*	*	*

Values are the same as for other women of comparative age.

Please note the following when using these charts: Each of the measurements found in the charts is in standard American measure. If you are outside of the United States, a conversion chart will help you determine your own measurement quantity. The preparation style listed for any item assumes that no additional ingredients, condiments, or seasonings were used in the preparation other than water, unless otherwise specifically noted. Brand names of any products are listed to provide a choice of foods and for reference. The use of the brand name does not in any way imply that I either endorse or detract from the named product, or that I recommend that you eat it or eliminate it from your diet choices. The use of any name also does not imply that it is the best or worst of its particular type of food, either. I simply chose those that I have included as a cross section of commonly found items.

My purpose is to provide intelligent choices in eating situations for today's busy lifestyles. Perhaps it would be better to eat a salad instead of a chocolate nut bar. But, if you're on the seventeenth floor of your building and starving because you already missed lunch, or your shipping manager has just informed you that you need to make three more deliveries before you can knock off for the day, the snack machine in the hall or out on the loading dock may be the only choice you have. One of the things that may surprise you is that some of those snack items may provide several times the punch of a cartload of salad, and may not always be a bad, short-term choice for quick nutrition.

The Best of Dairy: Diets with No Restrictions

With that in mind, let's take a look at our first category of persons and the foods that they should be eating to maintain adequate RDA of dietary calcium, those with no dairy restrictions. What are the best sources of dairy calcium? Which foods have you thought were great, but may be providing less nutrients than you could be getting from another choice? Let's examine some common dairy sources of dietary calcium, magnesium, and phosphorus and see which provide the best amounts of these essentials per serving.

Chart 15-2 on page 335 shows the levels of our three essential nutrients found in several commonly consumed dairy foods. All may be eaten by those with no dairy restrictions, but may not be easily digested by persons with lactose intolerance or milk allergy. We have learned in chapter 13 that even the lactose intolerant can ingest small amounts of these without discomfort or adverse effects, but they are probably not a good idea in any quantity for those who are milk, casein, or bovine serum albumin allergic.

These are some of the most common diary items found on your grocer's shelves. All of these items should be available in a commercial food store, unless otherwise noted. Those items may be unavailable at your local market. Check your health food store or nutritional center.

Sheep's milk per liquid cup is the big winner as far as the maximum amount of measured nutrients is concerned, followed by goat's milk. A cup of either nearly meets the entire daily DRI for most children. However, neither of these is probably readily available at your Mega Food Mart. Additionally, I would not advise IgG allergy positive patients to try these unless they have also been tested for sensitivity. Condensed and evaporated milk are excellent sources of these nutrients and are wonderful base ingredients for cooking.

It is also interesting to note that the low-fat and skim versions of both cow's milk and yogurt are higher in nutrient levels than the whole versions of either. This is good to keep in mind if you are considering weight or daily calorie reduction, but remember that children, particularly younger ones, need many of the elements found in milk fats for growth. Dry milks also contain high levels of nutrients, but read the labels carefully before considering them as an alternative to the liquid variety. Some dried milks have added processors or have had nutrients removed during processing. And, a cheerful

Chart 15-2 Nutrient Content of Liquid Dairy in Serving Measurements

Food Item	Serving	Preparation method	Ca	Mg	P
Cream, Half & Half	2 tbsp.	Low Fat	28 mg	2	24
Cream, Half & Half	2 tbsp.	Whole Fat	32	4	28
Cream, Non-Dairy	3.5 oz.	Liquid, Regular	4	2	59
Cream, Sour	2 tbsp.	Cultured	28	2	20
Cream, Whipped	2 tbsp.	Pressurized Can	6	ND	6
Eggnog, Non-Alcoholic	1 cup	Refrigerated Regular	330	47	278
Milk, Cow	1 cup	1% Fat	300	34	235
Milk, Cow	1 cup	2% Milk Fat	297	33	232
Milk, Cow	1 cup	Skim	302	28	247
Milk, Cow	1 cup	Whole	291	33	228
Milk, Cow, Buttermilk	1 cup	Whole	285	27	219
Milk, Cow, Canned	1 cup	Condensed, Sweetened	868	78	775
Milk, Cow, Canned	1 cup	Evaporated, Skim	738	68	496
Milk, Cow, Canned	1 cup	Evaporated, Whole	658	60	510
Milk, Cow, Chocolate	1 cup	1% Milk Fat	287	33	256
Milk, Cow, Chocolate	1 cup	2% Milk Fat	284	33	254
Milk, Cow, Chocolate	1 cup	Whole	280	33	251
Milk, Cow, Dry	1 oz.	Buttermilk	336	31	265
Milk, Cow, Dry	1 cup	Nonfat	356	31	274
Milk, Cow, Dry	1 cup	Skim	302	28	274
Milk, Cow, Dry	1 oz.	Whole	259	24	220
Milk, Goat HF	1 cup	Whole	326	34	270
Milk, Human **	1 cup	Whole	79	8	34
Milk, Ice Cream	1/2 cup	Chocolate, Hard	72	19	70
Milk, Ice Cream	1/2 cup	Vanilla, Soft	113	11	99
Milk, Ice Milk	1/2 cup	Vanilla, Soft	138	13	106
Milk, Sheep HF	1 cup	Whole	474	45	387
Yogurt	8 fl. oz.	Plain, Low Fat	415	40	326
Yogurt	8 fl. oz.	Plain, Skim	452	43	355
Yogurt	8 fl. oz.	Plain, Whole Milk	274	26	215
Yogurt, Frozen	1/2 cup	Soft Serve, Chocolate	106	19	100
Yogurt, Frozen	1/2 cup	Soft Serve, Vanilla	103	10	93

Key: Ca=Calcium, Mg=Magnesium, P=Phosphorus, ND=No Data Available, HF=Health & Nutrition Stores

** = Average Lactating Mother

note for you holiday revelers: Eggnog is loaded with good nutrients, although it certainly is not the most slimming beverage in the dairy case!

Sadly, no matter how good a mother we, or our spouses, might be, we fall short in these nutrient categories, even more so when we consider that a breast-fed baby does not normally drink a cup of breast milk at a feeding. Human breast milk, however, does provide so many other essential nutrients, not to mention the natural antibodies passed from the mother to the infant, that it still remains the best first food for a human infant. Human infants also require less DRI of all nutrients than older humans, thereby increasing the proportionate ratio of benefits to the infant, even though the numbers per serving are lower in relation to a similar-sized serving of other liquid food sources. And, psychologically, the bond that is forged between a lactating mother and breast-feeding child will last a lifetime, statistically increasing the growth and development potential of the breast-fed infant.

Dairy cheeses are an excellent source of calcium, magnesium, and phosphorus. Persons with no dairy restrictions can enjoy any number of these dairy products. To simplify the reference charts, Chart 15-3 shows the nutrient levels of common curd and soft cheeses only, as these may be enjoyed on a regular basis by persons with no dairy restrictions. Although you may also consume all other types of cheeses as well, I have listed the nutrient counts for semi-hard and hard cheeses in the section for those who are lactose intolerant, as those individuals can usually consume hard and semi-hard cheeses with little or no ill effect.

Again, I have listed only a cross section of the most popular or most nutritious cheeses here. For a more complete guide, I recommend that you purchase the vitamin and mineral food count book I discussed earlier in this chapter, and consult with your doctor or nutritionist. Remember, food is essentially a drug. Although we will explore that statement in more depth in the next chapter, I urge you to plan carefully before instituting sweeping dietary changes. Get yourself tested to determine whether or not you have milk allergies or dairy sensitivity before you begin to alter your diet in any major way. Additionally, a BCI analysis will reveal any existing deficiencies or excesses of these minerals in your body. Save this chapter until you know where you stand, systemically, and then use this and the next chapter to begin to plan your optimum nutritional intake.

Chart 15-3 Selected Nutrient Content of Common Curd and Soft Dairy Cheeses in Serving Measurements

Food Item	Serving	Preparation Method	Ca	Mg	P
Cheese, Soft	1 oz.	American, pasteurized	174 mg	6	211
Cheese, Soft	2 oz.	Bleu Cheese	300	14	220
Cheese, Soft	2 oz.	Brie	104	ND	106
Cheese, Soft	2 oz.	Camembert	220	12	196
Cheese, Curd	1/2 cup	Cottage, Large Curd	68	6	149
Cheese, Curd	1/2 cup	Cottage, 1% Low Fat	69	6	151
Cheese, Soft	2 oz.	Cream	46	4	60
Cheese, Soft	2 oz.	Edam	414	16	304
Cheese, Curd	2 oz.	Feta	280	10	192
Cheese, Soft HF	2 oz.	Goat HF	80	8	146
Cheese, Soft	2 oz.	Muenster	406	16	266
Cheese, Soft	2 oz.	Mozzarella, Whole Milk	294	10	210
Cheese, Soft	2 oz.	Mozzarella, Part Skim	366	14	262
Cheese, Curd	1/2 cup	Ricotta, Whole Milk	257	14	196
Cheese, Curd	1/2 cup	Ricotta, Part Skim	337	18	226

Key: Ca=Calcium, Mg=Magnesium, P=Phosphorus, ND=No Data Available, HF=Health & Nutrition Stores

Here we find some choices that may surprise you. This time, the big winners are two soft and very tasty cheeses, Edam and Muenster. Muenster is extremely popular and can be found in almost all grocery stores and delicatessens. You may want to consider choosing Muenster on your next sandwich instead of American, as a serving of this excellent dietary source contains nearly 35 percent of the DRI of calcium and

20 percent the DRI of phosphorus for young adults, and nearly 50 percent calcium and over 70 percent phosphorus daily DRI for adults, respectively.

Also, you will note that the part skim versions of both mozzarella and ricotta cheeses are higher in nutrient content than the whole milk version, but both versions are high in comparison to other cheeses, which is good news for lovers of Italian-style foods! Bleu cheese also comes up near the top of the list. Next time you're creating or ordering a salad, bleu cheese chunks may be a good thing to add for a quick 25 percent of your daily calcium DRI.

Unfortunately, in this nutrient contest, three old favorites do not score so well. American cheese, white or yellow, contains only average amounts of calcium and phosphorus, and dismal amounts of magnesium, as do our two other dietary standbys: cottage and cream cheese. Many diets swear by cottage cheese, and most restaurants offer it as a selection on their "diet plate" menus. However, as we can see, neither version of cottage cheese contains strong amounts of our nutrients. Many cooks substitute cottage cheese for ricotta when preparing Italian dishes, usually for cost considerations, as cottage is quite a bit less expensive. You may want to reconsider that decision, as nutritionally speaking, you are sacrificing value for price.

Cream cheese, although beloved by millions and consumed eagerly every morning with bagels, crackers, and toast, is the worst source of these nutrients in the soft cheese group. Perhaps a better choice would be spreadable Edam or Camembert. I'm not telling you to give up cream cheese. I am telling you that although marvelously tasty, it is not a primary source of dietary calcium, and you should keep that in mind when planning your diet. Flavored cream cheeses, particularly when mixed with pieces of lox or walnuts and raisins, may fare marginally better in these categories, but don't count on them as a source of the minerals we are concerned with in this chapter.

The previous two charts are only mildly interesting to you if you are milk allergic or one of the millions who suffer from lactose intolerance. For you, fluid milks and curd or soft cheeses are risky business and should be eaten only sparingly, if at all. You'll fare much better with the hard and semi-hard cheese group, which we'll examine next.

Dairy Choices for the Lactose Intolerant

Those of you who do suffer from dairy sensitivity or lactose intolerance will find these next two sections important. We will examine the nutrient count of the cheeses that fall into the hard and semi-hard groups. We have learned that several studies have proven most lactose intolerant persons *can* tolerate servings of these cheeses without experiencing ill effects. The actual amount of each cheese that you can tolerate will probably be determined by your own experimentation. Again, I advise you to work closely with your personal physician or nutritionist. They will be able to monitor you as you begin to try these excellent alternatives to fluid or soft cheeses.

Chart 15-4 illustrates the nutrient contents of the hard and semi-hard cheese groups.

Chart 15-4 Selected Nutrient Content of Common Hard and Semi-Hard Dairy Cheeses in Serving Measurements

Food Item	Serving	Preparation method	Ca	Mg	P
Cheese, Semi-Hard	2 oz.	Cheddar	408 mg	16	290
Cheese, Semi-Hard	2 oz.	Cheddar, Low Fat	236	10	274
Cheese, Semi-Hard	2 oz.	Cheddar, Low Sodium	400	16	274
Cheese, Semi-Hard	2 oz.	Goat	168	16	212
Cheese, Hard HF	2 oz.	Goat HF	508	30	414
Cheese, Semi-Hard	2 oz.	Gouda	396	16	310
Cheese, Hard	1 oz.	Parmesan, grated	390	14	229
Cheese, Hard	2 oz.	Swiss	544	20	342

Key: Ca=Calcium, Mg=Magnesium, P=Phosphorus, ND=No Data Available, HF=Health & Nutrition Stores

This time out, the most popular of our cheeses are also the high scores on the nutrient charts. Swiss rates the highest overall, providing all of the daily calcium required by an average three-year-old, and more than half for kids aged four to eight. A lunch-time sandwich with this universal favorite could be an excellent choice as a source of daily calcium and phosphorus. Again, goat cheese, in the hard variety, scores highly, but is not likely to be found down at the local grocery store.

Another high scorer is the single most popular cheese in the world. Cheddar is used in countless dishes, as a main ingredient, or as a topping. The low-sodium variety contains almost equal nutrient levels, but be aware that the low-fat version has had a large number of the important nutrients removed as well. Low-fat cheddar contains just over half of the calcium of the full-fat variety. Next time you're in the mood for a grilled cheese sandwich, why not consider substituting cheddar for American? It's more easily tolerated by the lactose intolerant, and contains almost four times as many nutrients as an equal serving of American cheese.

Those who are lactose intolerant should read this next section carefully. We will examine those foods that are the best substitutes for dairy calcium, and look at some foods that you may have thought were a good substitute, but that actually rate rather poorly when compared to some others that you may not be familiar with at all.

Life After Dairy—Finding Nutritional Supplements That Work for You

This is the section for those who, like myself, test IgG RAST positive for cow's milk allergy. I can sympathize with what you are feeling right now, especially if you have just been diagnosed. It seems to me that all that I did for the first few weeks after deciding to give up dairy products was to think about them. Everybody that I knew was eating cheese: on their burgers (which I couldn't have either), on their sandwiches, in their salads. I don't remember ever hearing so many ice cream trucks in the neighborhood, and, if I saw one more milk commercial, I was sure I would scream.

The good news is that the feeling does pass. Especially if you find new food friends to put into their place. In the next few charts we will explore alternatives to dairy: as part of your main courses, salads, and snacks. Some of these non-dairy sources of calcium, magnesium, and phosphorus may be completely foreign to you. Some may be surprising old favorites, and, some will amaze you.

First, let's look at the "non-dairy" substitutes. What are these? These are products made from foods that do not fall into the "dairy" group, or products not made from cow's milk. Read "non-dairy" labels carefully. Some of them may contain elements of milk, like casein. Others may contain the milk of other lactating animals, like goats, or sheep, which may contain elements that cause a reaction in dairy-sensitive people. I know I've said this before, but it bears repeating: consult with your doctor or nutritionist before you rush off and purchase these products. Although they may be perfectly healthy alternatives, your health care professional will help you decide which you will receive the most benefit from.

If you have undergone a BCI analysis, this advice becomes doubly significant. Even though it is important to replace the dietary nutrients you will lose when eliminating dairy, it is also imperative that you consider the levels of other elements in your system. Some of these foods may aid in bringing these levels into the normal ranges, but some may drive already high levels even higher, which can generate a whole new list of complications.

Chart 15-5 on page 342 examines the relative nutrient counts of popular non-dairy substitutes.

Some of these may be familiar to you; some may be brand new. There are many national brands of rice or soy milks and beverages like Rice Dream and VitaSoy. Others can be found in health food stores, or in some of the larger grocery store

Chart 15-5 Selected Nutrient Content of Common Non-Dairy Substitutes in Serving Measurements

Food Item	Serving	Preparation Method	Ca	Mg	P
Butter, Almond HF	2 tbsp.	Plain	86 mg	96	168
Butter, Cashew HF	2 tbsp.	Plain	14	82	146
Butter, Peanut	1/2 cup	Chunky Style	13	51	101
Butter, Peanut	2 tbsp.	Smooth Style	12	51	118
Butter, Sesame HF	2 tbsp.	Paste, Whole Seed	308	116	210
Butter, Sunflower Seed HF	2 tbsp.	Regular	38	118	236
Cheese, Vegetarian	2 oz.	Imitation Mozzarella	346	24	330
Cream, Sour	2 tbsp.	Non-Dairy	2	ND	26
Cream, Whipped	2 tbsp.	Non-Dairy	0	0	0
Egg, Imitation	1 oz.	Liquid	15	ND	34
Egg, Imitation	1 oz.	Powder	92	ND	136
Egg, Imitation	1 oz.	Vegetarian Egg Sub.	15.5	ND	25
Margarine	2 tbsp.	Blend, 40% Fat	82	8	64
Margarine	2 tbsp.	Regular, Plain	2	ND	2
Soy Beverage	8 fl. oz.	Eden Soy Extra	196	54	142
Soy Beverage	8 fl. oz.	Eden Soy Extra Vanilla	196	38	92
Soy Beverage	8 fl. oz.	Eden Soy Carob	68	43	105
Soy Beverage	8 fl. oz.	Eden Soy Original	82	55	143
Soy Beverage	8 fl. oz.	Eden Soy Vanilla	62	38	98
Soy Milk	1 cup	Fluid Regular	10	45	117

Key: Ca=Calcium, Mg=Magnesium, P=Phosphorus, ND=No Data Available, HF=Health & Nutrition Stores

chains. I have used Eden Soy products only to compare the relative nutrient levels of the different varieties available. Other brands contain similar counts.

Non-dairy substitutes do not need refrigeration and will be found on the shelves rather than in the refrigerated dairy case. After purchase, however, I recommend that you do refrigerate them. Most of them will taste better if they are chilled. Some butter substitutes will be found in the dairy aisle, others only in health food stores. Be careful when choosing one of these. Get into the habit of reading the nutritional labels. Note how little nutritional value is contained in margarine. Even when blended with animal fat, the value is not impressive. The systems of some people react poorly to the digestion of certain kinds of margarine. It can build up in the intestines. There are better choices.

Sesame butter, for instance, has a nutty flavor, almost like eating a crisp bread stick. It's also loaded with our three important nutrients. Note the serving size: only two tablespoons. Sesame butter can add an interesting taste twist to your baking, as well. Use it either as a spread, or as an ingredient substitute for butter in your favorite vanilla cookie recipe. It's tasty, and a terrific source of the nutrients you need. Almond butter is another good choice, especially for baking. The taste may be a little strong as a spread, unless used sparingly.

What about the substitutes for milk itself? How do these rate as nutritional replacements? We can discount non-dairy whipped toppings or spray creams, except in the area of taste. Some people prefer the taste of a non-dairy topping like Cool Whip to actual whipped cream. But, be aware: that's about as far as it goes. Don't look for nutritional value. It just isn't there.

Soy milk and soy beverages are a decent replacement for cow's milk as regards our specified nutrients. Yes, they do taste different from milk, but, so does Pepsi. They are not at all unpleasant, and some are delicious. You will have to try several different brands until you find the one that you like the best. Soy milk contains the least of our nutrients in the soy beverage group. The soy blend beverages, made from a mixture of rice and soy, are a much better selection, and have a richer flavor. Again, read labels, consult with your doctor or nutritionist, buy small samples, and experiment.

Remember, milk allergy does not always right itself and go away. You may have to make a non-dairy diet a lifetime choice, so choose your substitutes carefully to receive the maximum benefit and the most pleasurable eating experience. It's easy to replace an old food if you find a new one you really like. Also keep in mind that the most enriched soy beverage blends will still score short of the same quantity of milk. You will have to increase your portions in order to maintain the same level of nutrients.

If you are watching your weight, or have levels of other substances that are out of range in your system, increased portions may not be practical. You will have to consider alternate sources of calcium that are non-dairy in addition to these. The next series of charts will review alternate dietary sources of calcium, magnesium, and phosphorus. I have divided them into food types, for easy reference when planning a meal.

Let's begin with one of the best sources of alternate dietary calcium and phosphorus: fish, shellfish, and seafood. Fish is readily available in most areas, in a variety of species and serving styles. Many towns and cities have Japanese restaurants, where a large selection of fishes is always served. Raw bars have also become increasingly popular, and salad bars everywhere have crab legs, seafood salad, and chilled, cooked shrimp. How do these products of the sea compare as alternate sources?

Chart 15-6 compares the nutritional substitute value of a selection of fish and seafood.

Chart 15-6 Selected Nutrients Contained in Fish, Shellfish, and Seafood in Serving Measurements

Food Items	Serving	Preparation method	Ca	Mg	P
Abalone	4 oz.	Fried in Flour	42 mg	64	ND
Anchovy	2 oz.	Canned	104	31	113
Bass, Freshwater	4 oz.	Baked, Broiled, Micro	116	43	290
Bass, Striped	4 oz.	Baked, Broiled, Micro	ND	ND	ND
Bluefish	4 oz.	Baked, Broiled, Micro	10	48	330
Catfish, Farmed	4 oz.	Baked, Broiled, Micro	10	29	278
Catfish, Wild	4 oz.	Baked, Broiled, Micro	12	32	345
Clams, Hard Shell	20 Cherry	Boiled, Poached, Steamed	83	17	304
Clams, Hard Shell	20 Cherry	Breaded, Fried	119	27	353
Clams, Hard Shell	1 cup	Canned	148	30	540
Clams, Hard Shell	20 Cherry	Raw	83	17	304

Food Items	Serving	Preparation method	Ca	Mg	P
Cod, Atlantic	4 oz.	Baked, Broiled, Micro	10	35	253
Cod, Pacific	4 oz.	Baked, Broiled, Micro	10	35	253
Crab, Alaskan	1 lb.	Legs, Boiled, Steamed	67	ND	318
Crab, Blue	4 oz.	Canned	115	44	295
Crab, Dungeness	1.5 oz.	Boiled, Steamed	75	73	222
Fillet	4 oz.	Frozen, Breaded, 2 fillets	22	28	206
Fish, Perch, Ocean	4 oz.	Baked, Broiled, Micro	155	44	314
Haddock	4 oz.	Baked, Broiled, Micro	48	57	273
Haddock, Sticks	5 oz.	Frozen, Breaded, 6 sticks	30	35	255
Haddock, Vegetarian	3 oz.	Frozen, 2 pieces	15	ND	ND
Halibut	4 oz.	Baked, Broiled, Micro	68	121	323
Herring	4 oz.	Baked, Broiled, Micro	84	46	344
Herring	4 oz.	Kippered	95	52	369
Herring	4 oz.	Pickled	87	9	101
Lobster, Most Species	4 oz.	Boiled or Steamed	69	40	210
Lobster, Spiny	4 oz.	Boiled or Steamed	71	ND	260
Mackerel, Atlantic	4 oz.	Baked, Broiled, Micro	17	110	315
Mackerel, Jack	4 oz.	Canned, Drained	273	42	341
Mackerel, Pacific	4 oz.	Baked, Broiled, Micro	33	41	181
Mussels	4 oz.	Boiled, Poached, Steamed	37	42	323
Octopus	4 oz.	Boiled, Poached, Steamed	120	ND	316
Oyster, Atlantic	4 oz.	Baked, Broiled, Micro	ND	52	154
Oyster, Atlantic	4 oz.	Boiled, Steamed	102	108	230
Oyster, Atlantic	1 cup	Raw	112	118	336
Oyster, Pacific	4 oz.	Boiled, Steamed	18	50	276
Oyster, Pacific	5 oz.	Raw, 3 Medium	12	33	243
Perch	4 oz.	Baked, Broiled, Micro	116	43	291
Pike, Northern	4 oz.	Baked, Broiled, Micro	83	ND	320
Pike, Walleye	4 oz.	Baked, Broiled, Micro	160	43	305
Salmon, Atlantic	4 oz.	Baked, Broiled, Micro	17	ND	290
Salmon, Chinook	4 oz.	Baked, Broiled, Micro	32	ND	ND
Salmon, Chinook	4 oz.	Smoked	12	20	186
Salmon, Coho	4 oz.	Baked, Broiled, Micro	14	39	376
Salmon, Pink	4 oz.	Canned w/Bone	242	39	373
Salmon, Sockeye	4 oz.	Baked, Broiled, Micro	8	35	313

Food Items	Serving	Preparation method	Ca	Mg	P
Salmon, Sockeye	4 oz.	Canned w/Bone	271	33	370
Sardine, Atlantic	4 oz.	Can w/Bone, Soybean Oil	433	44	556
Sardine, Pacific	4 oz.	Canned in Tomato Sauce	272	39	415
Scallop, Vegetarian	3 oz.	Canned	5	ND	65
Sea Bass	4 oz.	Baked, Broiled, Micro	15	60	281
Sea Trout	4 oz.	Baked, Broiled, Micro	25	45	364
Shark	4 oz.	Batter, Fried	57	49	220
Shrimp	4 oz.	Boiled, Steamed, Poached	44	38	155
Shrimp	4 oz.	Breaded, Fried	76	45	247
Shrimp	4 oz.	Canned	67	46	264
Shrimp	4 oz.	Raw	60	40	232
Snapper	4 oz.	Baked, Broiled, Micro	45	42	228
Sunfish	4 oz.	Baked, Broiled, Micro	117	43	262
Swordfish	4 oz.	Baked, Broiled, Micro	7	39	382
Trout	4 oz.	Baked, Broiled, Micro	62	32	356
Trout, Rainbow	4 oz.	Baked, Broiled, Micro	ND	35	305
Tuna, Albacore	4 oz.	Canned, in Oil	5	39	303
Tuna, Albacore	4 oz.	Canned, in Water	24	56	373
Tuna, Light	4 oz.	Canned, in Oil	15	35	353
Tuna, Light	4 oz.	Canned, in Water	12	31	185
Tuna, Vegetarian	1/2 cup	Frozen	41	ND	83
Tuna, Yellowfin	4 oz.	Baked, Broiled, Micro	24	ND	245
Tuna, Yellowfin	4 oz.	Baked, Broiled, Micro	24	ND	245
Turbot	4 oz.	Baked, Broiled, Micro	26	74	187
Whiting	4 oz.	Baked, Broiled, Micro	70	31	323

Key: Ca=Calcium, Mg=Magnesium, P=Phosphorus, ND=No Data Available, HF=Health & Nutrition Stores

Almost all of the choices I have listed here are excellent sources of phosphorus, a nutrient found in every fish. Some are better choices than others. Shellfish, such as clams and oysters, contain the greatest amounts of our desired nutrients, and preparation in some cases actually increases the concentrations per serving. Perhaps as a result of their own diet, smaller fresh and saltwater pan or condiment fishes like anchovies, perch, sunfish, and herring have higher nutrient levels per serving than their larger cousins. Salmon, however, is the exception to this case, posting solid numbers per serving, as do mackerel and pike.

Sometimes, differences in origin can make a difference in nutrient content. Although there is not much difference in species of trout, for instance, there are almost twice as many nutrients found in a serving of Walleye pike as are found in the same size serving of Northern pike, and Jack mackerel has several times the calcium of its Atlantic relative. This is exactly why I recommend that you keep a nutritional count book handy. *The Complete Book of Vitamin and Mineral Counts* by Corinne T. Netzer is an excellent choice, full of thousands of foods of all types. Last, note that the vegetarian fish substitutes are no substitute source for our nutrients. Although I have listed only two varieties here, all of the vegetarian fish alternatives do not score well in these mineral classes. As a source of dairy nutrient replacement, I do not recommend any of them.

What about other food types, besides fish and shellfish? Grains are an excellent alternate source of dairy calcium, especially when presented as certain forms of cereals. Not all products made of grain, such as pasta, contain the same value. In fact, an average serving of even the most enriched variety of pasta has no more than 40 mg of calcium in a one-cup cooked serving, and the levels of magnesium and phosphorus are mediocre to below average at best. Let's take a look at some of the products made from grains that are good sources in the next chart, Chart 15-7 on page 348.

Bread, fresh or toasted, does not rate very highly when tested for our target nutrients, except for Navajo Indian fry bread. This delicious corn and maize pita-like item far outstrips its more common cousins in nutritional value. Readers in the southwestern United States and West Coast have a better chance of obtaining fresh samples of this Native American treasure than do their East Coast or Midwestern neighbors. However, bread crumbs do contain an appreciable amount of

Chart 15-7 Selected Nutritional Counts of Grains in Milligrams

Food Items	Serving	Preparation Method	Ca	Mg	P
Bread, Croutons	1/2 cup	Seasoned	38 mg	17	56
Bread, Crumbs	1 cup	Dry, Grated, Seasoned	119	45	160
Bread, French	1 slice	Fresh or Toasted	19	7	26
Bread, High Calcium	1 slice	Fresh or Toasted	130	7	15
Bread, Italian	1 slice	Fresh or Toasted	23	8	31
Bread, Navajo Indian HF	5" Round	Fried	210	15	141
Bread, Pita	6 1/2" Round	Fresh or Toasted	52	16	58
Bread, Pita, Wheat	6 1/2" Round	Fresh or Toasted	10	44	115
Bread, Pumpernickel	1 slice	Fresh or Toasted	22	17	57
Bread, Rye	1 slice	Seeded or Unseeded	23	13	40
Bread, Wheat	1 slice	Fresh or Toasted	20	24	64
Bread, White, Regular	1 slice	Fresh or Toasted	27	6	23
Cereal, Dry, Bran	1 cup	All Bran	200	240	288
Cereal, Dry, Bran w/Fruit	1 cup	Bran Flakes w/ Raisins	40	80	191
Cereal, Dry, Corn	1 cup	Corn Flakes	0	0	0
Cereal, Dry, Mixed Grain	1 cup	Mixed Grain Flakes	0	32	86
Cereal, Dry, Mixed Grain	3/4 cup	Mix Grain Flakes w/Honey	40	60	149
Cereal, Dry, Mixed Grain	1 cup	Mix Grain Flakes, Toasted	0	16	61
Cereal, Dry, Oat	3 oz.	Life	279	138	486
Cereal, Dry, Rice	1 1/4 cups	Crispy Rice	0	8	36
Cereal, Dry, Wheat	1 cup	Shredded, Small, Frosted	0	60	160
Cereal, Dry, Wheat	1 cup	Multi-Grain Blend	0	40	117
Cereal, Rolled Oat	1 pkt.	Instant Quaker Oats	170	39	140
Cereal, Rolled Oat	2/3 cup	Quaker Oats, Cooked	115	38	130
Cereal, Oat Bran	1 cup	Cooked	22	88	262
Cereal, Wheat Bran	1 cup	Crude	44	366	608
Corn, Tortilla	7" Round	Plain	44	16	79
Oatmeal	1 cup	Cooked	20	56	178
Rice, Wild	1/2 cup	Cooked	3	26	67
Wheat Germ	1/2 cup	Crude	22	136	478
Wheat Germ	1/2 cup	Toasted	26	182	650

Key: Ca=Calcium, Mg=Magnesium, P=Phosphorus, ND=No Data Available, HF=Health & Nutrition Stores the nutrients we need to replace, and you can find those anywhere, even in gas station quickie marts. When combined with selected items from the meat or fish charts, they are a quick, and relatively low-calorie way to add some extra nutrients when planning a meal.

Cereals can also be an excellent alternative supply, although not all of them. Corn flake cereals may be an old-time favorite, and a solid source of several other vitamins and minerals your body needs, but they contain no appreciable levels of our targets, nor does the snap, crackle, and pop of crispy rice cereals. On the other end of the scale, one of the best cereal sources is oatmeal and other rolled oat, cooked cereals. The instant varieties have been additionally fortified, and contain significant amounts of calcium, magnesium, and phosphorus. Although I have listed only one of them here for reference, there are many delicious varieties available for you to try. Easy to prepare, they are an excellent quick source of nutrition when you don't have the time to prepare a more complex meal.

Wheat germ and bran are good choices as well. Bran cereals score higher in these nutrients than almost any other cereal type. A single one-cup serving of Kellogg's All Bran contains twenty percent of the average DRI of calcium, about thirty-five percent of magnesium, and almost one hundred percent of the phosphorus daily requirements for women between the ages of nineteen and fifty. And, Quaker Life oat cereal contains about twenty to thirty percent of the daily DRI for calcium and magnesium, and exceeds the phosphorus requirement for both males and females under eighteen years of age. Read the labels carefully. Some of the most popular cereals on the market may not be as "healthy" or "nutritious" as their names claim. Again, a food count book is invaluable, as it will list most of the popular national brands by variety and brand name.

Once again, as with any of our alternate food choices, balance is the key to success. If you do not balance the mineral and nutrient levels in your system, it cannot function in an optimum state. Just because oatmeal is an excellent source of our target minerals, I am not suggesting that you eat oatmeal every day to the exclusion of all else. Oatmeal does not provide as high a content of other nutrients your body requires, such as vitamin C or iron, for instance. You need to choose a variety of foods in order to develop a balanced diet that meets your individual requirements. If you have an excess of iron in your system, you would want to limit the choices of those foods that may be high in calcium but may also be very high in iron, like some fishes. When you have brought your iron level back into line, you would want to consider adding some of the foods that are high in both nutrients to maintain an average level of each in your body.

Grain products, particularly flours, are a reliable alternative to dairy nutrient sources. Some, however, are far more valuable than others when it comes to securing our prime ingredients. Chart 15-8 on page 351 illustrates some of the more common flours, and how they stack up in nutrient value.

Notice the broad range of values found in these baking flours. Surprisingly, white self-rising flour contains the most of our target nutrients and is available in every grocery store. Enriched white, however, doesn't score nearly as well, nor does whole grain wheat flour, also known as brown flour. Cottonseed flour is the best of the alternate group per one-cup serving. Notice, however, that when the fat has been removed from cottonseed flour, the target nutrient levels are cut by two thirds. Combined in baking with self-rising white flour, the nutritional value of a roll or baked good almost doubles per serving. Carob flour scores highly and is a good alternate baking choice for those who wish to avoid the calories in chocolate and sugars. Soy flour does not rate as highly as the wheat family, but still measures appreciably better than other choices and is a good selection for those who are wheat-allergy positive. Plain, dark rye flour rates more highly than average and is excellent for baking any number of breads and rolls.

Chart 15-8 Selected Nutrient Content of
Common Flours in Serving Measurements

Food Item	Serving	Preparation Method	Ca	Mg	P
Flour, Buckwheat	1 cup	Plain	49 mg	301	404
Flour, Carob HF	1 cup	Plain	359	56	81
Flour, Corn	1 cup	Mesa Enriched	161	125	255
Flour, Corn	1 cup	Whole Grain	8	109	318
Flour, Cottonseed HF	1 oz.	Low Fat	135	203	451
Flour, Cottonseed HF	1 cup	Partially Defatted	449	677	1501
Flour, Cracker Meal	1 cup	Plain	27	28	120
Flour, Pancake, Mix	2.6 oz.	Two 4" Cakes, Unprepared	96	14	254
Flour, Peanut HF	1 cup	Defatted	84	222	456
Flour, Peanut HF	1 cup	Low Fat	78	29	ND
Flour, Rice, Brown HF	1 cup	Plain	18	177	533
Flour, Rice, White HF	1 cup	Plain	16	55	155
Flour, Rye, Dark HF	1 cup	Plain	72	318	809
Flour, Rye, Light HF	1 cup	Plain	21	72	198
Flour, Sesame HF	1 cup	High Fat	45	102	229
Flour, Sesame HF	1 cup	Low Fat	42	96	215
Flour, Soy HF	1 cup	Full Fat	175	364	420
Flour, Soy HF	1 cup	Low Fat	165	202	522
Flour, Sunflower Seed HF	1 cup	Plain	91	277	551
Flour, Wheat	1 cup	Whole Grain	40	166	415
Flour, Wheat, White	1 cup	Cake Flour	16	18	93
Flour, Wheat, White	1 cup	Enriched, All Purpose	18	27	135
Flour, Wheat, White	1 cup	Self Rising	422	24	744
Flour, Wheat, White	1 cup	Tortilla	228	23	233

Key: Ca=Calcium, Mg=Magnesium, P=Phosphorus, ND=No Data Available, HF=Health & Nutrition Stores

Some of these are old favorites, commercially available in all grocery stores. Others, like the rye flours, will be found in larger chain stores with gourmet baking aisles, and some, like sunflower and sesame flour, will be found only in health food stores. You can also obtain quantities of the more unusual flours from health food catalog suppliers or on the Internet at several health food distributor web sites. These ship the products directly to your home, an excellent idea if you are disabled, elderly, or live in a rural area that does not provide the more exotic foods found in health stores.

Another necessity in most cooking and baking dishes is oil. Whether as part of a salad dressing or as a baking ingredient or frying method, oil is a significant part of the average diet. As far as our nutrient replacement project is concerned, two tablespoons of corn, olive, peanut, safflower, hydrogenated soybean, or sunflower oils contain no measurable amounts of calcium, magnesium, or phosphorus. Choosing the type of oil you use will be a concern for other nutrients, but we will leave that discussion for the next chapter.

Are oils a better choice for replacement sources than the nuts and seeds that they originate from, or does it make that much of a difference? Chart 15-9 illustrates that they are not the better choice when it comes to these three nutrients. Without fail, the natural form of the oils, nut or seed, contains all of our targets, some in high quantities. I have also included the counts for other nuts not normally made into oils. Note that a small serving of these is a tasty way to put the desired minerals into your system, and they are easily included as a salad garnish, a nutritious snack, or an addition to baked goods.

Nuts are an excellent snack choice for several reasons. All nuts are nutritious, and even the higher-calorie varieties like cashew are a relatively low-calorie choice compared with some other snack foods that do not provide nearly as much nutritional benefit. I have included listings for each nut in their most popular commercially available preparation. Almost all of them can be found in a local grocery store and in all of the larger food stores.

Seeds are also exceptional sources of calcium, magnesium, and phosphorus. Seeds also make nutritious low-calorie snacks and are easy to add to salads or vegetable dishes for an interesting taste twist. Seeds are also terrific when baking, especially sesame, which combines high taste with relatively small serving size.

Chart 15-9 compares nuts and seeds as a source of alternatives to dairy.

Chart 15-9 Selected Nutrients in Common Nuts and Seeds in Serving Measurements

Food Item	Serving Size	Preparation Method	Ca	Mg	P
Nut, Almond, Blanched	1 oz.	Dried	70 mg	81	151
Nut, Almond, Blanched	1 oz.	Dry Roasted	80	86	156
Nut, Almond, Blanched	1 oz.	Oil Roasted	55	82	164
Nut, Almond, Unblanched	1 oz.	Dried	75	84	148
Nut, Almond, Unblanched	1 oz.	Oil Roasted	66	86	155
Nut, Brazil	1/2 cup	Unblanched, Shelled	123	164	420
Nut, Cashew	1/2 cup	Dry Roasted	31	178	335
Nut, Cashew	1/2 cup	Oil Roasted	27	166	277
Nut, Chestnut, European	1/2 cup	Roasted, about 8	21	24	72
Nut, Filbert	1/2 cup	Chopped	108	164	180
Nut, Filbert	3 oz.	Dry or Oil Roasted	165	252	276
Nut, Macadamia	1/2 cup	Dried	47	77	91
Nut, Mixed, w/ Peanuts	1/2 cup	Dry Roasted	48	154	298
Nut, Mixed, w/ Peanuts	1/2 cup	Oil Roasted	77	167	329
Nut, Mixed, w/o Peanuts	1/2 cup	Oil Roasted	77	180	323
Nut, Peanut, Spanish	1/2 cup	Oil Roasted	73	123	285
Nut, Peanut, Standard	1/2 cup	Dry Roasted	39	128	261
Nut, Peanut, Standard	1/2 cup	Oil Roasted	63	133	372
Nut, Peanut, Standard	1/2 cup	Raw, Shelled	67	123	274
Nut, Pecan	3 oz.	Dry Roasted	30	117	258
Nut, Pecan	1/2 cup	Oil Roasted	18	71	162
Nut, Pecan	1/2 cup	Raw, Shelled	20	69	157
Nut, Pistachio	1/2 cup	Dried	86	102	322
Nut, Pumpkin Seed	1/2 cup	Kernels, Roasted	49	606	1330
Nut, Sesame Seed	3 oz.	Kernels, Toasted	111	294	660
Nut, Sesame Seed	3 oz.	Whole, Toasted	843	303	543
Nut, Sunflower Seed	1/2 cup	Dried, Kernels	84	254	508
Nut, Sunflower Seed	1/2 cup	Dry Roasted, Kernels	45	83	739
Nut, Sunflower Seed	1/2 cup	Oil Roasted, Kernels	38	85	769
Nut, Walnut, Black	1/2 cup	Shelled, Chopped	36	126	290

Food Item	Serving Size	Preparation Method	Ca	Mg	P
Nut, Walnut, English	1/2 cup	Shelled, Pieces	57	101	190
Nut, Water Chestnut	1/2 cup	Chinese, Can, Sliced	3	3	14
Nut, Water Chestnut	1/2 cup	Chinese, Raw, Sliced	7	14	39
Olive, Manzanilla	1.6 oz.	About 10 Large	39	2	1
Olive, Sevilano	1.6 oz.	About 10 Jumbo	78	ND	ND

Key: Ca=Calcium, Mg=Magnesium, P=Phosphorus, ND=No Data Available, HF=Health & Nutrition Stores

You can clearly see that the original seeds or nuts of popular oils contain far more nutritional value than their processed products. Dried sunflower seeds are an above-average choice as a mineral source, whereas sunflower oil contains no appreciable levels of any of our target nutrients. The same is true for peanuts. Peanut oil measures no more than the sunflower or corn varieties, but peanuts, especially Spanish peanuts, rate substantial levels per serving in their natural form. A bag of roasted Spanish peanuts is a wonderful snack idea, full of value and delicious. They are an especially good selection for busy urban professionals. Roasted Spanish peanuts can be had from any number of sidewalk vendors in most large cities, or at fairs and carnivals across the country.

The clear winners in the nut and seed category are pumpkin and sesame seeds. Pumpkin seeds contain 300 percent to nearly 500 percent of the daily DRI for phosphorus for all ages and genders in a 1/2 cup serving. Add these to your pumpkin bread or muffins, or use them as a topping for pies or rolls. They are tasty and full of value. The same is true for sesame seeds. A lot of taste is packed into these small kernels. You will find throughout the nutritional charts in this book that sesame oil, butter, and flour all rate significantly in each category. Sesame seeds are loaded with the minerals we are concerned with here. Whether combined in salads, rolls, cakes, cookies, or as a stand-alone snack, sesame seeds are a splendid replacement for your lost dairy supplements.

We're beginning to see that dairy, although still the best source of dietary calcium, magnesium, and phosphorus in the ideal naturally occurring proportions, can be adequately replaced by alternate sources. But, are these the only alternatives? A balanced diet is more than seeded rolls. One-half cup of pistachio nuts may be nutritious and tasty, but they are hardly filling. High-nutrient breads and rolls are also sensible selections, but they do not help those who do not metabolize high-carbohydrate foods well. How about fruits and vegetables? How do they stack up in our dairy replacement project?

Fruit is an essential part of all human diets, rich in vitamin C, vitamin A, and other important nutrients, but fruit doesn't score highly in our specific minerals. Again, balance is the key. Do not discount fruit as a good food choice because it may not contain much calcium. In the next chapter we look at other vitamins, minerals, and nutrients that fruit does contain that are an essential part of the nutrients necessary for system balance.

Chart 15-10 illustrates the selected nutrient content of popular fruits.

Chart 15-10 Selected Nutrients in Common Fruits in Milligrams

Food Item	Serving	Preparation Method	Ca	Mg	P
Apple	1/2 cup	Dried, Sulfured	6 mg	7	17
Apple	Medium	Raw, Unpeeled	10	6	10
Apricot	1/2 cup	Dried, Sulfured	30	31	76
Apricot	1/2 cup	Fresh, Pitted	11	12	30
Avocado, California	Med., 8 oz.	Fresh	19	70	73
Avocado, Florida	Med., 8 oz.	Fresh	33	104	119
Blackberry, Fresh	1/2 cup	Trimmed	23	14	15
Blackberry, Frozen	1/2 cup	Unsweetened	22	17	23
Dates	2.9 oz.	About 10 Dates	27	29	33
Figs	1/2 cup	Dried, Uncooked	143	59	68
Figs	6.6 oz.	Fresh, about 10 Figs	269	111	128
Grapefruit, Red/ Pink	8.5 oz.	Fresh, 1/2 Large	13	10	11
Grapefruit, White	8.5 oz.	Fresh, 1/2 Large	14	11	9
Melon, Cantaloupe	1/2 fruit	5" Round Melon	28	28	45
Melon, Honeydew	8 oz.	Fresh, Sliced	8	9	13

Food Item	Serving	Preparation Method	Ca	Mg	P
Melon, Watermelon	1/2 cup	Fresh, Cubed	7	9	7
Milk, Coconut	1 cup	Grated w/ Water	39	89	240
Milk, Coconut	1 cup	Juice Only	58	60	49
Orange, California	1 medium	All Varieties	52	13	18
Orange, California	1 medium	Navel	56	15	27
Orange, California	1 medium	Valencia	48	12	21
Orange, Florida	1 medium	All varieties	65	15	18
Papaya	1/2 cup	Peeled, cubed	17	7	4
Peach	1/2 cup	Fresh, Sliced	5	6	11
Peach, Dehydrated	1/2 cup	Dried, Sulfured	22	33	94
Peach, Freestone	1/2 cup	Canned in Juice	8	9	22
Pear, Bartlett	1/2 cup	Canned in Juice	11	9	15
Pear, Bartlett	1/2 cup	Fresh, Sliced	10	5	9
Pear, Dehydrated	1/2 cup	Dried, Sulfured	30	30	63
Pineapple	1/2 cup	Chunks, Canned in Juice	17	18	8
Pineapple	1/2 cup	Fresh, Sliced, Chunks	6	11	6
Pineapple	1/2 cup	Frozen, Sweetened, Chunks	11	12	5
Prune	1/2 cup	Canned, Heavy Syrup	20	17	30
Prune	4 oz.	Dried, Cooked, Sweetened	24	22	37
Prune	4 oz.	Dried, Pitted	58	51	90
Raisins, Golden	1/2 cup	Dried	38	26	84
Raisins, Seeded	1/2 cup	Dried	21	22	55
Raisins, Unseeded	1/2 cup	Dried	36	24	70
Rhubarb	1/2 cup	Fresh, Chopped	52	7	9
Rhubarb	1/2 cup	Frozen, Cooked, Sweetened	174	15	10
Strawberry	1/2 cup	Fresh	11	8	14
Strawberry	1/2 cup	Frozen	12	8	10
Tangerine	1/2 cup	Canned	14	14	13
Tangerine	1/2 cup	Fresh	14	12	10

Key: Ca=Calcium, Mg=Magnesium, P=Phosphorus, ND=No Data Available, HF=Health & Nutrition Stores

Some fruits do rate significantly in our categories. In almost all varieties, the natural, dried form will rate the highest. Any of these can be added to prepared dishes for extra flavor, texture, and nutrition. They are easily obtained and prepared, and you can portion them out into small plastic food bags and take them with you to work, or place some dried fruits and nuts into a candy dish for those run-through snackers in your family.

Your grandmother probably told you that rhubarb was good for what ails you. Well, grandma, not surprisingly, was right. Rhubarb is a considerable source of our nutrient friends, especially the frozen variety, which makes it a convenient addition to fruit dishes.

Figs, dried or fresh, tally the richest counts in all categories. A staple of the diet of Mediterranean and Middle Eastern peoples for centuries, figs abound in flavor, texture, and nutrients. The Bible mentions John the Baptist as living in the wilderness on wild locusts and honey. Well, although "locust" is the common modern-day term for a winged insect, John was actually eating a type of wild fig, plentiful in the hills surrounding Galilee and still found in abundance in Israel, Egypt, and throughout Palestine today. And, although plums and apricots fall below average here, prunes and dried apricots calculate very well, as do the dried versions of peaches and pears. Larger grocery stores all carry the dried variety of these fruits, normally stocked in the produce section.

Oranges do very respectably in these categories. Valencia and navel varieties total the greatest values per serving, but all oranges place above average for the fruit group. Homeowners would do well to consider the addition of a few orange trees on the property in climate areas where this is feasible. Along with these minerals, oranges are a wonderful source of vitamins, and make a healthy snack choice for kids and adults, especially if grown right in your own yard. Fig trees, by the way, also thrive in a like climate, and make beautiful, large shade trees along with a valuable food source.

Last but not least in our fruit group is the beloved raisin. Probably one of the single most popular fruits, raisins are found in thousands of recipes. In their fresh form, grapes are not impressive sources for calcium, magnesium, or phosphorus.

But, when dried, raisins answer the nutrient call. Golden, from dried white grapes, rate the best here, but the dark varieties are close behind, seeded just edging out unseeded in the final tally. Rich in texture, each tiny fruit is additionally loaded with flavor and value. When considering a snack for kids, raisins are always a fine selection, especially for toddlers. Raisins are very easy for little fingers to handle and little teeth to chew. They are small, so choking dangers are greatly reduced.

Those of you who are watching your sugar and carbohydrate intake may wish to go easy on the amount of fruits you add to your overall diet or the quantity of fruit you consume at any one time. You would be better advised to include more vegetables when seeking to replace dietary nutrients formerly supplied by dairy. How do vegetables measure up in our nutrient categories?

Although I have researched the mineral values of almost two hundred different vegetables and their popular serving forms, for ease of reference, I have included only those that contain more than 20 mg. of calcium per average serving. For some selections, I have only included the commonly found form of the vegetable, which contains the highest rating in each category. For instance, green beans, when canned, contain only 18 mg. of calcium per serving, but a serving of the same vegetable in frozen, precut style contains 33 mg. per serving. Therefore, only frozen green beans are listed here.

For a complete listing of the relative amounts of minerals per serving, regardless of the preparation method or purchase style, and, at the risk of sounding like a broken record, I urge you to purchase a vitamin and mineral food count book. Get a paperback version, and take it with you to the grocery store until you become familiar with the nutrient level ranges of your different choices.

If you do not see your favorite vegetable listed in Chart 15-11, it simply means an average one-half cup serving contains less than 20 mg. of calcium in any form, and should not be considered a significant source of these nutrients in a dairy replacement diet.

Chart 15-11 Selected Nutrients in Common Vegetables Containing Greater Than 20 mg. of Calcium per Average Serving

Food Item	Serving	Preparation Method	Ca	Mg	Ph
Artichoke, Hearts	1/2 cup	Fresh, Boiled	38	51	72
Beans, Baked	8 oz.	Plain, Vegetarian	114	73	236
Beans, Baked	8 oz.	w/Pork	119	77	246
Beans, Black	1/2 cup	Boiled	24	60	120
Beans, Chickpeas	1/2 cup	Canned	39	35	108
Beans, Chickpeas	1/2 cup	Fresh, Boiled	40	39	137
Beans, Great Northern	1/2 cup	Canned	69	67	178
Beans, Great Northern	1/2 cup	Fresh, Boiled	60	44	145
Beans, Green	1/2 cup	Fresh, Boiled, Steamed	29	16	24
Beans, Green	1/2 cup	Frozen, Boiled, Steamed	33	16	21
Beans, Kidney, Red	1/2 cup	Canned	55	65	213
Beans, Kidney, Red	1/2 cup	Fresh, Boiled	25	40	125
Beans, Lima	1/2 cup	Canned	35	42	88
Beans, Lima, Baby	1/2 cup	Dried, Boiled	26	49	116
Beans, Navy	1/2 cup	Canned	62	61	176
Beans, Navy	1/2 cup	Dried, Boiled	64	53	143
Beans, Peas, Green	1/2 cup	Fresh, Boiled, Steamed	22	31	94
Beans, Peas, Snow	1/2 cup	Fresh, Boiled, Steamed	33	21	44
Beans, Peas, Snow	1/2 cup	Fresh, Trimmed	31	17	38
Beans, Peas, Snow	1/2 cup	Frozen, Boiled, Steamed	48	22	46
Beans, Pink	1/2 cup	Dried, Boiled	44	55	139
Beans, Pinto	1/2 cup	Dried, Boiled	41	47	136
Beans, Soybean, Dried	1/2 cup	Boiled	88	74	211
Beans, Soybean, Dried	1/2 cup	Dry Roasted	232	196	558
Beans, Soybean, Dried	1/2 cup	Roasted	119	125	312
Beans, Soybean, Kernels	1/2 cup	Roasted or Toasted	75	93	196
Beans, Soybean, Sprout	1/2 cup	Raw	23	25	57
Beans, Soybean, Sprout	1/2 cup	Steamed	28	28	63
Beans, White	1/2 cup	Canned	96	67	120
Beans, White	1/2 cup	Fresh, Boiled	81	57	102
Beans, Yellow	1/2 cup	Dried, Boiled	66	61	152
Broccoli, Fresh	6.3 oz.	Boiled, Spears	83	43	107
Broccoli, Fresh	1/2 cup	Chopped	21	11	29

Food Item	Serving	Preparation Method	Ca	Mg	P
Broccoli, Frozen	1/2 cup	Boiled, Chopped	47	19	51
Broccoli, Frozen	3 oz.	Boiled, Spears	42	17	46
Brussels Sprouts	1/2 cup	Fresh, Boiled	28	16	44
Cabbage, Green	1/2 cup	Boiled	23	6	12
Cabbage, Red	1/2 cup	Boiled	28	8	21
Cabbage, Sauerkraut	1/2 cup	Canned	36	15	23
Cabbage, Savoy	1/2 cup	Boiled	22	17	24
Cabbage, Chinese	1/2 cup	Boiled (Bok Choy)	79	9	25
Cabbage, Chinese	1/2 cup	Raw, Shredded (Bok Choy)	37	7	13
Carrot, Baby	1/2 cup	Frozen, Boiled	21	7	19
Carrot, Mature	1/2 cup	Boiled	24	10	24
Celery	1/2 cup	Chopped	32	9	19
Cucumber	1 medium	Raw, Sliced w/ Peel	43	33	60
Falafel	1 patty	Frozen, Regular Size	9	14	33
Hummus	1 cup	Regular	124	71	275
Kale	1/2 cup	Boiled	47	12	18
Kale	1/2 cup	Frozen, Boiled	90	12	18
Kale	1/2 cup	Raw, Chopped	46	12	19
Kale, Scotch	1/2 cup	Boiled	86	37	25
Kale, Scotch	1/2 cup	Raw, Chopped	70	30	21
Leeks	1/2 cup	Fresh, Chopped	30	14	18
Mustard Greens	1/2 cup	Fresh, Boiled	52	10	29
Mustard Greens	1/2 cup	Frozen, Boiled	75	10	18
Okra	1/2 cup	Fresh, Boiled	50	46	45
Okra	1/2 cup	Frozen, Boiled	88	47	42
Okra	1/2 cup	Raw, Sliced	41	28	32
Onion, Scallion	1/2 cup	Fresh, Chopped	36	10	18
Potato, All Purpose	1/2 cup	Mashed w/Whole Milk	28	19	50
Potato, All Purpose	1/2 cup	Microwaved in Skin	22	54	212
Potato, Sweet	1 medium	Baked w/Skin	32	23	62
Potato, Sweet	1/2 cup	Boiled w/o Skin	35	16	44
Potato, Sweet	1/2 cup	Canned, Mashed	38	31	67
Rutabaga	1/2 cup	Boiled, Mashed	41	20	48
Rutabaga	1/2 cup	Raw, Cubed	33	16	41
Sauce, Tomato	1/2 cup	Canned, Marinara	22	30	44

Food Item	Serving	Preparation Method	Ca	Mg	P
Sauce, Tomato	1/2 cup	Canned, Spaghetti	35	30	45
Seaweed, Agar	1 oz.	Dried	177	218	15
Seaweed, Kelp	3 oz.	Raw	144	102	36
Seaweed, Wakame	3 oz.	Raw	129	90	69
Spinach	1/2 cup	Boiled, Chopped	122	79	50
Spinach	1/2 cup	Frozen, Boiled, Leaf	139	65	46
Spinach	1/2 cup	Raw, Chopped	28	22	14
Spinach, New Zealand	1/2 cup	Boiled, Chopped	43	29	20
Squash, Acorn	1/2 cup	Baked, Cubed	45	43	46
Squash, Acorn	1/2 cup	Boiled, Mashed	32	31	33
Squash, Acorn	1/2 cup	Raw, Cubed	23	23	25
Squash, Butternut	1/2 cup	Fresh, Boiled, Cubed	42	30	27
Squash, Butternut	1/2 cup	Frozen, Boiled, Mashed	23	11	17
Squash, Crookneck	1/2 cup	Boiled, Sliced	24	.22	35
Squash, Pumpkin	1/2 cup	Canned, Drained	32	28	42
Swiss Chard	1/2 cup	Boiled	51	76	29
Tofu	1/2 cup	Firm	258	118	239
Tofu	1/2 cup	Regular	130	127	120
Tomato, Red	1/2 cup	Canned, Stewed	42	15	25
Tomato, Red	1/2 cup	Canned, Wedges	34	15	31
Tomato, Red, Paste	1/2 cup	Plain	46	67	104
Tomato, Sun Dried	1/2 cup	Oil Packed	25	45	77
Tomato, Sun Dried	1/2 cup	Plain	30	52	96
Turnip, Greens	1/2 cup	Boiled, Chopped	99	16	21
Turnip, Greens	1/2 cup	Frozen, Boiled	125	21	27
Turnip, Greens	1/2 cup	Raw, Chopped	53	9	12
Turnip, Yellow	1/2 cup	Boiled, Mashed	26	9	22

Key: Ca=Calcium, Mg=Magnesium, P=Phosphorus, ND=No Data Available, HF=Health & Nutrition Stores

Even in this abbreviated form, we can see that vegetables do provide a significant supply of our target minerals, in some forms and in some cases. For overall value, beans rate the most highly. Canned, baked beans score wonderfully well, in all varieties, from our old favorites made with pork pieces to the vegetarian style. Other legumes are just as healthy in our categories, particularly the red kidney, great northern, navy, and white varieties. A staple portion of the South American and Mexican diets, as well as the diet of many Native Americans, these beans provide an excellent source of alternate protein along with our selected minerals. A good choice for an overall balanced diet would be to include a bean-based entree as a main meal at least once a week.

Another superior alternative is the versatile soybean, in all forms. Tofu, made from soybean curd, has an extremely high count in all of our categories, and can be fashioned into just about anything, from burger patties to cubes for soups, like Chinese Hot and Sour. Southern, or soul food style cooking also shows great value in these categories. Okra, mustard greens, and turnip greens provide high mineral levels and also contain many other vitamins necessary to overall health.

The best source for all of our target nutrients, after beans, is leafy green vegetables, whether land or marine species. Popeye told us that he was "strong to the finish 'cause I eats me spinach . . ." Poor grammar, true, but great nutritional advice! Spinach, and its close cousin, Swiss chard, are packed with our big three. Other leafy greens, like Chinese bok choy cabbage and kale, in the Scotch or standard varieties, also contain significant amounts of dietary calcium, magnesium, and phosphorus. However, interestingly enough, when boiled, these three in particular almost double their nutrient counts per serving. Broccoli, long heralded as an excellent source, contains healthy levels in these categories, and rates much better than does the average vegetable, but not as well as the leafy greens or beans.

Marine greens deliver the highest counts, in all categories. Seaweeds are rich in all of our desired nutrients. Obtainable for home cooking from better health food stores and some fish markets, seaweed can be delicious when prepared correctly. A wonderful source for this excellent dietary choice can be found in Japanese restaurants. Many Japanese soups and sushi varieties are prepared with seaweed. Seaweeds can also be purchased in pill supplement form, if obtaining the fresh variety is difficult.

Now that we've examined the relative ratings of fruits and vegetables, what about meats? Vegetarian meals are not the choice of everyone, nor should they be. As we will learn in the next chapter, some blood types, and persons who do not easily metabolize carbohydrates require a certain amount of meat included in their diets.

Again, I have included only a cross section of some of the most popular cuts of meats in this chart. When shopping, your food count book is equally valuable in the meat department or at your butcher. A butcher is always a better choice as a meat supplier than the typical grocery store, as you can direct your butcher to trim or prepare your meats as you prefer, regulating the fat and bone content of each. Also, your local butcher will quickly become familiar with your personal preferences and will be able to trim your cuts to your specifications each time you order. Many butchers offer delivery as well, a convenience for the disabled or elderly.

Meats contain other important food values as well. They are arguably one of the best natural sources for protein for a human diet, for instance. Unless specifically directed to do so by your doctor or nutritionist, you should probably not exclude meats entirely from the average healthy diet.

All of the meat selections in this chart are illustrated as cooked with the skin or fat. Eliminating both, or either, may reduce calories for those who are controlling their weight, but, take note: elimination of the fat or skin may also eliminate other essential nutrients or dietary fats. As we learned from our milk studies in chapter 13, not all dietary fats are harmful. In fact, eliminating some of them may increase your risk for stroke or heart disease. I repeat: balance is the key to success. Balance means a return to optimum personal bests for your system nutrient and mineral levels. Your doctor or nutritionist can help you plan a diet that includes all of the desired elements while eliminating the undesirable, and you will experience far greater success on your personal road to a cure, or simply your best possible state of health.

Many times, however, patients with chronic or serious illnesses, such as MS patients, will be told to eliminate red meats from their diets, at least for a measurable period of time. I eliminated all red meat from my food intake for a year for just that reason. There are other, non-red meats, game meats, and poultry choices that will provide some of the same values, and in some cases, greater concentrations per serving.

Chart 15-12 illustrates the best alternatives to red meats in these categories. A reminder: if you do not see your favorite meat listed here, don't despair. It does not score significantly in these categories, but may provide excellent benefits in other areas.

Chart 15-12 Selected Nutrients in Common Meats and Comparative Vegetarian Meat Substitutes in Serving Measurements

Food Item	Serving	Preparation Method	Ca	Mg	P
Beef, Chuck	4 oz.	Pot Roast	11	23	254
Beef, Corned	4 oz.	Cured, Cooked	9	14	142
Beef, Ground, Lean	4 oz.	Broiled, Fried, Medium	12	24	179
Beef, Ground w/ Fat	4 oz.	Broiled, Fried, Medium	12	23	193
Beef, Organ Meats	4 oz.	Kidney, Simmered	19	20	347
Beef, Organ Meats	4 oz.	Liver, Pan Fried	12	26	523
Beef, Round, Bottom	4 oz.	Roasted	6	32	270
Beef, T-bone Steak	4 oz.	Broiled	9	28	209
Beef, Vegetarian	3.25 oz.	Canned, Steak	12	ND	86
Beef, Vegetarian	2.5 oz.	Frozen, Steak	49	ND	ND
Beef, Vegetarian	2.3 oz.	Hamburger, Frozen Patty	63	ND	ND
Chicken, Cornish Hen	1 bird	Roasted w/ skin	31	40	334
Chicken, Dark Meat	4 oz.	Leg, Fried, Broiled, Skin	15	27	204
Chicken, Dark Meat	4 oz.	Roasted w/ Skin	14	23	203
Chicken, Egg	1 large	Cooked, Fried, Hard Boiled	25	5	89
Chicken, Egg	1 large	Raw	25	5	89
Chicken, Egg	1 large	White Only	2	4	4
Chicken, Egg	1 large	Yolk Only	23	1	85

Food Item	Serving	Preparation Method	Ca	Mg	P
Chicken, Egg Imitation	1 oz.	Liquid	15	ND	34
Chicken, Egg Imitation	1 oz.	Powder	92	ND	136
Chicken, Egg Imitation	1 oz.	Vegetarian Egg Sub.	15.5	ND	25
Chicken, Organ Meats	4 oz.	Giblets, Simmered	14	23	260
Chicken, Organ Meats	4 oz.	Heart, simmered	22	23	226
Chicken, Organ Meats	4 oz.	Liver, Simmered	16	24	354
Chicken, White Meat	4 oz.	Breast, Fried, Broiled	18	34	264
Chicken, Vegetarian	5.2 oz.	Canned, Fried w/Gravy	15	ND	ND
Chicken, Vegetarian	3 oz.	Frozen Nuggets	41	ND	ND
Chicken, Vegetarian	3.4 oz.	Frozen, Sticks	20	ND	ND
Duck, Fresh or Frozen	4 oz.	Roasted w/ Skin	12	18	177
Goose	4 oz.	Roasted w/ Skin	15	25	306
Goose, Organ Meats	4 oz.	Liver, Raw	48	28	296
Ham, Regular	4 oz.	Cured, Whole, Roasted	8	22	243
Ham, Regular	4 oz.	Fresh, Shank, Roasted	7	24	271
Ham, Regular	4 oz.	Precooked, Canned, Roasted	9	19	276
Ham, Vegetarian	3.2 oz.	Frozen	10	ND	ND
Lamb, Ground	4 oz.	Broiled	25	27	228
Lamb, Leg	4 oz.	Roasted w/Fat	12	27	217
Lamb, Loin	4 oz.	Broiled, w/Fat	23	27	222
Lamb, Organ Meats	4 oz.	Kidney, Simmered	20	23	329
Lamb, Organ Meats	4 oz.	Liver, Pan Fried	10	26	484
Lamb, Rib	4 oz.	Broiled, w/Fat	22	26	202
Lamb, Shoulder	4 oz.	Broiled w/Fat	24	29	225
Lamb, Shoulder	4 oz.	Cubed, Broiled	14	35	254
Pork, Bratwurst	4 oz.	Fresh, Cooked	52	16	168
Pork, Kielbasa	4 oz.	Boiled, Steamed	48	20	168
Pork, Knockwurst	4 oz.	Boiled, Steamed	12	12	112
Pork, Loin, Top, Center	4 oz.	Roasted	11	22	254
Pork, Organ Meats	4 oz.	Chitterlings, Simmered	31	11	53
Pork, Organ Meats	4 oz.	Kidney, Simmered	15	20	272
Pork, Organ Meats	4 oz.	Liver, Pan Fried	11	16	273
Pork, Sausage	4 oz.	Fresh, Cooked	16	8	96
Pork, Sausage	4 oz.	Raw, Italian Style	20	15	141
Pork, Sausage, Vienna	4 oz.	Canned	12	8	56

Food Item	Serving	Preparation Method	Ca	Mg	P
Pork, Shoulder	4 oz.	Roasted	8	20	227
Pork, Spare Ribs	6.3 oz	Braised, 1 lb. Raw w/Bone	38	43	463
Pork, Tenderloin	4 oz.	Roasted	10	28	327
Pork/ Beef, Vegetarian	1.6 oz.	Hot Dog, Frozen, Deli Style	16	ND	36
Pork/ Beef, Vegetarian	4 oz.	Canned, Sausage, 5 Links	15	ND	ND
Pork/ Beef, Vegetarian	2.6 oz.	Frozen, Sausage, 2 Patties	30	ND	192
Pork/ Beef, Vegetarian	4 oz.	Frozen, Sausage, 5 Links	37	ND	135
Rabbit	4 oz.	Roasted	17	19	234
Rabbit	4 oz.	Stewed	23	23	256
Turkey, Breast Meat	4 oz.	Roasted w/ Skin	24	31	238
Turkey, Dark Meat	4 oz.	Roasted w/ Skin	37	26	222
Turkey, Drumstick	4 oz.	Roasted w/ Skin	36	26	226
Turkey, Ground	4 oz.	Cooked	20	20	161
Turkey, Light Meat	4 oz.	Roasted w/ Skin	24	29	236
Turkey, Organ Meats	4 oz.	Giblets, Simmered	15	19	231
Turkey, Organ Meats	4 oz.	Gizzard, Simmered	17	22	145
Turkey, Organ Meats	4 oz.	Heart, Simmered	15	25	232
Turkey, Organ Meats	4 oz.	Liver, Simmered	12	17	308
Turkey, Sausage	4 oz.	Links	45	13	160
Turkey, Wing	4 oz.	Roasted w/ Skin	27	28	223
Turkey, Vegetarian	4 oz.	Frozen, Smoked	10	ND	ND
Veal, Ground	4 oz.	Broiled	19	27	246
Veal, Leg, Top Round	4 oz.	Roasted, Lean w/ Fat	7	32	265
Veal, Loin	4 oz.	Roasted, Lean w/ Fat	22	28	240
Veal, Organ Meats	4 oz.	Kidney, Simmered	33	27	422
Veal, Ribs	4 oz.	Roasted, Lean w/ Fat	12	25	223
Veal, Shoulder	4 oz.	Roasted, Lean w/ Fat	31	28	244
Veal, Sirloin	4 oz.	Roasted, Lean w/ Fat	15	29	253
Veal, Vegetarian	5 oz.	Frozen, 2 Patties	52	ND	ND
Vegetarian Loaf	3.2 oz.	Frozen, Lentil Rice Loaf	21	ND	213
Vegetarian Loaf	3 oz.	Frozen, Nine Bean Loaf	27	ND	ND

Key: Ca=Calcium, Mg=Magnesium, P=Phosphorus, ND=No Data Available, HF=Health & Nutrition Stores

All beef contains a high amount of phosphorus, many cuts containing over 100 percent of the daily DRI for all ages and genders. Beef organ meats, particularly liver and kidney, are far and away the best sources from among all of the cuts. Believe it or not, liver, when prepared correctly, is a wonderful dish.

Veal cuts do not score appreciably higher in each category per serving when compared to adult cows, although they do rate somewhat higher than mature beef as a whole. The slight difference in concentration is not enough reason, at least in these categories, to cause you to purchase veal instead of less expensive beef, especially if you object to the way that most veal are raised. Vegetarian beef and veal alternatives, including the vegetarian loaf used as a meat loaf substitutes hardly compare to the real thing in any category. If you are directed to avoid red meats, choose another alternative from the meat group rather than these imitations to replace your target minerals.

Lamb, another popular red meat, is also an excellent phosphorus source and rates higher than beef in comparative cuts in all three categories. Again, lamb organ meats calculate greater totals than other cuts. Lamb's liver contains a whopping 484 mg. of phosphorus in a 4 oz. serving, more than 100 percent of the daily DRI for males 31 and older, the group requiring the most daily phosphorus, regardless of age or gender. A lamb shoulder chop of the same portion size delivers 225 mg. of phosphorus, more than 100 percent of the daily DRI for all children under 13, regardless of gender.

Pork, considered a "white" animal meat, and ham, a popular pork cut, rate only average as a meat source of calcium and magnesium, but roast cuts, particularly loin, shoulder, and tenderloin, contain high amounts of phosphorus. A delicious piece of news is that spare ribs score the highest of all of the cuts, save for, again, organ meats. Pork sausages also tally at greater levels per serving than the regular cuts, especially bratwurst, knockwurst, and kielbasa. Wonderful in German- and Polish-style dishes, they provide significant amounts of our mineral group.

Hams, specifically, score below average for calcium content and mediocre to average in magnesium per serving.

Phosphorus levels are high, however, and meet or exceed the daily DRI for kids under thirteen, both boys and girls. Ham sandwiches, when combined with a high calcium/magnesium hard cheese like Swiss, or Muenster for those with no dairy restriction, balance the nutrient scale, especially when served on a high-rating bread like dark rye or high-calcium white. Or, chunks of ham served in baked beans with corn bread will provide close to or actually over one hundred percent of the daily DRI of all three minerals in one serving, especially when combined with a nutrient-rich beverage.

Vegetarian pork substitutes do not fare well in the mineral ranking, with the exception of vegetarian pork sausage patties. These contain a fair amount of phosphorus and a slightly higher calcium concentration than do actual meats, but the magnesium count is so low as to be immeasurable. In the meat group category, vegetarian selections are not the best of choices.

Those of you who are red meat restricted, and those who may wish to avoid pork dishes for spiritual reasons will be interested in the poultry and game meats. Sorry, hunters: I was not able to obtain any reliable data on the mineral content of venison, so deer are not included here. Rabbit charts higher than average when compared to beef and pork cuts, especially in the calcium category. Duck scores about average for calcium and magnesium, but higher than average for phosphorus, as does goose. Goose liver, wonderful in paté, scores excellently in all three categories. When served on small corn tortilla chips, a single-serving snack will provide a significant amount of your daily DRI in all of our mineral categories.

For those of you with less exotic tastes, let's examine our two most popular poultry birds: chicken and turkey. For the purposes of these charts, all of the chickens and turkeys are considered farm-bred generic. Chicken selections are from hen cuts, and turkeys from tom cuts. All cuts are prepared with skin and some fat. Dark and white meat cuts of chicken score about the same in our three categories. Cornish hen, a small type of miniature chicken, did excellently. A single Cornish hen, served as an entree, provides one hundred percent of the daily DRI of phosphorus for all females, regardless of age, and for all males under the age of fourteen. Chicken liver also racks up high totals in each category. Paté from chicken liver is delicious, as is chicken liver and giblet gravy, made from the natural juices of the roasting bird.

Turkey, however, is a somewhat different story. Dark cuts do score measurably higher than breast or white cuts, and turkey liver does not score as highly as the body cuts, a reverse ratio from other types of meats. Turkey sausage, however, does outrank all other turkey cuts or products. These sausages are readily available in your grocer's meat counter, as is ground turkey. Pan fried in a small amount of oil, or included as a substitute for pork sausage in any number of dishes, turkey sausage is nutritious and tasty. Kids take to turkey sausage with more enthusiasm than they do to its chicken counterparts, and a four ounce serving of links gives kids eight and under one hundred percent of their daily DRI of phosphorus. If it is served with spinach and a sweet potato, for instance, the daily DRI in all three categories is significant, providing about twenty-five percent of the calcium and magnesium, and over one hundred percent of the phosphorus DRI.

Here again, in the chicken and turkey classes, the vegetarian substitute products simply do not provide even appreciable amounts of magnesium and phosphorus, although some calcium per serving is found. Unless you are specifically instructed otherwise, it is apparent that some meats should remain in the average healthy human diet. My apologies to all of the committed vegetarians out there, but a complete elimination of animal meats, fish and poultry, from the human diet is simply not indicated, nor can all minerals and nutrients found in meats be replaced by a strict vegetarian diet.

Finally, let's examine the egg. A better than average source of dietary calcium per serving, egg gets most of its value from the yolk. The white contains virtually no value in our selected nutrient categories. Although eating egg whites only is certainly lower in calories, a large portion of the nutritional value is stripped from the egg along with the calories when the yolk is removed. Unless an egg allergy is indicated, eating the egg whites only is not advised when nutrient replacement is the goal.

Egg substitutes also vary widely in value. Scoring even higher than real eggs is powdered egg mixture. Used for years by the military as a portable source of nutrition for soldiers, egg powder provides a substantial amount of the target minerals calcium and phosphorus, although it is not a significant source of magnesium. That's something to keep in mind while camping in the great outdoors, where food choices are necessarily limited. Powdered eggs have good mineral value and keep well without refrigeration. Normally in sealed containers or foil pouches, they are not tempting for nocturnal camp visitors like raccoons, chipmunks, and bears.

One final note on replacements for dairy. Milk also contains vitamin D. Most brands and grades of commercially available milk contain added vitamin D in the correct proportions necessary for maximum metabolization of the other nutrients. If you are not going to use dairy products, you will need to replace the vitamin D you lose by eliminating them. Otherwise, your body cannot metabolize the calcium you feed it, regardless of the source. It also does not efficiently handle magnesium and phosphorus if no vitamin D is present. Although your doctor or nutritionist can help you to determine what your exact daily DRI for vitamin D should be, here is a good proportional rule of thumb to follow when arriving at an adequate figure: For every thirty percent of daily calcium DRI your body ingests, you must also ingest twenty-five percent of the daily DRI of vitamin D in order to achieve maximum metabolization. In other words, if your daily DRI of calcium is 1000 mg., your daily DRI of Vitamin D is 5 IU. If 1 cup of milk contains 290 mg. of calcium, that is roughly twenty-nine percent of your daily requirement. You would need to supplement that intake with approximately 1.25 IU of vitamin D, or about twenty-five percent of your daily DRI in order to allow your body to most effectively utilize the milk nutrients. When choosing a vitamin D supplement, be certain to note the IU value in each capsule so that you are ingesting the correct amount for metabolization to occur.

Now that we're beginning to see the importance that food components play in overall optimum health, the next chapter will expand the picture to include other elements of food, namely the most important vitamins and minerals we have not covered here. Understanding how these elements are utilized by your body and how they affect you is crucial to recovering your health and eradicating disease from your system. We will examine the factors that determine the way your body metabolizes the food you eat: your blood type, your heritage, and your present nutrient levels. I will introduce you to the work of Dr. Barry Sears and Dr. Peter D'Adamo, and show you how you can combine their methods to determine a formula of food that is right for your body. It then becomes relatively easy to plan a diet that is the richest in nutrients while being the easiest for your body to digest and use efficiently.

In recognition of the busy and stressful lifestyle many of us live, I have included some of the most popular fast foods and quick supermarket meals, measuring their value against the more traditionally prepared meals. We'll find out what to choose when pressed for time, when unable to eat a "regular" meal, or when dining out in a restaurant. And, don't forget that snack machine in the hall. It might contain hidden nutritional treasures!

In conclusion, we can clearly see that indeed, there is life after dairy. Many other foods exist that can be used to substitute for dairy products. These foods, although maybe not providing as much calcium, magnesium, or phosphorus as dairy, in some cases do provide more per serving, or can be combined to create the same proportions as are found in milk and soft cheeses.

16

Making the Right Choices: Understanding the Role of Food in Creating a Nutrition Program That Works

As a Doctor of Naturopathic Medicine, I have long been aware of the importance of good diet and the value of natural substances in the role of optimum human health. Unfortunately, most people today give more attention to the foods that they feed to their pets than they do to what they feed themselves. Dogs, cats, and even fish, have special diets that have been scientifically formulated to provide the ideal balance of fats, proteins, carbohydrates, vitamins, and minerals. Pet owners go to great lengths to obtain those foods necessary to ensure their nonhuman companions enjoy good health and long life.

You can easily prove this interesting twist to human behavior with a simple experiment. Next time you're out enjoying a brisk walk, ask that fellow in the park what he feeds his radiant Irish Setter or playful Black Lab, and he will probably proudly list all of the premium foods that he provides for his happy and active animal. Or, ask your neighbor what she feeds that magnificent Persian or sleek Russian Blue, and she will most likely go to the cabinet and produce kitty's favorite meal, pointing out the elements on the label that maintain that bright eye and silky fur. People who keep fish are even more meticulous, not only choosing the proper type of food, but monitoring and maintaining water temperature, Ph balance, and tank filtration, glowing with pride as the visitor admires the results of their efforts.

Now, ask those same people what they feed themselves. I can almost guarantee that you'll be astounded by answers that range from the vague ("Oh, you know . . . just regular stuff, I guess"), to the careless ("Well, I don't always have the time to eat . . . "), to the ridiculous ("I eat guy stuff . . . steak, burgers, and beer," or "Well, I'm watching my weight, so I only eat a salad once a day . . . "). Almost none of them will launch into a discussion of proper nutrition. Those same individuals, so caring and diligent with their pet's food, will almost certainly be eating the wrong things themselves, and with far less concern for the consequences.

Those who live below the poverty line, in economically depressed conditions or on a fixed income like the disabled and the elderly, often do not have much of a choice. Their diets are determined by price. They eat what they can afford, cheaper foods low in nutritional value, or diets consisting of a disproportionate amount of one type of food. Game meats may be a staple in very remote areas, pastas and breads in urban impoverished homes. In these cases, nutritional education may make no appreciable difference. Knowing that certain foods are high in nutrients and better choices than others makes no difference when there are several mouths to feed and not enough money to make ends meet. I became quite familiar with this type of dietary dilemma while working in New York City. Parents knew that fruit juice was healthier than fruit drinks or Kool-Aid, but they could barely afford the latter.

The rest of us cannot hide behind that unfortunate excuse. I am willing to bet that every single one of us has been guilty

of eating the "wrong" foods, either chronically, or at least periodically. I have, even though I have a medical degree in nutrition. We all rationalize what we do in a myriad of ways. We call
it "indulging," "cheating," or just "enjoying ourselves" when we
overeat or consume foods that we know are unhealthy for us.
We are "watching our weight," "running late," or "staying
sharp" when we fail to eat at the proper times, or skip a meal
altogether. We blame stress, pressure, overloaded schedules,
client meetings, holidays, peer pressures, bad relationships,
bills, loss, fear of obesity, even our genetics ("Mom was always
thin as a rail," or "My Dad was a big guy . . . "). None of us want
to address the two main reasons humans of average or better
economic means eat poorly: ignorance and laziness. And,
none of us want to lay the blame where it belongs: at our own
two feet.

This chapter is meant to be a practical guide that will teach
you how to feed yourself properly. Although the methods that
I recommend here will primarily apply to MS patients, the
principles can be used for the establishment of a proper diet
for almost any individual. We examine the recommendations
of the eminent MS specialist and world-renowned author, Roy
L. Swank, M.D., and his special low-fat diet plan, published as
*The Multiple Sclerosis Diet Book: A Low Fat Diet for the Treatment
of MS*, which has been so successful in the management of
many MS cases.

We will also journey further and look beyond dietary management. I will show you how nutritional health requirements
are determined at the most basic human level, the individual
cell, by examining the work of Dr. Barry L. Sears. The practical application of his discoveries led to publication of his
highly regarded nutritional work, *The Zone: A Dietary Road
Map*, which has enjoyed growing popularity and an increasing
number of followers across the United States, including athletes, amateur, and professional sports teams and astronauts.

Through my own experience and success, I will build
upon both of these protocols by incorporating the work of

noted nutritional specialist Dr. Peter J. D'Adamo, who refines the principles of proper nutrition by blood type, choosing those foods which enhance and augment positive preexisting genetic factors. I review his valuable work, *Eat Right 4 Your Type: The Individualized Diet Solution to Staying Healthy*, and show you how you can formulate the optimum nutrition plan for your unique needs. We will examine more elements of the foods we saw in chapter 15 and look at some new ones to see how they may fit into our optimum nutritional plan.

Even though I can give you all of this knowledge and introduce you to important nutritional books and methodologies, I cannot give you the two most important factors that will determine your success at incorporating them into your lifestyle: determination and diligence. Only you can decide that you want to *live*, not merely exist. Only you can decide that you want to *work* at your health. If you want a feel-good, quick-result diet that will turn you from Quasimodo into Brad Pitt, don't look here. If you're seeking a plan that will take off weight and make you into Iman the supermodel, this is a great place to start, but not if you think that it will happen in thirty days or less. It won't.

Face it: there is no safe, quick diet that will magically drop those pounds or restore your health. Diet claims are everywhere, and people spend billions of dollars every year in their quest for the body of their dreams. Yet, a recent study shows that over sixty percent of Americans are dangerously overweight. Why?

> *Even though I can give you all of this knowledge and introduce you to important nutritional books and methodologies, I cannot give you the two most important factors that will determine your success at incorporating them into your lifestyle: determination and diligence. Only you can decide that you want to live, not merely exist. Only you can decide that you want to work at your health.*

Huge amounts of money are spent in research and production of supplements and nutritional aids to build bodies, lose weight, and replace elements lacking in our diets, not to mention the millions spent on advertising. Again, why? How is it that humans have walked upon this planet for untold thousands of years, living under conditions that we today would find appalling, and yet we now have to rely on pills and capsules to survive?

In my opinion, it is because we have progressed to the point where we have forgotten ourselves. In our quest to become "modern" and "civilized," we have lost sight of our true natures. The truth is, we are all still animals. The basic composition of the human body has remained virtually unchanged from time out of mind. Oh, we may be a little taller and larger than our great, great grandparents because adequate food is easier to obtain, and we may live a little longer and survive illness and injury more often because of advances in medical care, but intrinsically, human biology has not changed all that much in the last few thousand years.

Our eating habits, however, have changed drastically. Advances in food production, preservation, and preparation have radically altered our food intake. We receive the bulk of our nutritional information from commercial sources that couldn't care less if we eat right. In fact, they secretly hope that we don't, because if we did we wouldn't buy their products. And, when we do finally get our systems so out of balance as to leave us open for serious or chronic illness, most of the huge companies that produce vitamins and mineral supplements also make medical treatment drugs. An interesting thought.

So, what do we do? How do we determine exactly what our individual needs are, and how do we meet those needs in our daily diet? How can we incorporate the proper nutrition into our modern lifestyles? The first step to finding the answers to these questions is to look at one of the first protocols I followed in my search for my own personal optimum dietary intake, Dr. Swank's low-fat MS diet plan.

Treating MS through Nutrition—
The Protocols of Dr. Roy L. Swank

A retired Professor Emeritus of Neurology at Oregon Health Sciences University, Dr. Roy Lavar Swank has been specializing in the treatment and management of progressing multiple sclerosis for almost forty years. His ongoing research into the causes and effects of MS began in the post-World War II era, in August 1948, when he arrived at the Montreal Neurological Institute to study the disease on the invitation of the director of the facility at that time, Dr. Wilder Penfield.

Dr. Swank's initial research discovered what he believed were three primary keys to the illness: vascular restriction, geographical locality, and dietary fat intake. Based upon this foundation, his subsequent experiments, and those of others examining the filtration of substances found in human blood led to his development of a low-fat and food-restriction diet specifically for the treatment of MS patients. In December of 1948, Dr. Swank began what would become a thirty-six-year study of 150 MS patients in Montreal, Canada. The longevity of this study shows strongly that Dr. Swank is on the right track as far as management of the disease is concerned, because many MS patients around the world who are not following either Dr. Swank's protocol or some form of nutritional management do not live thirty-six years after diagnosis. In fact, many MS patients are reduced to a wheelchair state long before that length of time has passed.

The results of Dr. Swank's work were originally published in 1977, in his best-selling work, *The Multiple Sclerosis Diet Book*. Revised and reissued ten years later, in 1987, this comprehensive and practical guide to healthy eating for the MS patient includes the data accumulated from the Montreal study. If you have not had the opportunity to read this excellent and valuable book, I recommend that you obtain a copy.

After a twenty-year period, Dr. Swank's original study patients were evaluated, and the percentage rates of their relapses, performance, mortality, and degrees of disability as compared to other long-term ongoing patient studies were evaluated. In all categories, Dr. Swank's patients scored far better than those in other studies. For instance, a ten-year study of MS patients with varying initial degrees of disability conducted at the Mayo Clinic showed, although all of the participants were able to walk and work at the time the study was begun, after a ten-year period, only 50 percent were still able to do so (Maclean and Beckson 1951, 146:1367–1369). These patients were given no effective prescribed therapies. In comparison, only twenty-five percent of the patients on the Swank diet lost their ability to walk or work after the same period of time had elapsed.

Another important area where the Swank patients dramatically outscored other patients treated elsewhere was in the percentage of mortality. Compared to a mortality rate of twenty to twenty-eight percent in untreated control groups studied by Ragnar Miller (1949, 222:1–214) over a fifteen-year period, only six percent of the low-fat Swank patients died during the same period of time.

An even longer clinical study, conducted by eminent researcher R.S. Allison (1950, 73:103–120), and first published after twenty years of observation, showed that after two decades had elapsed, forty-three percent of the untreated patients studied had died, that number increasing to seventy-three percent after thirty-six years had passed. Only about ten percent of the Swank patients failed to survive after twenty years, and twenty-one percent were deceased after a comparative thirty-six-year span.

Dr. Swank's research also proved that, perhaps as important as the mortality rate improvement, patients following the Swank diet showed a marked reduction of disability symptoms. In fact, ninety-five percent of the MS patients who began to follow the Swank diet soon after the disease was initially diagnosed—when mild or no evident symptom disabilities were reported—either remained unchanged or significantly improved their physical health while following the Swank diet for twenty years or more.

What does Dr. Swank recommend to his patients that produces these undeniably positive results? Let's take a look at his recommendations, which include elimination of certain foods and restrictions of others. I will only examine these guidelines in summary. Dr. Swank gives a full and complete explanation of his reasoning for each in his excellent book. You can refer to the Bibliography or the resources section for more information on *The Multiple Sclerosis Diet Book*.

Red meats are forbidden entirely for the first year, and only three ounces per week are allowed after that time, except on rare or special occasions. Red meats can contain high amounts of saturated fats, a substance Dr. Swank advises be restricted or avoided. High levels of saturated fats clog the bloodstream, impeding circulation, especially in the peripheral vascular system. Reduced circulation limits the amounts of essential nutrients and minerals passed to other individual cells in the body. In all humans, this can lead to conditions that cause circulatory problems, including heart attack and stroke. In MS patients, impeded circulation also inhibits the delivery of substances necessary for the production of myelin, the main component of the cells that form the protective "sheath" layer of cells surrounding our central nervous system.

Dairy products are permitted, but all those which contain more than one percent butterfat must be eliminated, with specific exceptions only. Dr. Swank recommends that dairy, eggs, and poultry are good alternate sources of protein and most essential amino acids formerly supplied by meats in the diet. However, dairy may also contain high levels of saturated fats, especially in some of the richer milk products, some cheeses, and most animal fat butters, and are not a viable dietary choice for those who are lactose intolerant or have milk allergies.

The immediate reduction or virtual elimination of saturated fats is the primary objective of Dr. Swank's diet plan. The remainder of his diet protocol deals with this criterion, including the directive to restrict saturated fat intake at all times to fifteen grams or less per day. Saturated fats can produce a wax-like substance in the bloodstream, which collects on the walls of the arteries and veins, restricting blood flow and inhibiting distribution and absorption of substances by other cells in the body.

Unsaturated fats are likewise restricted on similar reasoning. On the Swank diet, unsaturated fat intake should fall between twenty and fifty grams per day and should never exceed the maximum figure. Additionally, daily supplementation of the diet by the inclusion of a multivitamin and a cod liver oil supplement is recommended to replace nutrients and oils that may become deficient by the dietary restrictions.

Indisputable research proves that Dr. Swank's recommended nutritional plan is significantly beneficial to the management of progressing multiple sclerosis, and should be seriously considered by the MS patient as a dietary regimen. I followed Dr. Swank's diet for almost two years. I found that my overall health and energy levels improved, and, through periodic BCI testing, found that several imbalances in my system substances began to be corrected.

However, I found that my nutrient imbalances were not correcting themselves as efficiently as I felt they could have been. I was searching for a way to cure my MS and not simply manage the condition and prevent its progression. I built upon the Swank foundation by incorporating other protocols into my daily dietary and nutritional plan as I became aware of them through further research.

We have already examined the directives for a zero dairy and zero sugar diet in chapter 6. After testing IgG RAST positive for cow's milk and chicken egg allergies, I incorporated these additional dietary restrictions into the principles of the Swank diet for nearly another year. I began to focus more on a vegetable- and grain-based diet, supplementing my daily food intake with prescribed vitamins and minerals.

I continued to explore the nutritional aspect of MS treatment with my own research, examining helpful substances ranging from ancient Asian herbal therapies to oil-based suppositories in an effort to restore the vitamin and mineral levels and proper ratios in my system. I began to research the functions of the body, reasoning that MS, if indeed a virus, as I firmly believe that it is, begins to affect the body on a much more basic level, beyond the destruction of the myelin sheathing and the appearance of lesions on the nervous system and in the brain. I am convinced that MS corrupts the function of the body at a cellular level. In order to attempt to determine what causes that corruption, I needed to first understand exactly what happens inside of a living cell in the course of daily, natural biologic function.

It was during the course of my research that I discovered the next valuable protocol in my regimen, the adjustment and production of substances within my own cells. It was at this time that I began to become familiar with the work of world-renowned scientist, Dr. Barry Sears, through his best-selling book, *The Zone: A Dietary Road Map*. His work was to completely change the way that I, even with all of my existing nutritional knowledge, was to view each substance that I put into my body. We will explore the work of Dr. Sears in this next section, and I will illustrate why I believe that the inclusion of his principles will help to further refine the individualized treatment of the MS-afflicted and aid in the restoration of optimal body function and health.

Breaking the Nutritional Code—The Healthy "Zone" of Dr. Barry Sears

One of the most important works on the basic nutritional needs of the human body has only been introduced recently. Even so, *The Zone: A Dietary Road Map*, the 1995 best-selling book by Dr. Barry Sears, has become the cornerstone of more than one publicly profiled nutritional regimen. The growing list of subscribers to the importance of Dr. Sears's work includes several organized teams and individually recognized athletes from a diverse number of amateur, collegiate, and professional sports. In addition, many doctors and nutritionists are offering seminars and training sessions to teach these principles. "Zone" bars and "Zone-friendly" restaurants have begun to spring up around the United States, as have services that will deliver pre-made "Zone" meals to the desiring customer.

What accounts for this growing popularity? We already know that people, especially Americans, are "diet" crazy. Dr. Sears promises that if you follow his nutritional regimen, you will certainly lose weight. Is this just another "get thin quick" book like so many others, espousing radical dietary changes that promise to produce "the ultimate you"? Or, has his research produced something more? Before we dismiss his claims of attaining, and remaining in, an optimum state of health, let's examine briefly exactly what Dr. Sears has to say on the subject of nutrition, and food intake, and how they ultimately determine the function of the human body.

Barry Sears, Ph.D., received his doctorate in biochemistry from Indiana University, where he specialized in examining the molecular structure of lipids, basic fats. He originally began to study the effects of these and other substances on the human body as an admitted means of self-preservation. With an immediate family history of heart attacks and other cardiac malfunctions, Dr. Sears was concerned with his own prognosis for longevity, especially after the untimely demise of his own father at the age of fifty-three from a heart attack.

Dr. Sears began to take his research beyond the realm of pure science as he set out to investigate the effects that these compounds had on the human system. Reviewing a study conducted at Mount Zion Hospital in San Francisco, California by researchers Sanford Byers and Meyer Friedman, Dr. Sears noted that rats fed a high-saturated-fat diet developed atherosclerosis, or hardening of the arteries. These same rats, however, when injected with the same phospholipid compounds Dr. Sears had worked with during his doctorate dissertation, showed complete reversal of their physical condition, eliminating entirely the adverse effects of the saturated fats. Later studies, although initially conducted to disprove these findings, merely served to further strengthen the conclusion, including a large 1975 study conducted by one of the largest American manufacturers of medical drugs, Upjohn Laboratories.

Far from becoming a welcome hallelujah in the fight against heart disease and related cardiac conditions, the results of this study were largely ignored. Dr. Sears attributes this curious reaction to the fact that as phospholipids are part of the basic components of every human cell, and therefore a naturally occurring substance, no company could obtain a patent on medications or drugs containing phospholipids as their primary ingredient. Since no patent could reasonably be obtained, drug companies had no vested financial interest in further research, as the expense would not produce any appreciable or projected revenue as a result. Heart disease, stroke, and heart attack, however, create millions of dollars in revenue from the medications required to treat them.

Cynical? Possibly. True? Almost certainly. Fortunately, Dr. Sears continued his research, driven largely by his own biological clock. He developed and patented synthetic phospholipid molecules, offering to associate with Upjohn to produce them for public use. Their greatest objection was to the fact that Dr. Sears's medication was an injectable, a traditional death knell to common usage in almost all widely prescribed medications, the obvious exception being, of course, insulin.

Undeterred, Dr. Sears pursued his research, focusing on converting his synthetic phospholipid injectables into pill form. Through a fortunate partnership with David Yessair of the drug manufacturing company Arthur D. Little, Dr. Sears was able to use his phospholipid technology in combination with Yessair's water-insoluble anti-tumor drugs to produce new and far less toxic anti-cancer drugs than had formerly been available. A blessing to cancer and autoimmune

patients, Dr. Sears's combination of the phospholipid technologies with these anti-cancer formulas would go on in the
early 1980's to produce AZT, one of the only approved drugs
prescribed in the treatment of AIDS.

It was during this time that the Nobel Prize for Physiology
and Medicine was awarded in 1982 to scientists Sune Bergstrom
and Bengt Samuelsson of the Karolinska Institute of Stockholm,
Sweden, and to John Vane of the Royal College of Surgeons in
England. The prize was given for their research in two important
areas of scientific medical study: a powerful class of hormones
called "eicosanoids," and their discovery that these eicosanoids
are affected by aspirin, solving the enduring mystery as to why
this simple yet effective medication was able to relieve pain,
reduce fever, and slow or arrest an occurring heart attack.

Eicosanoid hormones are, in the words of Dr. Sears, the
"master switches" that control virtually every function of the
human mechanism, including the cardiovascular, immune,
and fat storage systems. Dr. Sears further postulated that
many afflictions such as heart disease, diabetes, cancer, and
autoimmune dysfunction, including MS, could be caused by a
severe imbalance of these eicosanoid hormones. Therefore,
restoring and maintaining the eicosanoid balance could be
the key to the prevention and even the primary treatment for
the reversal and treatment of these same diseases. There are
awesome implications to this theory if it is indeed true.

In *The Zone*, Dr. Sears goes on to explain that his theory is not
only true, but relevant to our daily lives by practical application.
He began to apply his theories to human nutrition by examining
the elemental essentials of each food item: proteins, carbohydrates, and fats. His goal was to discover how to affect eicosanoid
production at the individual cellular level by using food to manipulate and maintain an optimum eicosanoid balance, thereby preventing or reversing the effects of these diseases.

Dr. Sears initiated this phase of his research by viewing
food from a unique perspective: as a drug as powerful, addictive, and dangerous as any other drug. He further applied

standard drug delivery principles to food, reasoning that each item must be ingested in mathematical, defined proportions in order to attain maximum effectiveness, just as an anesthesiologist determines through mathematical formula the proper amount of medication needed by a 235-lb. male to bring the patient in comfort and safety through a three-hour surgical procedure, a dosage that would be, for instance, different from that necessary to take a 110-lb. woman through a root canal. Through personal and clinical experimentation, Dr. Sears developed a series of adjustments and refinements, a precise scientific formula to determine the optimum amount of each food component necessary to achieve optimum eicosanoid balance.

Perhaps one of the reasons I admire Dr. Sears so greatly is his motivation and methodology that resulted in this nutritional breakthrough. Much like myself, Dr. Sears refused to accept the predicted diagnosis that he would succumb in his forties or early fifties to the heart attacks that hit every one of his uncles and killed his father. He refused to accept that which seemed to be a foregone conclusion, just as I refused to accept the fact that once I had MS, my life was basically circling the drain as I waited to die, crippled and decrepit. And, much the same as I, Dr. Sears tested his theories of food and its relation to eicosanoid balance on the subject whose reaction he could monitor and control most closely: himself.

Encouraged by the positive results obtained through experimenting on himself, Dr. Sears expanded his clinical testing to include the members of his family. Again, the results were positive and promising. Ranging farther afield, Dr. Sears convinced the coaches of the Stanford University men's and women's swim teams, Skip Kenney and Richard Quick, respectively, to apply his Zone principles to the diets of the team members.

The results of the experiment were astonishing: Stanford swimmers came home from the 1992 Barcelona Olympics with eight gold medals. Since that time, Stanford swimmers have dominated American swimming championships. Not surprisingly, a Zone diet is a required part of their team's training regimen.

One of the most interesting "side effects" of a Zone-based nutrition plan is not only does it manipulate and control eicosanoid balance, it also helps the body shed excess weight. Although this was certainly not the focus of Dr. Sears's initial research, it is indeed a logical outcome of restoring body system balance. Just as Dr. Sears's phospholipids flushed the vascular system of artery-hardening substances, eating a Zone favorable diet also flushes the system, removing toxins and deposits of harmful substances, including excess stored body fat, making it one of the safest and most effective weight-loss tools available to those seeking to restore optimum health and vitality.

So, what are the basic principles of the Zone? The Zone balanced diet has met with vociferous opposition from some of the leading "diet doctors" in our country, as its principles absolutely fly in the face of conventional weight-loss programs. Let's look at what they are, and how they may augment, or radically differ from the "conventional wisdom" on weight loss and nutrition.

"Eating fat does not make you fat." This single statement is a stake driven through the heart of every major diet purveyor or weight-loss institution operating in the world today, where "low fat, no fat" has become the almost hysterical mantra of the obese. And, while they are still reeling in horror, Dr. Sears's research has proven that high-carbohydrate, low-fat, and low-protein diets actually do more harm than good. The excess carbohydrates ingested in these unbalanced diets are converted and stored in the human system as excess body fat. This is not at all good news for diet centers that feed their customers required pre-packaged and usually very high-carbohydrate, low-protein foods, or for the food companies that produce the large lines of "diet" foods in your grocer's frozen food section. Millions of pounds of these products are sold every year to poor souls seeking to achieve a healthy, sleek body.

Restricting calories does not make weight loss any easier. In fact, it may make it increasingly more difficult. When calories are restricted below the amount necessary for your body to perform basic vital functions, the prevailing wisdom is that you will force your body to burn your stored fat as energy. In fact, just the opposite is true. When calories are severely limited, biochemical signals are sent throughout your body that tell it to hold on to its existing stored resources, your fat, for dear life, releasing only what is necessary to maintain basic function. This is an instinctive survival reaction, something along the lines of a bear hibernating in the deep winter. Persons who begin these diets do initially lose weight, simply as a result of a smaller food intake. However, after a certain time, weight loss will level off, and a point will be reached where further weight loss, if achieved, will be from the destruction of muscle tissue, not body fat, raising a whole new crop of undesirable complications.

Diets based on choice restriction and calorie limits usually fail. Boredom is a major reason. This is an important point, not only for those persons seeking to lose weight, but also for the MS patient facing dietary restrictions. Human beings were not given their excellent sensory organs, so well suited to appreciating the myriad differences in smell and taste, in order that they should live entirely on lettuce, celery sticks, and rye crisp. Although kitty may love the same food day in and day out, human beings would certainly go mad if subjected to that routine. Diets that severely limit food choices usually fail simply because people get bored with eating the same six or seven things.

Weight loss is not a question of "will power." If you pay attention to *what* you are eating, it does not necessarily matter *how much* of it you consume. Of course, common sense should be exercised, as in all things, especially in the case of the MS patient seeking to correct system element or ratio imbalances. This is good news for those who have always thought that obesity and the failure to correct it were a result of a character flaw. You can eat fresh fruit every day of your life in an effort to stay healthy, but if your body does not metabolize citrus foods well, you may as well be eating pure sugar, or even cardboard, for all the good that it will do you in your efforts to achieve health or lose weight.

All foods can be either good or bad. It is not the composition of any food that makes it healthy or unhealthy, but the ratio of the components in that food, the proteins, carbohydrates, and fats, and their relation to other foods in your diet or meal that make them either beneficial or detrimental to your optimum state of well-being.

The biological effects of food have remained unchanged for forty million years. Dr. Sears concurs with my views expressed earlier in this chapter. The human body has a pre-set biological response to food that has remained virtually unchanged since the days of our primitive ancestors. Whether your beliefs are Creationist or Evolutionist, the bottom line remains the same. A human body will process certain types of food in specific ways, regardless of the preparation or packaging methods used by "modern science" (Sears and Lawren 1995).

This is all well and good, certainly, but how does it relate to MS patients, or other autoimmune disease sufferers? The answer to that lies with the eicosanoids, the components of our cells so thoroughly researched by Dr. Sears and his colleagues. Let's examine how eicosanoids affect our body systems and how their imbalance may determine the virulence of your MS symptoms. We'll also examine how correcting those imbalances may help to arrest the progress of the disease and actually begin to heal and reverse the existing damage already done.

Eicosanoids are "superhormones," referred to collectively as paracrine hormones. They are manufactured by the body naturally, and they are found in every cell. Eicosanoids do not stay resident in your system, and they are not dependent on your bloodstream in order to reach individual cells and perform their specific functions. Depending upon their place of origin in your body, they are given a variety of group names to differentiate between them and their separate functions. Each group has a specific and individual function, acting as catalysts that trigger other necessary processes.

How do these elements play such an important role in our system maintenance and balance? Like all hormones, eicosanoids operate as control systems, a series of cellular checks and balances that maintain optimum cell health. The combination of the foods that you eat will all produce eicosanoids of some sort and in some quantity. There are two distinct types of these hormones, simply referred to as "good" or "bad." In your cardiovascular system, good eicosanoids promote clean blood flow and good circulation. Bad eicosanoids promote blood clumping, causing clots that can lead to numbness, paralysis, heart attack, or stroke. They also affect all of other the major functions of your body's involuntary systems.

Good eicosanoids prevent blood clumping, promote clean and healthy veins and arteries, prevent overproduction of system antibodies, stimulate your immune responses and promote the body's natural healing processes, help in the production of anti-inflammatory agents, and decrease pain. Bad eicosanoids do just the opposite. You must remember that both of these groups must be kept in balance because you can also have too much of a good thing when it comes to eicosanoids. Too many good blood eicosanoids can cause low blood pressure, which can cause the body to go into shock. Too many bad blood eicosanoids constricts the arteries, which can lead to heart attack. And, perhaps most important to MS patients, good eicosanoids aid in the production and utilization of neurotransmitters, including myelin.

The importance of keeping these groups in balance, therefore, becomes glaringly apparent. But do you have to be a scientist in order to maintain this delicate balance? Dr. Sears doesn't think so, and, through experience, neither do I. The trick to maintaining the balance of eicosanoids in your system is relatively simple, but it does require that you radically alter your thoughts about the food that you eat.

All of us know, from birth, that when we are hungry, we must have food. Of course. But which food? How do we determine what we should eat, when we should eat, and how much we should eat in order to maintain a good/bad eicosanoid balance, and consequently, optimum health? In order to do this, you must alter your perceptions about food.

Every single food item on this planet is a sum of its individual parts. In other words, each edible substance is composed of specific, mathematically measurable amounts of proteins, fats, carbohydrates, vitamins, and minerals. Each of these substances, when ingested in the proper amounts and proportions, will create the proper ratio of good/bad eicosanoids, supply the correct amount of your body's required nutrients, and therefore promote healing, system balance, and, ultimately, optimum health and biological performance. In order to understand this principle, you must first understand the nature of foods. How do we do that? By a series of comparison questions and their answers.

For instance: What other substances in life have these properties? What other compounds enter the body that produce other good or bad effects according to their proportions and amounts? If you are either an MS patient or autoimmune disease sufferer, you already know the obvious answer. Drugs. Whether prescribed medicinally or available publicly, like alcohol, nicotine in tobacco, or varieties of "recreational" or "street" substances, drugs are the answer to these questions.

Look at your bottles of medications. Each has a specific dosage, and clear instructions as to the method of ingestion, injection, and the time intervals necessary for optimum benefit. Follow the directions, and the prescribed substance should produce the intended benefit. Deviate from those instructions, and the drug will be rendered ineffective, addictive, or possibly even lethal, as in the case of accidental or deliberate overdose.

Here's the shocker, folks: *food is a drug*. Food is the single most powerful and unregulated drug in the world. Anyone past the preschool age can eat virtually anything that they desire, in any amount, at any time, and completely without professional advice or supervision. The exceptions, of course, are those persons institutionalized, incarcerated, in a contained military environment, or under in-hospital care. All the rest of us are free, however, to do just about what we please.

Those of you who are parents may think that you are the person who controls what your children eat, but *are* you? Completely? No matter how healthy a meal you may be giving your children at home, what about when they aren't with you? Remember school lunches? Not always the most nutritious fare, even with the advanced knowledge of food groups we have today. "Brown bag" lunches may give you a measure of control over your child's diet when not at home, but kids can trade their food. Face it, children have so many opportunities to eat unwisely in our modern society and with our active lifestyles. School parties, sports games, field trips, even meals at another child's home where the parents may not be as nutritionally aware as yourself. Finally, no matter how conscientious a parent you are, there are times when we work overtime or are simply running late. We all have the number for the pizzeria that delivers in our address book.

Stop and think for a moment. Food *is* a drug. And we humans use it for all of the things that drugs are used for. We drink tea to calm down, coffee to wake up, eat chocolate for comfort, chicken soup for a cold, mountains of pasta before a marathon. We eat candy for quick energy, take cod liver oil for indigestion, prune juice for constipation, cranberry juice to clean our urinary systems, and on and on.

The practice of using food for emotional satisfaction is as old as human history. Grandma always had some food or drink remedy to offer, no matter what you might be suffering from, and you always felt better after Mom made you just the right thing when you were ill. Certainly, a lot of the remedy can be attributed to the healing powers of love and emotional bonds between human beings. But the bulk of the cure may actually have been in the components of the foods that we ingested.

Now, if food is a drug, then it becomes clear that every one of us should strive to treat it as a drug, by measuring the proportions of the foods that we put into our bodies. Ideally, all food should be measured in proper proportions. Some people may have the time and the means to precisely measure their food. Most of us, however, are late for the kid's soccer practice, stuck in traffic, or working on the seventeenth floor with the cafeteria in the basement and the candy machine in the hall. We're out on a dinner date, at lunch with a client, at a club meeting or at the ballpark, on a camping trip with the scouts. We can't measure our food portions.

So, what do we do? Dr. Sears has developed a simple solution to the problem with his Zone diet plan. Really, it should be referred to as the Zone *meal* plan, as weight loss is really a side effect and not the primary focus of his nutritional guidelines. Reasoning that all food is actually the sum of its collective parts, Dr. Sears classifies these parts into three types: proteins, carbohydrates, and fats. Foods from each one of these categories are required by your body each day in order to stimulate and maintain a balanced production of good and bad eicosanoids, thereby restoring and sustaining optimum health.

Dr. Sears has proven that elements from each of these categories are contained in finite quantities within each edible substance, no matter what the origin. For example, consider a simple red apple—medium, raw, and unpeeled. That tasty and popular fruit is actually composed of the following substances: 21.1 grams of carbohydrates, 3.7 grams of fiber, 1/2 gram of fat, 3/10 of a gram of protein, zero cholesterol, no B_{12}, 30 IU of vitamin A, 159 mg. of potassium, 10 mg. each of calcium and phosphorus, 6 mg. of magnesium, 3 mg. of vitamin C, 1.6 mg. of vitamin BC, 1 mg. sodium, .06 mg. each of copper and manganese, 1/2 mg. of zinc, 1/4 mg. of iron, 4 micrograms of niacin, 3 mcg. of B_6, 1 mcg. each of thiamine and riboflavin, 81 calories, and enough water to hold it all together into the familiar fruit form. Whew! Had no idea, did you? Well, neither did I, until I began to research the medicinal properties of food.

So, we see that each food we choose to eat is composed of measurable proportions of many elements. Once you begin to understand the nutritional components of food, you can utilize Dr. Sears's optimum nutrition formula. Dr. Sears has developed a mathematical formula to calculate what amounts of proteins, carbohydrates, and fats you should eat each day in order to remain in the Zone of optimum bodily performance. Breaking down the measurable content of these three elements into "blocks," Dr. Sears shows you how to calculate the amount of blocks of each substance that you need to eat at any given time to maintain your position in the Zone. He does this simply by teaching you how to calculate your present lean body mass and percentage of overall body fat, using a common home weight scale and tape measure.

After you have determined these percentages for your existing body, you can then calculate how many blocks of each category you will need each day to either adjust your body and change it from its present condition into a Zone healthy body, and how much of each you will need in order to maintain an optimum Zone balance once your body reaches the correct percentage proportions for optimum health.

I am not going to reproduce the calculations here. Dr. Sears is far better equipped to explain his research and its significance and practical application than am I. His book also contains worksheets that you can use to calculate your own body measurements, tables that help you to convert your measurements into accurate percentages, lists of recommended and discouraged foods, and a host of healthy and tasty recipes that will keep you in a Zone-friendly state. *The Zone: A Dietary Road Map* includes recommendations for food on the run, listing popular fast foods that are actually Zone-friendly and a good alternative for those times when you cannot prepare your own meals. I have also included contact information for Dr. Sears in the resources section.

Even though I have experienced a great deal of success in my nutritional efforts by applying Dr. Sears's Zone methods to the foods that I eat, I still wanted to be certain that I was eating the correct foods, to ensure that I was obtaining maximum benefit and therefore expediting my healing. Quite by happy accident, I came across another book that I also found to have much potential benefit in my quest for a nutritional cure for my MS: *Eat Right 4 Your Type: The Individualized Diet Solution to Staying Healthy*, by Dr. Peter J. D'Adamo. I used this new information and incorporated it into the Zone-friendly foods that I was already eating for optimum health.

> *I believe that using all of these important nutritional works in combination with your individual system nutrient levels as determined by a BCI analysis is the key to success when it comes to the special nutritional needs of the MS patient in the fight to overcome the disease, and afterwards, in order to maintain a healthy system and prevent a relapse, reoccurrence, or other undesirable complications.*

In this next section, I will explore Dr. D'Adamo's work, and explain why combining it with both Dr. Sears's Zone and Dr. Swank's MS diet may be the way to allow your body to begin to heal you from within. I believe that using all of these important nutritional works in combination with your individual system nutrient levels as determined by a BCI analysis is the key to success when it comes to the special nutritional needs of the MS patient in the fight to overcome the disease, and afterwards, in order to maintain a healthy system and prevent a relapse, reoccurrence, or other undesirable complications.

Staying True to Type—
Your Nutritional Bloodline

Now that we are beginning to understand the importance of proper nutrition in the role of healing and maintaining proper health, let's take a look at how refining the process even further can give us the edge in our fight to rid our bodies of MS, or any number of diseases. Let's examine the science behind the theory of blood-type-specific nutrition, and one of the leading experts in this field of study, Peter J. D'Adamo, N.D.

The statement could accurately be made that Dr. Peter J. D'Adamo was born into his field. Son of widely respected naturopathic physician and author James D'Adamo, N.D., Peter entered the field of naturopathic medicine in his father's footsteps. The elder D'Adamo had begun to study the varied effects of using the same vegetarian and low-fat diet plan for health promotion given to individuals in the late 1950's. Dr. James D'Adamo noted that, although some of the patients did extremely well on this type of nutritional plan, others experienced only mediocre or no results, and some actually got worse. He began to formulate the theory that blood, as the major life-sustaining component in the human body, may have something to do with the predicted success or failure rate of certain individuals. This belief was strengthened over the years as he continued to collect clinical data from his patients.

Finally, in 1980, Dr. James D'Adamo published his clinical findings in a book entitled *One Man's Food.* Two years later, his son Peter, then in his senior year of study for his naturopathic degree at John Bastyr College in Seattle, Washington, began to research existing scientific and medical literature to attempt to scientifically prove his father's subjective theory of correlation between blood type and ability to tolerate and utilize certain foods in the diet. He found the confirmation he was seeking by discovering existing research that proved his father's theories.

Dr. Peter D'Adamo initially discovered that persons with Type O blood were associated with peptic ulcers, a condition that resulted from the production of too much stomach acid. Second, and conversely, stomach cancer caused by too little stomach acid was found more highly in persons with Type A blood, as were more cases of pernicious anemia, a condition resulting from a B_{12} deficiency. B_{12} needs sufficient stomach acid in order to be adequately utilized by the human system. Therefore, Dr. Peter D'Adamo reasoned that there was indeed a scientific connection between blood type and human system function. He decided that after receiving his degree this would be his primary area of interest. In 1996, after nearly fifteen years of scientific and clinical research, Dr. Peter D'Adamo published his own work on blood types and nutrition entitled *Eat Right 4 Your Type: The Individualized Diet Solution to Staying Healthy*.

Dr. D'Adamo explains how scientific and historical research supports the contention that blood type is genetic and inherited. Unlike racial type, blood type originated through the course of human development. Blood Type O is the oldest, originating with ancient man. Type A developed largely upon the development of an agrarian society. Type B came later, as humans began to migrate northward into colder climates. Only in fairly recent human history has a fourth type, AB, emerged. The newest and rarest of blood types, AB was created by the mingling of the blood of Type A agrarian peoples and the Type B blood of northern Mongolian and Asian invaders. As with any occupational force, a certain amount of fraternization occurred, producing offspring that mingled the two blood types together to produce a unique third type, AB.

Blood type is a true blueprint of who you are as an individual, regardless of your racial origin or physical characteristics. Your blood type contains many individualized factors which define each human being as unique, such as the DNA code, or genetic fingerprint. Dr. D'Adamo further explains how each blood type originated, and how because of its origin it requires specific nutrients for optimum function in the body. I will summarize his research here.

Blood Type O is known as the "universal donor." All blood contains components known as antigens, elements that sense and attack foreign invaders. Type O blood contains both type A and type B antigens. That means it will detect and reject type A or B blood when introduced into the system. However, because it contains all of the elements of the other blood types, it can be introduced into all of those systems and become acclimated. Blood Type O is the oldest and original human blood type. Because it dates back to man's earliest history on the continent of Africa, the food that Type O persons require for optimum health is of a high-protein, low-carbohydrate nature, as the bulk of the primitive human diet was obtained by the hunting and killing of other mammals. Type O people thrive on diets high in meat and vegetables, and low in starches, sugars, and grains.

Blood Type A was the second to emerge, as ancient populations increased and people began to migrate to other areas of the world. Type O was still found in the majority of the population, as humans began to branch out into other areas in search of an adequate meat supply. Skin pigment and bone mass began to lighten as humans began to enter colder climate areas. Shorter days and the lack of the strong African sun made lighter skin pigment types more likely to survive, as they are better able to absorb vitamin D_3 from the sun in a shorter period of time. As people grew more numerous and began to concentrate in larger populations, alternate sources of food began to be investigated. Soon humans had discovered how to grow the food they needed, settling in communities as opposed to the nomadic hunter lifestyle. Their diets began to include more grains, fruit, nuts and beans, and less bulk from animal sources. Today, Type A persons flourish on a largely vegetarian diet.

Blood Type B first began to appear in the Caucasian and Mongolian peoples of northern Asia and the Himalayas. These were warlike people, surviving on both hunted meats and conquering raids on more peaceful, agrarian societies. As the warriors pushed southward and westward into lower Asia and Western and Northern Europe, Type B blood began to appear in these areas, as the raiders mingled with the local populations. Because their diets contained such a variety of foods, today's Type B person does best on a diet that consists of a balance of meats, fruits, and grains.

Type AB blood is the newest and rarest of blood types. Known as the "universal recipient," it is able to acclimate the other three types into its system, because it contains no antibodies that would reject any of them. But, because it also contains multiple blood antigens, it will be rejected by all other blood types when introduced into those systems. Type AB blood is thought to be less than one thousand years old, appearing first around the time of William the Conqueror as peoples of different backgrounds began to mingle and multiply. This blood type combines the characteristics of both Type A and Type B, causing some interesting nutritional dilemmas. For instance, although Type AB persons are genetically able to digest meat, a heritage received from their Type B ancestors, they often lack sufficient stomach acid necessary to digest red meat adequately, a characteristic typical of the agrarian Type A. Therefore, Type AB can more easily digest white meats and seafood, and should consider restricting or eliminating the amount of red meats in their diets.

Dr. D'Adamo explores the correct foods and proper quantities of each needed for individual blood types to thrive. He also explores the different personality types that seem to be prevalent according to type, the different exercise requirements for each, and the predisposition or ability to resist certain types of ailments and diseases. His excellent book includes meal plans and recipes that the readers can follow when beginning to eat correctly for their genetic composition. I highly recommend that you obtain a copy of this excellent book. I have included contact information for Dr. D'Adamo in the resources section.

Recalling the patients I have treated over the years with nutrition and BioCybernetics, and the imbalances present in their systems, Dr. D'Adamo's data made perfect sense to me. I reviewed my own remaining imbalances and began to consider the benefits of incorporating this new information into my existing nutrition plan. The Swank diet, alone and then in combination with the zero dairy and sugar protocol, had noticeably improved my condition. I had more energy, and no new symptoms of MS had presented. But, the BCI analyses continued to show imbalances.

Dr. Sears's impressive credentials, thorough research, and documented results convinced me to begin the Zone directives. After following this protocol, I began to see marked improvement in my imbalances and element ratios. I attribute this change to the re-inclusion of foods restricted on the Swank and Zero Dairy, Zero Sugar plan. Restriction of fat, particularly saturated fat, was helpful in keeping my immune system focused on the MS, and after testing positive for milk allergies, the elimination of dairy reduced the stress on my system further as it did not have to devote resources to allergic reactions. However, the fact remained that those restrictions prevented my body from receiving some of the essential raw materials necessary to restore my system balance permanently.

The Zone diet protocol reinstated those raw materials. By directing the consumption of measured blocks of proteins, carbohydrates, and fats, my body was again receiving all of the elements necessary for healthy system function. As subsequent analyses showed, those elements which were not improving now began to right themselves.

So, why incorporate the work of Dr. D'Adamo into my diet regimen, especially if the Zone was working for me? On the face of it, the adjustment may seem superfluous. My nutritionist training, however, directed me to include any protocol that would further refine my optimum dietary intake. Refining my diet to include those foods which were the easiest for my body to utilize was an obvious positive. There are other factors proven by Dr. D'Adamo's research that additionally weighted the scales in favor of this final refinement. His clinical research showed that Type A persons were prone to diseases like cancer, heart attack, diabetes, and malfunctions of the immune system. I have Type A blood and was afflicted with MS, a disease often classified as an autoimmune disorder.

I am not aware of any study regarding the predominant blood type of MS patients. If such a study exists, I would welcome the opportunity to review it. If you have participated in, or have knowledge of such a study or clinical trial, I invite you to contact me. Should such a study prove that MS is contracted more often by one blood type than others, it may explain why MS cuts across racial and gender lines. It may also explain why some members of a family may contract this affliction, while others do not, or why the disease progresses rapidly in some, while in others progress is slow or arrested for long periods of time.

One important factor that you must remember throughout all of your nutritional planning is that it is essential for you to continue to receive the RDA and DRI of daily nutrients, regardless of how you alter the source. You also need to consider the results of your personal system substance analysis.

This may sound impossibly complicated, but it is in reality quite simple and largely common sense. Let me give you a practical example: Suppose your blood type is A, like mine, and you are structuring your diet to be Zone-friendly and blood-type specific. You have a BCI analysis and your results show that you have an excessively high amount of iron in your system. Utilizing your BCI data, you would want to limit the number of iron-rich foods you consume, like certain beans, legumes, and grains, even though your optimum diet is suited

to those foods. As periodic retesting shows your levels returning to normal, you can then begin to reintroduce those foods
into your diet. During the period of excess, your BCI counselor, nutritionist, or physician can help you to choose alternate foods or recommend supplements that will maintain the
correct intake of the other essential nutrients, besides iron,
that are found in the foods you are limiting.

You need to remember that food is a drug. As such, it may
react either positively, negatively, or be nullified by other food
drugs introduced into the system in conjunction. Keep in
mind that just as all prescription drugs do not come in the
same strengths, not all foods contain the same concentration
of vitamins, minerals, or other essential elements.

Let's look at a general example: Eating beans instead of
steak may provide an almost equal amount of protein per serving, but beans alone will not provide the proper amount of fat
necessary to keep the elements in proportion, nor will they
provide certain vitamins and amino acids that are only available in animal flesh. You can choose to eliminate meat from
your diet, but you *must not eliminate* the nutrients that would
be found in meat, and in the proportions the serving would
contain. You must utilize alternate companion food choices
with supplements, especially if you are beginning a restrictive
plan like the Swank diet or the Zero Dairy, Zero Sugar protocol. You need to begin to look at food as a combination of
components instead of as individual items.

Here's an interesting allegory that may help you begin to
alter your perceptions about food. A friend of mine has always
loved music, and in fact sang in school, church, and amateur
groups often in her younger years. She possesses a large and
eclectic collection of records, tapes, and CDs. Even though
she loved many different pieces, she has often said that until
she began to share her life with a talented drummer, she never
really *heard* music. Her companion taught her to listen to each
individual instrument by explaining where the cues were that
each musician used to connect themselves to the others and

perform the piece. Now, each time she listens to any type of music, she hears the individuals while appreciating the song as a whole.

Begin to view your food in the same way, as the sum of its parts. I have told you that one of the benefits of a Zone and blood-type-specific diet is weight control. Weight gain can become a problem for many MS patients, especially as your mobility begins to decrease, or as a result of the use of conventional drugs like Betaseron. I want to give you one final example to illustrate the importance of food in the correct combinations and address the problem of weight gain and obesity in general.

If your blood type is B, your optimum diet recommends that you eat lots of vegetables, and meats of certain kinds are beneficial, but you may not do as well with pastas and breads. A BCI analysis reveals that you have a vitamin A deficiency, and low reserves of the B family of vitamins. You are physically overweight, so you want to avoid high-calorie food choices. It sounds straightforward, but in the case of MS patients or others with serious illness, this may be difficult to do without the development of personal discipline. Sometimes indulgence, especially in the beginning, may be strangely unavoidable.

Let me show you what I mean. Dr. D'Adamo's work on the heredity of blood types reveals that our attitudes about food are as ancient as our origins. Earlier, I touched upon the fact that food is used in human society more than as a means to survive. This becomes even more relevant to the MS patient as we consider the psychological ramifications of food.

It is natural for any human to become frightened, angry, or depressed when faced with a major life crisis or devastating diagnosis, like MS, and to seek comfort in those circumstances. One of the most ancient means of comfort is food. Our ancestors hunted and gathered food to bring to sick or injured community members who could not provide for themselves. The person would have died without their help. The practice has continued, the originating reason long forgotten, becoming instead a way to show love and support. Think about it. A sick person always receives "cheery" food: candy, cakes, pies, and cookies. People love and like you. They feel bad about your condition, and they genuinely want to show their sympathy by bringing you a lovely food gift to cheer you up.

From the time of infancy, food has meant comfort and safety. The presence of food implies that everything will be all right. The "comfort food" appears, and you begin to eat it, overindulging in high-calorie, low-nutrient items that taste wonderful but do not help you to fight the virus or properly nourish your system. Occasional lapses may be unavoidable, especially in cases of food gifts brought by family members. The problem begins when the pattern becomes excessive, when you no longer work it off, or eat other foods to balance the indulgences. You begin to gain weight and damage your internal balance and your body's ability to use immune and healing systems to fight your affliction and restore your health. Combine that with the adverse effects that may occur with the use of conventional drug treatments, and you can find yourself in serious physical trouble.

You need to be aware of and avoid this cycle at all costs. I am not recommending that you engage in highly stressful physical exercise or push yourself beyond a reasonable threshold of pain. I am, however, urging you to remain in control of your situation. Explain the importance of proper nutrition to your family and those close to you. Show them how the Zone and your specific-blood-type foods help you to regain your health. Encourage them to bring you food gifts that enhance your diet regimen instead of detracting from it. You will find that most of them will be eager to help you. And, in those cases where you do receive an improper food, develop your personal discipline. Learn the art of friendly refusal. Learn to resist temptation by keeping your focus on your goal. Remember always that continued optimum nutrition will equal optimum health. With practice, you will discover that you can maintain your nutritional plan and achieve the results you seek.

Let's review what we have learned so far. We know that our system balance is the result of the proper levels and relationship ratios of vitamins, nutrients, minerals, and elements. We know that the Zone diet is a nutritional plan that provides the proper combination of those substances from food. And, we have learned that our blood types cause us to use certain foods more efficiently than others. Now, in the final sections of this chapter we will examine the vitamin and mineral counts of several different types of food. These charts provide a practical illustration of several food choices and show you how to maximize the nutritional benefits you receive each time you eat. You can refer to these charts and those in the previous chapter when planning your meals.

Finding Nutritional Treasure—The Hidden Vitamin Value of Foods

When most people think of vitamin-rich foods, they picture a salad. How correct is this perception? Let's look at the relative vitamin content of several types of meats, grains, and vegetables. I have even included some restaurant "fast" foods and snacks to see how they stack up in the vitamin and mineral category. I'll explain more about those later.

These charts should be used for reference only. Compiled through the utilization of existing nutritional information available from a variety of U.S. government agencies, food and dairy councils, manufacturers' labels, and published food guides like the ones I have recommended to you, they should be viewed as guidelines. The size of the portion served, the method of seasoning, and preparation can affect the amounts of the vitamins and minerals found in each portion as represented here.

Nutrient and calorie counts can also differ between manufacturers, or brand names. The brands that I have listed are examples only, and the information listed is publicly available. The use of any brand name item does not mean I recommend or necessarily discourage eating it, or that I prefer one brand over another. I simply used nationally known brands wherever possible to allow the largest group of readers to picture the food item clearly when reading the charts.

This having been said, let's look first at what is thought to be the most vitamin-rich group of foods, the vegetable group. If you do not see your favorite vegetable listed here, it means that either that item did not have sufficient measurable amounts of the nutrients we are concerned with, or complete data on the item were not available. It does not necessarily indicate that your particular favorite food, or preparation style, does not contain nutrient value. Refer to a food count book, or read the nutrition labels printed on the product in question.

Chart 16-1, beginning on page 406, shows the relative vitamin content of several common vegetables.

We can see that the best sources of vitamin A are the dark green, leafy vegetables and vegetable greens like broccoli, kale, spinach, and mustard or turnip greens. Tomatoes, technically a fruit, also score highly, as do kelp and certain members of the squash family. Sweet potatoes score well in all categories, but their close cousins, yams, don't do nearly as well. Another oft-neglected but nutritious "old-fashioned" vegetable is the rutabaga, a good source of vitamin A and dietary fiber. Dark green and leafy vegetables are also an excellent source of vitamin BC, or folacin, which is especially important to MS patients. We have already explored in detail the benefits of the B family of vitamins to the MS patient in chapter 12.

Each vegetable is strong in a particular area, while only trace elements or no appreciable amounts of a particular vitamin or mineral are found in other categories. Eating portions of these vegetables in combination with other plant-based foods will allow you to maximize your nutrient intake. For a more complete listing of how all vegetables measure up in these categories, obtain a food count book and use it until you begin to know from experience which foods contain the most nutrient value per serving.

Chart 16-1 Relative Vitamin Content of
Common Vegetables Measured as Indicated

Food Item	Serve Size	Prep.	A IU	C Mg	TH Mg	RB Mg	NI Mg	B$_6$ Mg	BC Mcg	B$_{12}$ Mcg
Alfalfa	1/2 cup	Sprout	26	3	.03	.04	.16	.01	12.2	0
Artichoke Heart	3 oz.	Frozen	131	4	.05	.13	.73	.07	95	0
Asparagus	4 spears	Fresh	485	10	.11	.11	.97	.11	132	0
Beans										
Baked	8 oz.	Veg.	217	ND	.19	.08	.54	.17	30.4	0
Baked	8 oz.	Frank	349	5	.13	.13	2.04	.10	68.1	.77
Baked	8 oz.	Pork	405	4	.12	.09	1.01	.15	82.4	.05
Chickpeas	1/2 cup	Dried	22	1	.1	.05	.43	.11	141.0	0
Green	1/2 cup	Canned	389	5	.03	.06	24	.04	21.8	0
Green	1/2 cup	Fresh	413	6	.05	.06	.38	.04	20.6	0
Green	1/2 cup	Frozen	359	6	.03	.05	.28	.04	ND	0
Red Kidney	1/2 cup	Dried	0	1	14	.05	.51	.11	114.1	0
Lentils	1/2 cup	Dried	8	2	.17	.07	1.05	.18	178.9	0
Lima, Baby	1/2 cup	Dried	0	0	.15	.05	.6	.07	136.4	0
Lima, Fordhook	1/2 cup	Frozen	162	11	.06	.05	.91	.10	ND	0
Navy	1/2 cup	Dried	2	1	.18	.06	.48	.15	127.3	0
Pea, Green	1/2 cup	Canned	653	8	.1	.07	.62	.05	37.7	0
Pea, Green	1/2 cup	Fresh	478	11	.21	.12	1.62	.17	50.7	0
Pea, Green	1/2 cup	Fresh	461	29	.19	.10	1.51	.12	47	0
Pea, Green	1/2 cup	Frozen	534	8	.23	.08	1.18	.09	46.9	0
Pea, Snow	1/2 cup	Frozen	133	18	.05	.1	.45	.14	ND	0
Pea, Split	1/2 cup	Boiled	7	ND	.19	.06	.87	.05	63.6	0
Pink	1/2 cup	Dried	0	0	.22	.05	.48	.15	141.3	0
Pinto	1/2 cup	Dried	2	2	.16	.08	.34	.13	146.2	0
Soybean	1/2 cup	Roast	172	2	.09	.13	1.21	.18	181.5	0
Soybean	1/2 cup	Kernel	108	1.2	.05	.08	.95	.16	121.3	0
Beets	1/2 cup	Fresh	30	3	.02	.03	.28	.06	68.0	0
Broccoli	6.3 oz.	Spear	2498	134	.1	.2	1.03	.26	89.0	0
Broccoli	1/2 cup	Chop	1082	58	.04	.09	.45	.11	39.0	0
Broccoli	1/2 cup	Frozen	1741	37	.05	.75	.42	.12	51.9	0
Broccoli	3 oz.	Spear	1741	37	.05	.08	.42	.12	28.0	0
Brussels Sprouts	1/2 cup	Fresh	561	48	.08	.06	.47	.14	46.8	0
Brussels Sprouts	1/2 cup	Frozen	459	36	.08	.09	.42	.23	79.0	0

Item	Serve Size	Prep.	A IU	C Mg	TH Mg	RB Mg	NI Mg	B$_6$ Mg	BC Mcg	B$_{12}$ Mcg
Cabbage										
Green	1/2 cup	Boiled	99	15	.04	.04	.21	.09	15	0
Savoy	1/2 cup	Boiled	649	12	.04	.02	.02	.11	ND	0
Savoy	1/2 cup	Raw	350	11	.03	.01	.11	.07	ND	0
Chinese	1/2 cup	Boiled	2183	22	.03	.05	.36	ND	ND	0
Chinese	1/2 cup	Raw	1050	16	.01	.03	.18	ND	ND	0
Carrot, Baby	1/2 cup	Can	10055	2	.01	.02	.4	.08	6.7	0
Carrot, Baby	1/2 cup	Frozen	12922	2	.02	.03	.32	.09	7.9	0
Carrot, Mature	1/2 cup	Boiled	19152	2	.03	.04	.40	.19	10.8	0
Carrot, Mature	1/2 cup	Raw	15471	5	.05	.03	.51	.08	7.7	0
Cauliflower	1/2 cup	Boiled	87	45	.04	.06	.42	.13	26	0
Cauliflower	1/2 cup	Raw	76	44	.04	.05	.37	.11	29	0
Celery	1/2 cup	Chop	80	4	.03	.03	.19	.05	17	0
Chicory	1/2 cup	Raw	3600	22	5	.09	.45	ND	ND	0
Collard Greens	1/2 cup	Boiled	1745	8	.01	.03	.19	.03	4	0
Corn, Yell/Wht	1/2 cup	Boiled	178	5	.18	.06	1.32	.05	38.1	0
Corn, Yell/ Wht	1 ear	Boiled	167	5	.17	.06	1.24	.05	35.7	0
Cucumber	1 med.	Raw	112	3	.01	.01	.12	.02	7	0
Eggplant	1/2 cup	Boiled	31	1	.04	.01	.29	.04	6.9	0
Kale	1/2 cup	Boiled	4810	27	.03	.05	.33	.09	8.6	0
Kale	1/2 cup	Frozen	4130	16	.03	.07	.44	.06	9.3	0
Kale	1/2 cup	Raw	3026	41	.04	.04	.34	.09	10	0
Kale, Scotch	1/2 cup	Boiled	1296	34	.03	.03	.52	.09	8.6	0
Kale, Scotch	1/2 cup	Raw	1054	44	.02	.02	.44	.08	ND	0
Lettuce, Endive	1/2 cup	Fresh	513	2	.02	.02	.1	.01	35.5	0
Lettuce, Iceberg	1/2 cup	Fresh	198	3	.03	.03	.12	.01	33.6	0
Lettuce, Romaine	1/2 cup	Shred	728	7	.03	.03	.14	ND	38	0
Mushroom	1/2 cup	Boiled	0	3	.06	.23	3.48	.07	14.2	0
Mustard Greens	1/2 cup	Fresh	2122	18	.03	.04	.30	ND	ND	0
Mustard Greens	1/2 cup	Frozen	3352	10	.03	.04	.19	.08	ND	0
Okra	1/2 cup	Fresh	460	13	.11	.04	.70	.15	36.5	0
Okra	1/2 cup	Frozen	473	11	.09	.11	.72	.04	134	0
Okra	1/2 cup	Raw	330	11	.1	.03	.50	.11	43.9	0
Onion, Scallion	1/2 cup	Fresh	193	9	.03	.04	.26	ND	32	0
Onion, All	1/2 cup	Frozen	36	3	.02	.03	.15	.07	14.1	0

Food Item	Serve Size	Prep.	A IU	C Mg	TH Mg	RB Mg	NI Mg	B_6 Mg	BC Mcg	B_{12} Mcg
Pepper, Chili, Hot	1/2 cup	Raw	578	182	.07	.07	.71	.21	17.5	0
Pepper, Chili, Hot	1/2 cup	SunDr	4900	5.8	.01	.23	1.6	.15	9.5	0
Pepper, Sweet	1/2 cup	Boiled	403	51	.04	.02	.33	.16	11	0
Pepper, Sweet	1/2 cup	Raw	316	45	.03	.02	.26	.12	11	0
Pepper, Yellow	1/2 cup	Raw	124	95	.02	.01	.46	.09	14	0
Potato, White	1 med.	Baked	0	26	.22	.07	3.32	.70	22.2	0
Potato, White	1/2 cup	Boiled	0	18	.14	.03	1.96	.41	13.6	0
Potato, White	1/2 cup	Mashed	20	7	.09	.04	1.17	.25	8.6	0
Potato, White	1/2 cup	Micro	0	12	.10	.02	1.27	.25	9.7	0
Potato, Sweet	1 med.	Baked	24877	28	.08	.15	.69	.28	25.7	0
Potato, Sweet	1/2 cup	NSkin	27968	28	.09	.23	1.05	.40	18.2	0
Potato, Sweet	1/2 cup	Can	19268	7	.03	.12	1.22	ND	ND	0
Potato, Sweet	1/2 cup	Frozen	14441	8	.06	.05	.49	.16	19.6	0
Potato, Yam	1/2 cup	Boiled	0	8	.07	.02	.38	.16	10.9	0
Rice										
Brown, L. Gr.	1/2 cup	Cook	0	0	.09	.02	1.5	.14	4	0
Brown, M. Gr.	1/2 cup	Cook	0	0	.10	.01	1.3	.15	4	0
White, Instant	1/2 cup	Cook	0	0	.06	.04	.72	.01	3	0
White, L. Gr.	1/2 cup	Cook	0	0	.06	.04	.72	.01	3	0
White, S. Gr.	1/2 cup	Cook	0	0	.15	.02	1.39	.06	2	0
Rutabaga	1/2 cup	Boiled	674	23	.10	.05	.86	.12	19	0
Rutabaga	1/2 cup	Raw	406	18	.06	.03	.49	.07	14	0
Sauce, Tomato	1/2 cup	Marin.	1202	16	.06	.07	1.99	ND	ND	0
Sauce, Tomato	1/2 cup	Plain	1195	16	.08	.07	1.4	ND	ND	0
Sauce, Tomato	1/2 cup	Spag.	1528	14	.07	.07	1.87	ND	ND	0
Sauce, Tomato	1/2 cup	Mush.	1165	15	.09	.13	1.54	ND	ND	0
Sauce, Tomato	1/2 cup	Onion	1038	16	.09	.16	1.52	ND	ND	0
Seaweed, Kelp	3 oz.	Raw	99	ND	.01	.04	.13	ND	51	ND
Seawd, Wakame	3 oz.	Raw	306	3	.06	.18	1.35	ND	ND	0
Spinach	1/2 cup	Boiled	7371	9	.09	.21	.44	.22	131.2	0
Spinach	1/2 cup	Frozen	7395	12	.06	.16	.40	.14	102.1	0
Spinach	1/2 cup	Raw	1880	8	.02	.05	.20	.06	54.4	0
Squash										
Acorn	1/2 cup	Baked	437	11	.17	.01	.90	.2	19.1	0
Acorn	1/2 cup	Boiled	315	8	.12	.01	.65	.14	13.8	0

Food Item	Serve Size	Prep.	A IU	C Mg	TH Mg	RB Mg	NI Mg	B_6 Mg	BC Mcg	B_{12} Mcg
Acorn	1/2 cup	Raw	238	8	.10	.01	.49	.11	11.7	0
Butternut	1/2 cup	Fresh	7141	15	.07	.02	.99	.13	19.6	0
Butternut	1/2 cup	Frozen	4007	4	.06	.05	.56	.08	ND	0
Crookneck	1/2 cup	Boiled	259	5	.04	.04	.46	.09	18.1	0
Crookneck	1/2 cup	Raw	220	5	.03	.03	.30	.07	14.9	0
Zucchini	1/2 cup	Can	615	3	.05	.05	.60	ND	ND	0
Zucchini	1/2 cup	Frozen	483	4	.05	.05	.43	.05	8.8	0
Zucchini	1/2 cup	Raw	221	6	.05	.02	.26	.06	14.4	0
Swiss Chard	1/2 cup	Boiled	2762	16	.03	.08	.32	ND	ND	0
Swiss Chard	1/2 cup	Raw	594	5	.01	.01	.07	ND	ND	0
Tomato										
Red	1/2 cup	Stewed	710	17	.06	.05	.91	ND	ND	0
Red	1/2 cup	Wedg	757	19	ND	.07	.04	.88	ND	
Red	1/2 cup	Fresh	892	28	.08	.07	.90	.11	16	0
Red	1/2 cup	Raw	561	17	.05	.04	.57	.07	13.5	0
Red, Paste	1/2 cup	Plain	3234	55	.20	.25	4.22	.50	ND	0
Red, Puree	1/2 cup	Reg.	1701	44	.09	.07	2.14	.19	ND	0
Sun Dried	1/2 cup	Oil	707.5	56	.11	.21	2.0	.17	12.5	0
Turnip, Greens	1/2 cup	Boiled	3959	20	.03	.05	.3	.30	85.3	0
Turnip, Greens	1/2 cup	Frozen	6540	18	.04	.06	.38	.38	32.3	0
Turnip, Greens	1/2 cup	Raw	2128	17	.02	.03	.17	.07	54.4	0
Watercress	1/2 cup	Raw	799	7	.02	.02	.03	.02	ND	0

Key: A = Vitamin A, C = Vitamin C, TH = Thiamine, RB = Riboflavin, NI = Niacin, B6 = Vitamin B6, BC = Vitamin BC, (Folacin), B12 = Vitamin B12, ND = No Data Available, HF = Health Food Store

Chart 16-2 on page 410 illustrates the vitamin content of several common fruits.

Although all fruits post significant amounts of vitamins A and C, orange or dark-colored fruits score the highest, especially tangerines, apricots, prunes, and cantaloupe, an orange-fleshed melon. Fruits do contain a high amount of natural sugars, which can be considerations when choosing foods to add to your diet if you have also been diagnosed with diabetes or hypoglycemic conditions, or if you are on a restricted diet and are concerned with calories from sugar.

Chart 16-2 Relative Vitamin Content of Common Fruits Measured as Indicated

Food Item	Serve Size	Prep.	A IU	C Mg	TH Mg	RB Mg	NI Mg	B₆ Mg	BC Mcg	B₁₂ Mcg
Apple	Medium	Unpeeled	30	3	.01	.01	.04	.03	1.6	0
Apricot	1/2 cup	Dried	4706	2	.01	.10	1.94	.10	4.50	0
Apricot	1/2 cup	Pitted	2024	8	.02	.03	.47	.04	6.70	0
Avocado, Calif.	8 oz.	Fresh	1059	14	.19	.21	3.32	.48	113.3	0
Avocado, Florida	8 oz.	Fresh	1860	24	.33	.37	5.80	.85	161.9	0
Banana	Medium	Peeled	92	10	.05	.11	.62	.66	21.8	0
Blackberry	1/2 cup	Syrup	280	4	.04	.05	.37	.05	33.9	0
Blackberry Fresh	1/2 cup	Trimmed	119	15	.02	.03	.29	.04	ND	0
Figs	6.6 oz.	10 Figs	248	2	.13	.17	1.3	.42	14.1	0
Grapefruit, Pink	8.5 oz.	1/2 Large	318	47	.04	.03	.24	.05	15	0
Cantaloupe	1/2	5"Melon	8608	113	10	.06	1.53	.31	45.5	0
Watermelon	1/2 cup	Cubed	293	8	.06	.02	.16	.12	1.7	0
Watermelon	1 slice	Medium	1762	47	.39	.1	.96	.69	10.4	0
Orange, Calif.	1 med	All	269	70	.11	.05	.37	.08	39.7	0
Orange, Calif.	1 med	Navel	256	80	.12	.06	.41	.1	47.2	0
Orange, Calif.	1 med	Valencia	278	59	.11	.05	.33	.08	46.7	0
Orange, Florida	1 med	All	302	68	.15	.06	.6	.08	26.1	0
Papaya	1/2 cup	Peeled	1410	43	.02	.02	.24	.01	ND	0
Peach	1/2 cup	Fresh	455	6	.01	.04	.84	.02	2.9	0
Peach	1/2 cup	Dried	1731	4	ND	.17	3.5	.05	ND	0
Peach, Freestne	1/2 cup	Canned	473	4	.01	.02	.72	ND	ND	0
Pineapple	1/2 cup	Chunks	48	12	.12	.02	.36	ND	ND	0
Prune	1/2 cup	Syrup	933	3	.04	.14	1.01	ND	ND	0
Prune	4 oz.	Dried	323	3	.02	.11	.77	.23	.1	0
Prune	4 oz.	Dried	2253	4	.09	.18	2.22	.3	4.2	0
Rhubarb	1/2 cup	Fresh	61	5	.01	.02	.18	.02	4.3	0
Rhubarb	1/2 cup	Frozen	83	4	.02	.03	.24	.02	6.4	0
Tangerine	1/2 cup	Canned	1056	43	.1	.04	ND	ND	ND	0
Tangerine	1/2 cup	Fresh	897	30	.1	.02	.16	.07	19.9	0

Key: A = Vitamin A, C = Vitamin C, TH = Thiamine, RB = Riboflavin, NI = Niacin, B₆ = Vitamin B₆, BC = Vitamin BC (Folacin), B₁₂ = Vitamin B₁₂, ND = No Data Available, HF = Health Food Store

Sometimes, products made from the whole, natural food item score more highly than the naturally occurring version. Fruit juices are an excellent example, although not all of them are high in our target nutrients. Look at the next chart, which examines the relative nutrient value of some popular beverages.

Chart 16-3 compares vitamin content of common beverages.

Some fruit beverages score highly, as do some powdered drink mixes. Surprisingly, fast food shakes also do very well in our categories, but beware! These are also loaded with calories and sugar. Coffee contains trace elements of niacin, but nothing else of value, and is full of caffeine. Teas also contain

Chart 16-3 Relative Vitamin Content of Common Beverages Measured as Indicated

Food Item	Serve Size	Prep.	A IU	C Mg	TH Mg	RB Mg	NI Mg	B_6 Mg	BC Mcg	B_{12} Mcg
Beer	12 fl. oz.	Light	0	0	.03	.11	1.4	.12	14.7	.02
Beer	12 fl. oz.	Regular	0	0	.02	.09	1.6	.18	21.4	.06
Drink Mixes										
Malted Milk	8 fl. oz.	w/ Milk	376	2	.2	.54	1.28	.18	22	1.04
Malted Milk	3/4 oz.		68	0	.11	.14	1.07	.08	10	.16
Orange	3 tsp.	Breakfast	0	22	.04	.01	0	0	ND	0
Shake	10 fl. oz.		263	1	.16	.69	.46	.14	9.9	.97
Shake	10 fl. oz.	Vanilla	368	2	.13	.52	.52	.15	9.2	1.01
Juice										
Grape	6 fl. oz.	Bottle	12	.01	.05	.07	.5	.13	4.8	0
Grapefruit	6 fl. oz.	Unsweet	12	54	.08	.04	.43	.04	19.2	0
Orange	6 fl. oz.	Conc.	144	73	.15	.04	.38	.08	81.6	0
Papaya	6 fl. oz.	Nectar	210	5	.01	.01	.28	.02	3.6	0
Peach	6 fl. oz.	Nectar	480	10	.01	.02	.54	ND	ND	0
Pear	6 fl. oz.	Nectar	2	2	.01	.02	.24	ND	ND	0
Pineapple	6 fl. oz.	Canned	6	20	.1	.04	.48	.18	43.2	0
Tangerine	6 fl. oz.	Sweet	786	41	.11	.04	.19	.06	ND	0
Tomato	6 fl. oz.	Plain	1012	33	.09	.06	1.23	.2	36.1	0
Vegetable	6 fl. oz.	V-8 Style	2130	50	.08	.05	1.32	.26	ND	0

Key: A = Vitamin A, C = Vitamin C, TH = Thiamine, RB = Riboflavin, NI = Niacin, B_6 = Vitamin B_6, BC = Vitamin BC (Folacin), B_{12} = Vitamin B_{12}, ND = No Data Available, HF = Health Food Store none of these vitamins we seek. Neither do table wines, of any variety, or any carbonated soda. Beer does contain rather good amounts of folacin, or vitamin BC, per serving, but the alcoholic content may be a prohibitive consideration, especially if you are currently taking any number of medications, which may interact adversely. The big winners in these categories are clearly the nectar juices, and tomato or vegetable blend juices. Overall, the best choice of juice is a mixed vegetable style, but take note that some of you may experience digestive problems due to the high acidic content.

Throughout these charts, you will see that I have included some "fast" foods, sometimes termed "junk" foods. You may be surprised to see that I have listed them, especially as I am a naturopath and a nutritionist. My reasons for doing so are twofold. First, my recent education into the components of foods has shown me that not all "fast" food is worthless. Dr. Sears contends that no food item is "bad" food. While I agree with that statement in principle, I believe that, whenever possible, a more natural food should be chosen over a processed or prepared type. Additionally, as you will see in later charts, some of these "junk food" snacks do contain a significant amount of vitamins and nutrients, such as the shakes listed above.

Second, although I am a doctor, I am also a realist. Many MS patients will not have access to the healthier or more natural forms of some foods. You may have to rely on someone else to drive you or do the shopping for you depending on the state of your illness. It may not be possible to obtain items from a farm stand or health food store. Lifestyle is also a consideration. Many patients carry a full schedule of daily activities. Whether they are employed full time or at home raising children, time constraints may make it impossible to eat correctly at each meal. One of the principles of the Zone is that food eaten at regular intervals is essential to metabolism function. It is actually worse to skip a meal entirely because you can't "eat right" than to choose a less than ideal food. Therefore, I have included these foods as the better choices in those situations. I do not recommend that you make a steady diet of any of them, but they can provide a temporary solution when no viable alternative is available.

In keeping with that viewpoint, other foods are part of our everyday meals, which we may not pay much attention to unless we are watching our weight, like butter, spreads, and condiments. I have not included a comparison chart, but we should discuss them briefly. Of the butter and spread choices, margarine contains the highest concentration of vitamin A, but no appreciable amounts of our other nutrients. Margarine is also a largely indigestible substance, so you may want to consider that its detriments outweigh the benefits of including it in your meal planning. Animal fat, vegetable oil, and nut-based butters also do not score at all well in these target vitamins, although they do provide other necessary fats for our diet.

Condiments are another overlooked source of some essential nutrients. A cup of plain barbecue sauce, for instance, contains over 2100 IU of vitamin A. Jalapeno peppers, pimentos, and salsa also hold over 1000 IU of vitamin A each per 1/2-cup serving. Salt contains none of our desired vitamins, but salt substitute scores 186 IU of vitamin A in a one-teaspoon serving. Cayenne pepper is loaded with vitamin A, having almost 750 IU in one teaspoon, but common black pepper does not score nearly as well. Other commonly used condiments contain no appreciable amounts of the desired vitamins per serving.

Grains and the flours made from them are a primary staple in the diet of many cultures today. How do these food items stack up in our quest for essential vitamins? Chart 16-4 illustrates their relative values.

Chart 16-4 Relative Vitamin Content of Common Grains Measured as Indicated

Food Item	Serve Size	Prep.	A IU	C Mg	TH Mg	RB Mg	NI Mg	B_6 Mg	BC Mcg	B_{12} Mcg
Cereals, Dry										
Bran	1 cup	All Bran	1500	30	.76	.86	10	1	ND	3
Bran w/Fruit	1 cup	Raisin Bran	1500	0	.76	.86	10	1	ND	3

Food Item	Serve Size	Prep.	A IU	C Mg	TH Mg	RB Mg	NI Mg	B₆ Mg	BC Mcg	B₁₂ Mcg
Corn	1 cup	Corn Flakes	750	15	.38	.43	10	1	ND	0
Mixed Grain	1 cup	HlthCh. Flake	500	0	.53	.6	7	.7	ND	2.1
Mixed Grain	¾ cup	Mueslix	750	0	.38	.43	5	.5	ND	1.2
Mixed Grain	1 cup	Special K	750	15	.53	.6	7	.7	ND	0
Rice	1¼ cups	Rice Krispies	750	15	.38	.43	5	.5	ND	0
Wheat Bran	1 cup	Crude	1250	15	.38	.43	5	.5	ND	1.5
Cereals, Cooked										
Oat	1 pkt.	Inst. Oatmeal	1237	0	.44	.21	3.64	.47	122	ND
Oat Bran	1 cup	Cooked	750	15	.38	.43	5	.5	ND	0
Oatmeal	1 cup	Rolled Oats	38	0	2.26	.05	.3	.05	9	0
Flour										
Buckwheat	1 cup	Plain	0	0	.5	.23	7.38	.7	64	0
Carob	1 cup	Plain	15	.01	.06	.48	1.95	.38	29.9	0
Corn	1 cup	Mesa Enriched	ND	0	1.63	.86	11.2	.42	28	0
Corn	1 cup	Whole Grain	ND	0	.29	.09	2.22	ND	30	ND
Cracker Meal	1 cup	Plain	0	0	.8	.54	6.56	ND	ND	0
Pancake Mix	2.6 oz.	Two 4" cakes	12	0	.08	.08	.65	.04	ND	.07
Peanut	1 cup	Defatted	0	0	.42	.29	16.2	.3	148	0
Rice, Brown	1 cup	Plain	0	0	.7	.13	10.0	1.16	25	0
Rice, White	1 cup	Plain	0	0	.22	.03	4.09	.69	6	0
Rye, Dark	1 cup	Plain	0	0	.4	32	5.47	.57	77	0
Sesame	1 cup	High Fat	20	0	.76	.08	3.80	.04	8.7	0
Sesame	1 cup	Low Fat	18	0	.72	.08	3.56	.04	8.2	0
Soy	1 cup	Full Fat	102	0	.49	.99	3.67	.39	293	0
Soy	1 cup	Low Fat	35	0	.33	.25	1.90	.46	361	0
Wheat	1 cup	Whole Grain	0	0	.54	.26	7.64	.41	52	0
Wheat, White	1 cup	All Purpose	0	0	.98	.62	7.38	.06	33	0
Wheat, White	1 cup	Self-Rising	0	0	.84	.52	7.29	.06	53	0
Wheat, White	1 cup	Tortilla	0	0	.82	.55	6.46	.04	ND	0
Misc. Grains										
Rice, Wild	½ cup	Cooked	0	0	.04	.07	1.06	.11	22	0
Wheat Germ	½ cup	Crude	66	0	.96	.42	2.82	.32	212	.05

Key: A = Vitamin A, C = Vitamin C, TH = Thiamine, RB = Riboflavin, NI = Niacin, B6 = Vitamin B6, BC = Vitamin BC (Folacin), B12 = Vitamin B12, ND = No Data Available, HF = Health Food Store

Note the high range of differences between whole grains and their respective products. Most dry grain cereals contain enough vitamin A per single serving to meet or exceed the daily DRI of all females and children, and between seventy-five percent and 150 percent of the DRI for males. Bran, wheat bran, and oat cereals score the strongest in all categories. When these grains are processed into flours, however, they do not contain appreciable amounts of vitamin A, but become instead good sources of niacin. The exception in the flour category is soy flour, which scores well in all categories, except for vitamin C. Wheat germ is also a good source of our target nutrients, especially folacin, or vitamin BC. An addition of one or two tablespoons of wheat germ to your dry or cooked morning cereal is an easy way to boost your meal value.

Before we examine our next group of foods, meat and poultry, let's review dairy foods again. We now know that your blood type has a great deal to do with determining your optimum diet. If you do not test positively for milk allergy, and it is applicable to your blood type, you should consider including dairy products in your daily nutrition plan. Dairy is probably one of the best natural sources for all of these nutrients, plus calcium, magnesium, and phosphorus. Cow's milk products commercially available have additionally been fortified with other nutrients, most noticeably vitamin D. Dairy foods are rich in a number of essential amino acids your body requires for the processing of other nutrients and the manufacture of good eicosanoids, making these products a good choice for persons who can easily handle them in their systems. To obtain a complete listing of all of the vitamins and nutrients found in dairy products, including the milks and cheeses from goats and sheep, consult a food count book and read the individual product labels.

Non-dairy alternatives, including frozen and powdered varieties, do not contain anywhere near the nutritional value of real dairy, and should not be looked to as an adequate substitute, unless you are careful to supply the lack with the addition of daily supplements to your diet.

Chart 16-5 reviews the relative vitamin counts of animal meats, poultry, and eggs.

Chart 16-5 Relative Vitamin Content of Meats, Poultry, and Eggs Measured as Indicated

Food Item	Serve Size	Prep.	A IU	C Mg	TH Mg	RB Mg	NI Mg	B_6 Mg	BC Mcg	B_{12} Mcg
Beef										
Chuck	4 oz.	Pot Roast	0	0	.08	.27	3.55	.32	10.2	3.31
Corned	4 oz.	Cured, Cooked	0	18	.03	.19	3.44	.26	ND	1.85
Ground, Lean	4 oz.	Broiled, Med.	0	0	.06	.24	5.85	.29	10.2	2.66
Ground, Lean	4 oz.	Fried, Med.	0	0	.06	.25	5.43	.32	10.2	2.57
Ground, Reg.	4 oz.	Broiled, Med.	0	0	.03	.22	6.54	.31	10.2	3.32
Ground, Reg.	4 oz.	Fried, Med.	0	0	.03	.23	6.61	.27	10.2	3.07
Heart	4 oz.	Simmered	0	2	.16	1.75	4.62	.24	2.3	16.22
Kidney	4 oz.	Simmered	1407	1	.22	4.6	6.83	.59	111.1	58.17
Liver	4 oz.	Pan Fried	40943	26	.24	4.69	16.37	1.62	249.5	126.8
Porterhouse	4 oz.	Broiled	0	0	.11	.25	4.59	.4	7.90	2.44
Round, Bot.	4 oz.	Roasted	0	0	.09	.25	4.25	.39	12.50	2.90
T-Bone Steak	4 oz.	Broiled	0	0	.11	.25	4.63	.39	7.90	2.44
Chicken										
Cornish Hen	1 bird	Roast w/Skin	363	2	.25	.57	19.01	.99	9	1.12
Cornish Hen	1 bird	Roast w/o Skin	70	1	.08	.24	6.70	.38	2	.32
Dark Meat	4 oz.	Leg, Fried, Skin	103	0	.1	.26	7.33	.38	9	.35
Dark Meat	4 oz.	Roast w/ Skin	118	0	.11	.27	7.76	.36	9.1	.34
Dark Meat	4 oz.	Roast, No Skin	61	0	.07	.22	6.50	.35	7.9	.31
Dark Meat	4 oz.	Thigh, Fry, Skin	61	0	.06	.15	4.31	.21	5	.19
Egg	1 large	Fried	394	0	.03	.24	.04	.07	18	.42
Egg	1 large	Hard Boiled	280	0	.03	.26	.03	.06	22	.56
Egg	1 large	Raw	317	0	.03	.25	.04	.07	23	.50
Egg	1 large	White Only	TR	0	TR	.15	.03	TR	1	.07
Egg	1 large	Yolk Only	323	0	.03	.11	ND	.07	24	.52
Giblets	4 oz.	Simmered	8427	9	.1	1.08	4.65	.39	426.5	11.5
Heart	4 oz.	Simmered	32	2	.08	.84	3.18	.36	90.7	8.27
Liver	4 oz.	Simmered	18569	18	.17	1.98	5.05	.66	873.2	21.99
White Meat	4 oz.	Breast, Fry, Skin	57	0	.09	.15	15.58	.66	4.5	.39
White Meat	4 oz.	Roast w/o Skin	33	0	.07	.13	14.09	.68	4.5	.39

Food Item	Serve Size	Prep.	A IU	C Mg	TH Mg	RB Mg	NI Mg	B_6 Mg	BC Mcg	B_{12} Mcg
Duck	4 oz.	Roast w/Skin	238	0	.2	.31	5.47	.2	6.8	.34
Duck	4 oz.	Roast w/o Skin	87	0	.29	.53	5.78	.28	11.3	.45
Goose	4 oz.	Roast w/Skin	79	0	.09	.37	4.73	.42	2.3	ND
Lamb										
Ground	4 oz.	Broiled	0	0	.11	.26	7.60	.16	21.5	2.96
Leg	4 oz.	Roasted w/Fat	0	0	.11	.31	7.43	.18	24.9	3.03
Leg	4 oz.	Roasted w/o Fat	0	0	.12	.32	7.25	.19	27.2	3.07
Loin	4 oz.	Broiled, w/Fat	0	0	.11	.28	8.05	.15	20.4	2.8
Loin	4 oz.	Broiled, w/o Fat	0	0	.12	.32	7.77	.18	27.2	2.86
Kidney	4 oz.	Simmered	516	14	.4	2.35	6.79	.14	91.9	89.47
Liver	4 oz.	Pan Fried	29482	15	.4	5.21	18.92	1.08	453.6	97.18
Tongue	4 oz.	Braised	0	8	.09	.48	4.18	.19	3.4	7.14
Rib	4 oz.	Broiled, w/Fat	0	0	.1	.25	7.94	.12	15.9	2.88
Rib	4 oz.	Broiled, w/o Fat	0	0	.11	.28	7.43	.17	23.8	2.99
Shoulder	4 oz.	Broiled w/Fat	0	0	.1	.29	7.31	.14	21.5	3.37
Shoulder	4 oz.	Broiled w/o Fat	0	0	.11	.32	6.97	.16	26.1	3.53
Shoulder	4 oz.	Cubed, Broiled	0	0	.08	.25	7.18	.11	19.3	3.18
Pork										
Ham, Reg.	4 oz.	Cured, Roasted	ND	ND	.68	.25	5.06	.43	3.4	.73
Ham, Reg.	4 oz.	Fresh, Roasted	9	.01	.65	.34	5.05	.44	5.7	.78
Ham, Reg.	4 oz.	Can, Roasted	0	16	.93	.29	6.01	.34	5.7	1.2
Liverwurst	4 oz.	Most Varieties	15936	12	.28	1.72	10.68	.36	TR	22.76
Loin, Ctr Rib	4 oz.	Roasted	9	0	.67	.32	5.56	.4	9.1	.64
Loin, Top	4 oz.	Roasted	9	0	.72	.35	6.07	.45	10.2	.62
Chitterlings	4 oz.	Simmered	0	0	0	.09	.11	ND	ND	ND
Kidney	4 oz.	Simmered	295	12	.45	1.8	6.56	.52	46.5	8.63
Liver	4 oz.	Pan Fried	20409	27	.29	2.49	9.57	.65	184.8	21.17
Sausage	4 oz.	Fresh, Cooked	0	0	.4	.12	2.36	.16	ND	.88
Shoulder	4 oz.	Roasted	9	ND	.61	.36	4.52	.37	4.5	.94
Spare Ribs	6.3 oz	Braised, 1lb.	18	ND	.72	.68	9.69	.62	7.0	1.91
Tenderloin	4 oz.	Lean, Roasted	8	ND	1.07	.44	5.34	.48	6.8	.62
Rabbit	4 oz.	Roasted	0	0	.08	.18	7.50	.42	10.2	7.38
Rabbit	4 oz.	Stewed	0	0	.07	.19	8.12	.39	10.2	7.38
Turkey										
Breast Meat	4 oz.	w/Skin, Roasted	0	0	.06	.15	7.22	.72	6.8	.41

Food Item	Serve Size	Prep.	A IU	C Mg	TH Mg	RB Mg	NI Mg	B_6 Mg	BC Mcg	B_{12} Mcg
Dark Meat	4 oz.	w/Skin, Roasted	0	0	.07	.27	4	.36	10.2	.41
Drumstick	4 oz.	w/Skin, Roasted	0	0	.07	.27	4.04	.37	10.2	.41
Ground	4 oz.	Cooked	0	0	.04	.14	3.95	.32	5.0	.27
Light Meat	4 oz.	w/Skin, Roasted	0	0	.06	.15	7.13	.53	6.8	.4
Giblets	4 oz.	Simmered	6845	2	.05	1.03	5.11	.37	391.2	27.3
Gizzard	4 oz.	Simmered	210	2	.04	.37	3.48	.14	59	2.2
Heart	4 oz.	Simmered	32	2	.08	1	3.69	.36	89.6	8.1
Liver	4 oz.	Simmered	14267	2	.06	1.61	6.74	.59	755.2	53.9
Wing	4 oz.	w/Skin, Roasted	0	0	.06	.15	6.5	.48	6.8	.39
Veal										
Ground	4 oz.	Broiled	0	0	.08	.31	9.11	.44	12.5	1.44
Leg, Top Rnd	4 oz.	Roasted, w/ Fat	0	0	.07	.37	11.43	.35	18.1	1.34
Loin	4 oz.	Roasted, w/Fat	0	0	.06	.32	10.05	.39	17.0	1.41
Kidney	4 oz.	Simmered	759	9	.22	2.26	5.25	.2	23.8	41.84
Ribs	4 oz.	Roasted, w/Fat	0	0	.06	.31	7.92	.28	14.7	1.66
Shoulder	4 oz.	Roasted, w/Fat	0	0	.08	.39	7.18	.29	13.6	2.06
Sirloin	4 oz.	Roasted, w/Fat	0	0	.07	.4	10.06	.36	17.0	1.61

Key: A = Vitamin A, C = Vitamin C, TH = Thiamine, RB = Riboflavin, NI = Niacin, B6 = Vitamin B6,

BC = Vitamin BC (Folacin), B12 = Vitamin B12, ND = No Data Available, HF = Health Food Store, TR=Trace

All animal meats are the best sources of concentrated vitamin A, niacin, riboflavin, B_6, folacin (BC), and B_{12} available naturally to the human diet. Note that the highest concentrations of nutrients are in the organ meats of all animal species, with astronomical numbers in most categories. I know that liver and animal hearts may not be your favorite foods, but for pure nutritional value, they certainly should be. Next time you serve roasted chicken or turkey, consider making a natural juice gravy with the giblets, heart, and gizzard of the bird. Add a little soy flour to thicken the mixture, and you have a nutrient-packed condiment!

It is important to note that almost all of the nutritional value of eggs is found in the yolk. Yes, egg yolks do contain cholesterol, but the amount is relatively low compared to the vitamins and nutrients found in the versatile egg. I often ate eggs before being diagnosed with MS, but after testing positive for hidden egg allergy, I do not eat them now. I do recommend eggs for those who can eat them as an excellent nutrient source.

For those with more exotic tastes or hunters in the family, duck, goose, and rabbit also score well in these categories. They can be a nice change of pace from everyday foods. Interesting note: the strong numbers found in a portion of roasted or braised rabbit drop sharply when included in stew, so you may not wish to choose that preparation style.

Some blood types, like my Type A, should not overload their diet with meats, especially red meats. Dr. Swank recommends that all red meats be avoided for at least one year. As meats do contain so many essential vitamins, minerals, and nutrients, not to mention their essential amino acids and fats, you need to find a good replacement if you are going to eliminate them from your diet entirely. Vegans, those who consume a strictly vegetarian diet, should also take note of the nutrient numbers in the previous and following charts. Some vegans include fish and shellfish in their diets, while others eschew all foods save those of plant origin. Those individuals should be certain to develop a daily supplement regimen that replaces the elements found in animal and poultry meats, especially the essential amino acids. These are essential to the manufacture of good eicosanoids, which in turn promote and strengthen the healing system. Your nutritionist or medical professional can educate you on the best substitutes.

How do fish and shellfish measure up in our vitamin competition? Let's take a look at some of these choices in Chart 16-6.

Fortunately for those for whom meat is either restricted, not recommended, or eliminated by choice, several breeds of fish and shellfish do the job quite nicely. With the exception of bluefish, tuna, and rainbow trout, the highest concentrations of vitamin A, and in fact all of our target nutrients, are found in the smaller food fishes, like sardines, mackerel,

Chart 16-6 Relative Vitamin Content of
Fish and Shellfish Measured as Indicated

Food Item	Serve Size	Prep.	A IU	C Mg	TH Mg	RB Mg	NI Mg	B$_6$ Mg	BC Mcg	B$_{12}$ Mcg
Fish										
Bluefish	4 oz.	Baked, Broiled, Micro	540	0	.07	.11	8.23	.53	2.3	7.05
Catfish, Farm	4 oz.	Baked, Broiled, Micro	57	1	.48	.08	2.85	.18	7.9	3.18
Cod, Atlantic	4 oz.	Baked, Broiled, Micro	52	1	.1	.09	2.85	.32	TR	1.19
Mixed Fillet	4 oz.	Breaded, 2 Fillets	120	TR	.14	.20	2.42	.06	20.8	2.04
Haddock	4 oz.	Baked, Broiled, Micro	71	0	.05	.05	5.25	.39	ND	1.57
Mixed Sticks	5 oz.	Breaded, about 6 Sticks	150	TR	.2	.25	2.4	.1	20.5	2.5
Halibut	4 oz.	Baked, Broiled, Micro	203	0	.08	.10	8.08	.45	TR	1.55
Herring	4 oz.	Baked, Broiled, Micro	116	1	.13	.34	4.68	.39	TR	14.9
Herring	4 oz.	Kippered	145	1	.14	.36	4.99	.47	TR	21.21
Herring	4 oz.	Pickled	1153	TR	.04	.16	TR	TR	2.7	4.84
Mackerel, Atl.	4 oz.	Baked, Broiled, Micro	204	.01	.18	.47	.78	.52	ND	21.54
Pike, North	4 oz.	Baked, Broiled, Micro	92	4	.08	.09	ND	.15	ND	ND
Pike, Walleye	4 oz.	Baked, Broiled, Micro	92	4	.08	.09	ND	.15	ND	ND
Salmon, Atl.	4 oz.	Baked, Broiled, Micro	57	4	.39	.15	9.12	.73	38.6	3.18
Chinook	4 oz.	Smoked	100	TR	.03	.11	5.35	.32	2.2	3.7
Salmon, Coho	4 oz.	Baked, Broiled, Micro	223	2	.11	.13	8.38	.64	15.9	3.59
Salmon, Pink	4 oz.	Canned w/Bone	62	0	.03	.21	7.41	ND	17.5	ND
Sockeye	4 oz.	Baked, Broiled, Micro	237	TR	.24	.19	7.56	.25	ND	6.58
Sockeye	4 oz.	Canned w/Bone	200	0	.02	.22	6.21	ND	11.1	ND

Food Item	Serve Size	Prep.	A IU	C Mg	TH Mg	RB Mg	NI Mg	B$_6$ Mg	BC Mcg	B$_{12}$ Mcg
Sardine, Atl.	4 oz.	Can, Soy Oil	254	0	.09	.26	5.95	.19	13.4	10.14
Sardine, Pac.	4 oz.	Can, Tomato Sauce	414	1	.05	.26	4.76	.14	27.6	10.2
Swordfish	4 oz.	Baked, Broiled, Micro	155	1	.05	.13	13.4	.43	TR	2.29
Trout, Rnbo.	4 oz.	Baked, Broiled, Micro	325	4	.27	.91	9.97	.45	27.2	5.64
Tuna, Alba.	4 oz.	Canned, in Water	22	0	.01	.05	6.58	.25	2.3	1.33
Tuna, Light	4 oz.	Canned, in Water	64	0	.04	.08	15.1	.4	4.5	3.39
Whiting	4 oz.	Baked, Broiled, Micro	129	0	.08	.07	1.89	.2	17	2.95
Shellfish										
Lobster	4 oz.	Boiled or Steamed	99	ND	.01	.07	1.21	.09	12.6	3.53
Lobster, Spiny	4 oz.	Boiled or Steamed	99	ND	.01	.07	1.21	.09	12.6	3.53
Clams, Hard	20	Cherrystone Steamed	646	ND	TR	.48	3.8	TR	TR	112.1
Clams, Hard	20	Cherrystone Fried	568	ND	TR	.46	3.88	TR	TR	75.71
Clams, Hard	1 cup	Canned	646	ND	TR	.48	3.8	TR	TR	112.1
Clams, Hard	20	Cherrystone Raw	540	ND	TR	.38	3.18	TR	TR	89.0
Crab, Alask.	1 lb.	Legs, Boiled, Steamed	39	0	.07	.07	1.8	TR	TR	TR
Oyster, Atl.	4 oz.	Boiled, Steamed	204	7	.21	.21	2.82	.14	15.8	39.71
Oyster, Atl.	1 cup	Raw	248	9	.25	.24	3.42	.46	24	48.25
Shrimp	4 oz.	Canned	TR	0	.03	.04	3.12	.13	2	1.37
Shrimp	4 oz.	Raw	TR	0	.04	.04	2.88	.12	.32	1.32

Key: A = Vitamin A, C = Vitamin C, TH = Thiamine, RB = Riboflavin, NI = Niacin, B6 = Vitamin B6,

BC = Vitamin BC (Folacin), B12 = Vitamin B12, ND = No Data Available, HF = Health Food Store, TR = Trace

herring, and whiting. Surprisingly good news for today's active lifestyle, both mixed fish breaded fillets and sticks contain high amounts of our desired vitamins per serving. Clams and oysters are the best choices of the shellfish group and the best overall choice for the essential element B$_{12}$.

Now that we've examined a cross section of all of the foods that you can find naturally and prepare at home, what about those times when you are not at home? No matter how carefully we may plan, or how aware we may be that good nutrition is a vital part of our war against MS, there are times when the demands on our time simply do not allow us to stop and eat a "proper" meal. What should we do in those circumstances?

Believe it or not, not all "fast food" is synonymous with "junk food." Although fast food is for the most part highly processed and prepared under circumstances over which you have no control, there are some choices that you can make that are better than others, and will provide you with sufficient nutrition for an emergency or special occasion meal. Again, as a naturopath and nutritionist, I caution you against making these quick meals a steady part of your diet. Although the percentages are not reflected in these charts, many of them do contain an inordinate amount of fats or sugars and are very high in calories. As a realist and a doctor with many years of clinical experience, I know that patients have lapses, or get into situations where these foods may be the only available choices. If you must eat them, these charts will show you which of them are the best of the lot.

The next chart examines the relative nutrient contents of popular fast food and quick meal items. It is important to remember in this category especially that these are only guidelines, chosen for example only. These types of meals can vary widely between manufacturers and restaurant franchises. I have tried to use national food chains and name brands whenever possible so that the greatest number of readers can picture the listed item easily. Use of any brand name product or franchise menu item does not indicate a preference of any kind for one restaurant chain over another.

Most national franchises have a nutrition list, much like a package label, that they will be glad to give to you if you ask them. Fast food restaurants are also becoming more and more sensitive to the nutrition concerns of their customers and will prepare your selected sandwich or entree without ingredients or condiments at your request. If you do not see your favorite fast food listed here, it simply means that compared to the other items on the chart, it did not score very highly in these categories. Perhaps most surprising, quite a few of these quick meals are "Zone friendly" as well, some just as they are, some with slight and easily made modifications. Refer to Dr. Sears's book, *The Zone: A Dietary Road Map*, for specific listings of Zone-compatible foods in this category.

Chart 16-7 illustrates the relative nutrient content of common fast food and take-out items.

Chart 16-7 Relative Vitamin Content of Take-Out Foods Measured as Indicated

Food Item	Serve Size	Prep.	A IU	C Mg	TH Mg	RB Mg	NI Mg	B_6 Mg	BC Mcg	B_{12} Mcg
Bread Muffins,										
Blueberry	2 pcs	Toaster Type	188	0	.12	.18	1.2	ND	ND	0
Corn	6 oz.	Corn, Large	354	TR	.48	.57	3.48	.15	ND	0
Mix	4.8 oz.	Blueberry	150	.01	.3	.51	3.3	ND	ND	0
Mix	4.8 oz.	Bran	300	0	.24	.36	5.7	ND	ND	0
Mix	4.8 oz.	Corn	270	.01	.27	.27	2.4	ND	ND	0
Waffle	2.4 oz.	Frozen, 2 4"	400	0	.13	.16	1.46	.3	12	.83
Fast and Take-Out Foods—Prepared										
Breakfast Items										
Biscuit	Reg	w/ Egg, Ham	874	.05	.68	.6	2	.26	32	1.2
Biscuit	Reg	w/ Egg, Sausage	635	.05	.5	.46	3.6	.2	40	1.4
Croissant	Reg	w/ Bac, Egg, Chs	472	2	.35	.34	2.19	.12	35	.9
French Toast	4.2 oz.	Frozen, 2 pcs	472	.05	.58	.5	3.91	.05	30	.4
Hash Browns	Reg	Fried	18	6	.08	.01	1.07	.17	8	.02
Lunch or Dinner Items										
Burger	6.9 oz.	Bacon Chsburger	406	2	.32	.42	6.63	.31	33	2.3
Burger	5.9 oz.	Big Mac Style	398	2	.35	.28	8.05	.18	23	1.9
Burger	8 oz.	Whopper Style	311	3	.42	.38	7.28	.33	36	2.4
Burrito	7.7 oz.	Bean	332	2	.62	.62	4.06	.31	118	1.1
Burrito	10.7oz.	w/Beef, Cheese, Chilis	972	4	.62	1.24	8.34	.38	58	2.1
Chicken	1 thigh, 1 drum	Fried	222	0	.14	.43	7.21	.33	10	.83
Chicken	2 lt. meat pcs	Fried	192	0	.14	.3	11.98	.57	9	.67

Food Item	Serve Size	Prep.	A IU	C Mg	TH Mg	RB Mg	NI Mg	B6 Mg	BC Mcg	B12 Mcg
Crab Cakes	4.2 oz.	Deep Fried	626	.01	.12	.14	2.34	.3	20	8.8
Nachos	9 oz.	Ch, Bean, Beef,								
		Pepper	3401	5	.24	.69	3.35	.41	39	1.0
Pizza	1 slice	Cheese	382	1	.18	.16	2.48	.04	59	.33
Pizza	1 slice	Cheese, Pepperoni	524	2	.21	.17	1.96	.09	27	.36
Potato	10.4 oz.	Baked w/cheese	834	26	.22	.22	3.35	.72	28	.2
Potato	12 oz.	Baked Cheese, Broc.	1695	49	.26	.26	3.58	.8	61	.3
Potato	Reg	French Fries	22	4	.1	.03	1.72	.2	25	.09
Potato	1 cup	Mashed w/ Gravy	33	.01	.07	.04	.96	.19	7	.04
Roast Beef	4.9 oz.	Arby's Style Sndwch	210	2	.38	.31	5.86	.27	40	1.2
Salad	1½cup	Chef Salad	1053	17	.41	.39	5.97	.43	100	.84
Salad	¾ cup	Coleslaw	337	8	.04	.03	.08	.11	39	.18
Salad	1 cup	Potato Salad	285	3	.18	.33	.78	.42	72	.36
Salad	1½cup	Seafood w/Lett.	6245	38	.3	.21	3.56	.35	100	1.7
Submarine	8 oz.	Hero, Italian								
		Cold Cuts	425	12	1	.8	5.5	.13	54	1.1
Submarine	9 oz.	Tuna Salad	188	4	.46	.35	11.33	.23	58	1.6
Soups Ready to Serve and Condensed										
Bean, Blck	1 cup	Condensed	506	1	.08	.05	.53	.09	24.7	.02
Beef, Chunky	1 cup	Ready to Serve	2611	7	.06	.15	2.71	.13	13.4	.61
Chick Nood	1 cup	Condensed	711	ND	.05	.06	1.39	.03	2.2	ND
Chick Veg.	1 cup	Condensed	2656	1	.04	.06	1.23	.05	ND	ND
Chick, Chunky	1 cup	Ready to Serve	1299	1	.09	.17	4.42	.05	4.6	.25
Clam, Manh.	1 cup	Ready to Serve	3292	12	.06	.06	1.85	.26	9.3	7.9
Cr. Potato	1 cup	Condensed	288	0	.03	.04	.54	.04	3.0	ND
Minestrone	1 cup	Condensed	2337	1	.05	.04	.94	.1	16.1	0
Tomato	1 cup	Condensed	688	67	.09	.05	1.42	.11	14.7	0
Vegetable	1 cup	Condensed	3005	1	.05	.05	.92	.06	10.6	0
Veg. Beef	1 cup	Condensed	1891	2	.04	.05	1.03	.08	10.6	.31

Key: A = Vitamin A, C = Vitamin C, TH = Thiamine, RB = Riboflavin, NI = Niacin, B6 = Vitamin B6,

BC = Vitamin BC (Folacin), B12 = Vitamin B12, ND = No Data Available, HF = Health Food Store

Surprisingly, quite a few fast food choices are high in our selected vitamins. In the breakfast category, corn muffins and biscuit sandwiches are the best of your choices. They rate much more highly than others, including the muffin-type sandwiches and pancakes or French toast. Note that hash browns, although part of almost every breakfast "value meal," really don't have very much to offer in our categories. Birds like them, though. You may want to consider sharing that part of your next fast food breakfast with them.

Lunch and dinner fast food items or quick meals offer another group of decent temporary choices when you are pressed for time or away from home. The big winners are salads, especially seafood salad with lettuce. Chef's salad is a good choice, low in calories and high in nutrients. Chef's salads do have eggs, so be careful if you are prone to allergic reaction.

Burger franchises have some meal choices which are surprisingly good, and on a par with one another. The best are the bigger sandwiches, with or without cheese. Both Whopper and Big Mac burgers offer high nutrient counts, but, beware! These are very high in fat, which is not recommended for persons on a restricted diet or those watching their weight.

Better choices, overall, are the Mexican food franchises. Burritos and nachos not only contain our desired nutrients in impressive quantities, they also contain needed proteins, good carbohydrates, and the proper proportion of fats. These are really relatively healthy meals, and probably your best fast food selections. Although I have listed only a couple of them here, the entire line of Mexican foods contains a fair amount of nutrients. Get a nutrient sheet from your local franchise, or pick up a food count book that lists commercial restaurant foods. You'll be surprised at what these may have to offer in the way of nutritious emergency meals on the go.

For those of you who are looking for something without meat, try a baked potato, available as a side order from some of the better burger and chicken franchises. These may not be suitable for some of you, particularly Type O people, but they are great for Type A's like me.

Last, there are good temporary alternatives for those of you who cannot leave the job site in order to eat, or bring a lunch from home and store it where you work. Try soup. Both the ready-to-eat and condensed varieties have some good choices. And, should you have a company cafeteria, their bulk soup contains about the same proportional nutrients as the ones that I have listed here.

Ready-to-serve varieties, particularly Manhattan clam chowder and chunky-style beef soups, are your best overall choices, but other chunky varieties are quite respectable in the vitamin category. Good old-fashioned tomato soup is the winner in the condensed varieties. Prepare this at home, put it into a thermos, and take it with you. Pop it into the break room microwave at lunch. Add a few corn or tortilla chips, and you've got a healthy and nutritious midday meal.

The final chart in this section will no doubt cause raised eyebrows from others in the medical and health professions. It reviews what is commonly termed "junk" food, including desserts, snacks, and candy. Most nutritionists and doctors will counsel you to stay strictly away from these foods. They are almost all high in fat, sugars, or contain processing elements. Dr. Sears, however, considers some of them to be Zone-friendly because of the proportions of their respective elements, and acceptable in a pinch. Although I may not choose to eat them myself, nor would I recommend that you do so, I know that sometimes it just can't be helped. I would rather see a patient eat one of these foods on a very occasional basis than skip a meal, slow the metabolism, and stop the production of good eicosanoids.

The chart shows some popular styles of nationally known vended snacks, common coffee shop and coffee truck offerings. Brand names, when listed, are for example only and do not indicate a preference or imply that I recommend you eat the item. Slight count variations may occur according to manufacturer. Note that several of the categories may not have counts for each item. Data were either not available for that nutrient, or amounts varied too widely according to manufacturer in order to be accurately included. Read all labels and choose carefully, as quantity, quality, and serving size may vary. Remember also that most of these foods are extremely high in calories per serving.

Chart 16-8 reviews some of the most common snacks, desserts, and candies.

Chart 16-8 Relative Content of Snack Foods Measured as Indicated

Food Item	Serve Size	Prep.	A IU	C Mg	TH Mg	RB Mg	NI Mg	B_6 Mg	BC Mcg	B_{12} Mcg
Cake										
Cheesecake	4 oz.	Plain	ND	ND	.04	.24	.24	.08	16.0	.2
Chocolate	5 oz.	w/ Choc. Frosting	ND	ND	.04	.18	.74	ND	ND	ND
Coffee	4 oz.	w/ Cinn., Crumbs	ND	ND	.24	.28	1.92	.04	36.0	ND
Fruit	4.5oz.	Old Fashioned	ND	ND	.06	.12	1.02	.06	3.0	ND
Pound	4 oz.	Plain	688	ND	.16	.28	1.48	ND	ND	ND
Devil's Food										
Snack	3.6 oz.	w/Creme Filling	16	ND	.22	.30	2.42	ND	ND	ND
Sponge										
Snack	3 oz.	w/Creme Filling	121	0	.14	.12	1.04	.03	11.2	.16
Sponge	3 oz.	Plain	118	0	.18	.20	1.46	.04	10.0	.18
Yellow	4.6 oz.	w/ Van. Frosting	80	0	.12	.10	.64	ND	ND	ND
Candy										
Generic	3 oz.	Milk Chocolate	90	ND	.06	.3	.3	ND	ND	ND
Granola Bar	2 oz.	Peanut But., Soft	TR	0	.07	.04	.89	.03	9	.06
Granola Bar	2 oz.	Plain, Soft, Uncoat.	0	0	.08	.05	.15	.03	7	.11
Hershey	3 oz.	Golden Almond	125	ND	.05	.45	.9	ND	ND	ND
Hershey	1.9 oz.	Rolo Caramels	33	ND	.03	.14	.05	ND	ND	ND
Mars	1.4 oz.	Chunky	25	.01	.04	.16	.76	ND	ND	ND
Mars	1.74oz.	M & Ms Peanut	TR	ND	.03	.1	1.6	.09	27	ND
Mars	2.15 oz.	Milky Way	127	1	.02	.14	.21	.03	5	.27
Mars	2.16 oz.	Snickers	72	ND	.03	.11	1.82	.11	24	.25
Nestlé	2.16 oz.	Butterfinger	40	ND	ND	.03	2.01	.04	19	ND
Nestlé	2.8 oz.	Kit Kat	85	1	.05	.2	.32	.04	0	.49
Nestlé	1.4 oz.	Nestlé Crunch	23	ND	.02	.11	.2	.03	4	ND
Nestlé	1.5 oz.	Raisinets	17	ND	.04	.09	.18	ND	ND	ND

Food Item	Serve Size	Prep.	A IU	C Mg	TH Mg	RB Mg	NI Mg	B$_6$ Mg	BC Mcg	B$_{12}$ Mcg
Reese	1.6 oz.	Reese's PB Cups	31	ND	.02	.09	1.79	.04	12	.21
Cookies										
Homemade	2 oz.	Brown Edge Van.	80	0	.01	.04	.2	ND	ND	ND
Refrig.	2 oz.	Chocolate Chip	34	0	.1	.1	1.12	ND	ND	ND
Refrig.	2 oz.	Peanut Butter	26	0	.1	.1	2.36	ND	ND	ND
Refrig.	2 oz.	Sugar	20	0	.12	.08	1.36	ND	ND	ND
Chips & Snacks										
Chips, Corn	3 oz.	Nacho Flavor	315	3	.12	.15	1.23	.24	12.0	ND
Tortilla Chips, Corn	3 oz.	Plain	162	0	.06	.15	1.02	.24	ND	0
Tortilla Chips, Corn	3 oz.	Ranch Flavor	219	ND	.09	.21	1.23	ND	ND	0
Tortilla Chips, Corn, Yellow	3 oz.	Plain	81	0	.03	.12	1.02	.21	18.0	0
Chips, Potato	3 oz.	BBQ, All Types	186	30	.18	.18	3.90	.54	72.0	0
Chips, Potato	3 oz.	Plain, Reg. Varieties	0	27	.15	.18	3.27	.57	39.0	0
Chips, Potato	3 oz.	Plain, Light Variety	0	21	.18	.24	5.94	.57	ND	0
Chips, Potato	3 oz.	Sour Crm & Onion	144	33	.15	.18	3.42	.57	54.0	ND
Cracker, Butter	1.2 oz.	About 10 Round	70	0	ND	.01	.3	ND	ND	ND
Cracker, Rye	2.5 oz.	About 3 Triples	ND	ND	.33	.21	1.2	.21	33.0	0
Cracker, Saltine	1 oz.	About 10 Crackers	0	0	.16	.18	1.72	.02	4.0	0
Cracker, Wheat	1 oz.	About 10 Crackers	0	0	.1	.10	1.0	.01	0	0
Popcorn	1 cup	Caramel w/Pnuts	24	0	.02	.06	.72	.07	ND	0
Popcorn	1 cup	Cheese Flavor	27	.1	.01	.03	.16	.03	1.4	0
Popcorn	1 cup	Plain, Salt, Oil Pop	20	0	.01	.02	.10	.02	1.7	0
Popcorn	1 cup	Plain, Unsalt, Air Pop	16	0	.02	.02	.16	.02	2.0	0
Pretzels	3 oz.	Plain, Salt	0	0	.39	.54	4.47	.09	TR	0
Pastry										
Danish	2.3 oz.	Cheese	ND	ND	.14	.19	1.42	ND	ND	ND
Danish	2.3 oz.	Cinnamon	ND	ND	.2	.17	1.86	ND	ND	ND

Food Item	Serve Size	Prep.	A IU	C Mg	TH Mg	RB Mg	NI Mg	B_6 Mg	BC Mcg	B_{12} Mcg
Donut	3 oz.	Creme Filled	ND	ND	.29	.13	1.91	ND	ND	ND
Donut	2.1 oz.	Honey Glazed	ND	ND	.22	.13	1.71	.03	13.0	0
Donut	3 oz.	Jelly Filled	ND	ND	.27	.12	1.82	ND	ND	ND
Donut	1.7 oz.	Plain	27	ND	.10	.11	.87	.03	4.0	ND
Toaster	2 pcs	Blueberry	1004	ND	.30	.38	4.10	.4	84.0	ND
Toaster	2 pcs	Br. Sugar Cinn.	986	ND	.38	.58	4.58	.42	80.0	ND
Toaster	2 pcs	Cherry	1000	ND	.30	.34	4.00	.4	ND	ND
Toaster	2 pcs	Choc., Frosted	1000	ND	.30	.34	4.00	.4	ND	ND
Toaster	2 pcs	Strawberry	1004	ND	.30	.38	4.10	.4	84.0	ND
Pie										
Apple	1 slice	Per Recipe	154	4	.04	.03	.33	.05	5.0	0
Blueberry	1 slice	Per Recipe	175	ND	.01	.04	.38	.05	ND	0
Boston Cre	1 slice	Per Recipe	350	0	.14	.32	.90	ND	ND	ND
Cherry	1 slice	Per Recipe	ND	ND	.03	.04	.25	.05	10.0	0
Coconut Cre	1 slice	Per Recipe	58	0	.03	.05	.13	ND	ND	0
Lem Mering	1 slice	Per Recipe	198	4	.07	.24	.73	.03	10.0	ND
Peach	1 slice	Per Recipe	123	ND	.07	.04	.23	.03	ND	0
Pecan	1 slice	Per Recipe	198	1	.10	.14	.28	.02	7.0	ND
Pumpkin	1 slice	Per Recipe	ND	ND	.06	.17	.20	.06	17.0	ND

Key: A = Vitamin A, C = Vitamin C, TH = Thiamine, RB = Riboflavin, NI = Niacin, B_6 = Vitamin B_6, BC = Vitamin BC (Folacin), B_{12} = Vitamin B_{12}, ND = No Data Available, HF = Health Food Store, TR = Trace

Well, there you have it, a good cross section of "grab it and go" foods. Surprisingly, some of them are not too bad. Some have more nutrients per serving than an equal serving of many fruits or vegetables. But, again, I caution you. These are not calorie-conscious foods! Most of them are also high in sugars and fats and can throw your nutritional balance out of line if they become a steady part of your diet.

But, if you are stuck, choosing some form of food is certainly preferable to skipping a meal, especially if you want to remain in the Zone. In the cake category, pound and sponge cakes score the best, although coffee and plain cheesecake score well in the folacin (BC) category. Refrigerated peanut butter cookies are the best choice for fast snacks you can make at home and take with you. All cakes contain eggs and sugar, and some, like the pound, coffee, and cheese varieties, contain butter and other dairy products. These should not be eaten in any circumstance by those with egg or cow's milk allergy. Some individuals can also have an adverse reaction to peanuts and peanut butter, so avoid those choices if you have tested positive for this type of allergy.

Far and away the best choices in chips are the corn family, especially nacho tortilla chips. Barbecue potato chips are the healthiest selection from the potato family, and pretzels have good levels of niacin per serving and are low in fat or fat free. Popcorn, widely touted as a perfect "diet" food, really doesn't offer much in the way of nutrition as regards our selected nutrients, nor do Danish or doughnuts. Toaster pastries score better. Two pieces of most of the varieties provide the DRI for vitamin A for males and exceed the requirements for females for all ages, except for pregnant or lactating mothers. Pies can vary widely, according to the quality and quantity of ingredients used in preparation, but, generally, Boston cream, lemon meringue, and pecan pie are your most nutritious choices. Note, however, that these are also very high in calories, and in the case of the Boston and pecan varieties, high in sugar. Boston cream contains eggs and dairy, and meringue is made from egg whites and sugar. Try to avoid cakes and pies when possible, or accept only the smallest polite piece when impossible to do otherwise.

Finally, how about candy? Unfortunately, most candies do not contain appreciable amounts of our nutrients, as they are largely composed of sugars. Chocolate bars with nuts, or nuts and raisins are your best choices, followed by chocolate-coated wafers or peanut butter and chocolate cups. Note that the granolas, long heralded as healthy snacks, generally have more fat and sugar than any appreciable nutritional value, unless fortified with additional nutrients by the manufacturer. Although I used specific brand names in comparison, all of these types of candy have basically the same value. Again, I certainly do not recommend candy as a regular part of your daily diet, but, when you're faced with grabbing something or skipping a meal, some of them can provide a few nutrients while giving you that quick energy boost.

In conclusion, I urge you to use all of the charts represented here in a commonsense manner. You can fool yourself into thinking that a diet consisting largely of fast food and snacks is providing all of your essential vitamins and minerals, and indeed may well be. But, what it is also providing is an undesirable excess of certain food components, like sugars and fats, and high caloric intake that can easily lead to weight gain. Eating these foods repeatedly additionally creates a deficiency in other essential elements, like amino acids or some vitamins that are damaged or nullified by certain methods of cooking or processing.

Instead, I recommend that you use the natural, unprocessed forms of food whenever possible. Choose your preparation style carefully to maximize the nutrient count per serving. Select foods that are most efficiently metabolized by persons with your blood type. Pick up a food count book to compare the relative values of the foods in your recommended groups. Combine different items from these to meet the requirements of your Zone plan. And, include supplements to adjust for any system deficiencies or additional dietary restrictions that your doctor or nutritionist may recommend.

If you follow these methods and choose your food drugs carefully, you should start to see your system imbalances begin to right themselves at last. Through periodic BCI testing, you can refine your dietary intake to reflect your needs as your imbalances decline. When all of your system levels have been restored to normal ranges and relationships, you can continue to follow this nutrition plan to maintain your optimum state of health.

The first section of the final chapter will summarize the steps on my five-year journey to find a cure for my MS. The last portion contains the resources section, where you can obtain the contact information for the medical professionals who have assisted me, various suppliers of products, supplements, nutrients, and bees, and places where you can learn more about multiple sclerosis and the treatments I used successfully.

17

The 9 Effective Steps: A Successful Plan for Reversing Multiple Sclerosis

This final chapter will help you to follow the same steps that I have taken on my journey to victory. Here you will find listings for each of the doctors, physicians, clinical nutritionists, and other healing professionals who have assisted me with treatment and healing modalities throughout the five-year period. I will review the steps that I have found most successful in my journey to wellness—alternative medicines that heal naturally, without the undesirable side effects possible with conventional medical treatments.

I still continue to work to remove all traces of the lesions left upon my nervous system by this devastating disease. I take the Calcium2-AEP orotates to bring my remaining excess levels of calcium back into an acceptable range, and I continue with the Sphingolin Myelin Basic Protein as an added protection against any resurgence of the disease. I also continue to make adjustments in the natural protocols that will remove all traces of EBV from my body. I periodically undergo BCI analyses as my system element levels return to optimum range.

I maintain a daily nutritional plan using the Zone diet of Dr. Sears, specifically modified for my particular blood type as recommended by Dr. D'Adamo. I have become so familiar with the requirements of both experts that even when dining at a social occasion, I can continue to easily choose foods that maintain the proper balance of nutrients my body requires. I also take daily nutritional and vitamin supplements to maintain my present level of excellent health.

It is my sincerest hope that detailing my own experiences will make it easier for you to decide to give these healing protocols a try. On the other hand, even though many of the therapies I underwent caused fear and concern before I decided to attempt them, nothing that I have ever done has ever scared me as badly as the "possible side effects" section of conventionally prescribed MS drug pamphlets.

As you review the material in this final chapter, remember always: this is *your* health, and *your* life. No one, not your doctor, your spouse, parents, children, or friends should decide your method of treatment. You should work closely with your chosen medical professional to determine a course of treatment that will be most beneficial to your particular case. Let everyone else who is close to you offer comfort, support, sympathy, and advice, but please, for your own sake, let the final decision rest solely with you. Understand that there will always be opposition to any new or unconventional treatments, and often, the objections of those close to you stem from a very real and caring fear that you will come to some harm.

It is natural for you to feel some fear on your own, especially when considering BVT or injection therapies. I, too, was afraid, and that is one of the primary reasons I have written this book. It is my sincerest hope that detailing my own experiences will make it easier for you to decide to give these healing protocols a try. On the other hand, even though many of the therapies I underwent caused fear and concern before I decided to attempt them, *nothing* that I have ever done has ever scared me as badly as the "possible side effects" section of conventionally prescribed MS drug pamphlets.

However, I stress this one last time: This does not mean I recommend in any respect that you go it alone! I am a doctor in two fields. I have almost two decades of experience with conventional and alternative medicine, and yet I regularly consult other medical professionals in the course of my continued treatment and wellness regimen. If your doctor is not versed in these healing modalities, why not bring him your copy of this book? If he or she still recommends conventional drugs, then you, and only you, have a decision to make regarding your future course of treatment.

Let's review the nine healing modalities I have found to be most effective in ridding my body of multiple sclerosis:

1. **BioCybernetics Analysis:** I urge you to consider having a BCI Analysis *before* beginning any method of treatment! The tests are not expensive, and the complete picture of the vitamin, nutrient, mineral, and metal element levels in your body will give you an excellent and reliable foundation on which to build your personal healing plan. In the resources section, I have provided contact information for myself and the BCI team headed by Clinical Nutritionists Bob Santoro and Al Weyhreter.

2. **Chelation therapy:** If your BCI tests reveal that you have unacceptably high levels of toxic or heavy metals in your system, especially mercury, consider heavy-metal chelation to remove these excesses. Chelation can be costly, but an increasing number of health insurance providers do recognize it as a viable and approved treatment method.

3. **Silver or mercury amalgam filling removal:** Whether or not you have high levels of metal in your body, think about having your poisonous fillings replaced with biologically friendly materials such as porcelain. I also encourage you to read Dr.

Hal Huggins's and Dr. Thomas Levy's book. Contact information for their offices is included in the resources section.

4. **Apitherapy and bee venom treatment:** This is a very courageous step. Remember, BVT is only a portion of apitherapy, the use of all products of the hive. BVT has been repeatedly successful in aiding the restoration of mobility and the lessening or eradication of many MS symptoms. Whether you decide to try working with live bees or collected venom, I have provided plenty of contact information for you in the resources section. I have listed contact information for Dr. Theodore Cherbuliez, Dr. Bradford S. Weeks, Mrs. Pat Wagner, Ferris Apiaries, and the American Apitherapy Society.

5. **Sphingolin Myelin Basic Protein supplement:** I still continue to take this pure form of myelin concentrate each day, to prevent any remnants of the disease from doing further damage to my nervous system. If you decide to try only one of these healing protocols, this should be the one. Even if you are following conventional medical treatments, this additional myelin can do nothing but help you, as the virus will attack it instead of your natural myelin. Contact information for the supplier of SMBP, Emerson Ecologics, is listed in the resources section.

6. **Vitamin and nutrient therapy:** The daily use of vitamin, mineral, and nutrient supplements has enabled me to consistently increase my health by restoring my system level balances and ratios. For instance, the Calcium 2-AEP orotates have been instrumental in reducing my excess levels of calcium and restoring essential calcium to other mineral ratios. Again, this is an area where a BCI analysis is essential. Your personal supplement requirements will be determined by your specific excesses or deficiencies. Several reliable supplement suppliers are listed in the resources section.

7. **Personal nutrition plan:** Determine your blood type if not already known, and obtain both Dr. Sears's and Dr. D'Adamo's books. Make a list of your recommended blood-type-friendly foods and use them to form optimum Zone combinations. Ensuring that your body receives the proper amount of nutrients necessary to repair existing damage, replace deficiencies, correct excesses, convert raw materials, and manufacture healing substances will enable your system to arrest the development of the virus and begin to reverse its effects.

8. **Allergy testing and dietary restrictions:** If you have a weight problem, or your MS is at a severe stage, you may also want to consider Dr. Swank's low-fat diet plan. Remember to take EFA supplements to replace the essential fatty acids that you will no longer be receiving through your diet while on the Swank plan. Additionally, I recommend that you receive an IgG RAST test for hidden allergies to cow's milk, eggs, and wheat. If your results are positive, you should consider implementing the Zero Dairy, Zero Sugar protocol. This protocol is also helpful with weight control. Again, remember to add the proper amount of supplements necessary to maintain an adequate supply of nutrients to your system.

9. **Regular Exercise:** Exercise is essential to maintain your muscle tone and body strength. Walk, jog, run, bike, swim, play tennis, racquetball, ski, ride horses, mow the lawn. Play a game of basketball, or take up Irish dancing. If exercise in the conventional sense is too boring, find something more creative to do that will hold your interest, increase your cardiovascular activity, and flex and tone your muscles. If you are in a severe state of depletion, develop an isometric exercise routine. Remember, it is harder to restore a body the more depleted it becomes.

Last, please remember: *You can do this!* MS need not be a dark hallway, a journey into oblivion. Contrary to conventional wisdom, there are other options.[1] It all depends on your personal decision. Will you resignedly accept your fate, or fight for your life? I'd like to conclude with the same thought that began my story, my personal mantra for victory:

"If you are ever diagnosed with a life-threatening disease, you must pursue, with all of your might, every doctor, of all varieties, with every healing modality known to them, and never give up, until you find the ones that heal you."

I wish you joy, inner peace, and courage as you face your future, challenged but unafraid. Most of all, I hope that you will undertake your own journey to wellness, your personal life quest that will bring you out from the ranks of the MS-afflicted. I truly feel that if you diligently apply these things that I have learned, you will no longer be known as an "MS victim." At the end of your own journey, you will have become an MS victor! May God bless, keep, and guide you always as you discover your own path to health.

---

[1]Hyman Engelberg, M.D., has been studying the effects of heparin since 1940. His book, *Your Heart's Best Friend,* published in 1987, was written for those who have had a heart attack or Transient Ischemic Attack (TIA). In his book, Dr. Engelberg talks about how heparin cleans the plaque off the main vessels that feed the heart.

According to Dr. Engelberg, heparin has many actions, but for the MS patient, heparin prevents relapses. The MS patient would need to drink a half glass of water containing either 1cc four times a week or 1/2cc every day for a duration determined by a physician.

This treatment must be prescribed by an M.D. If doctors or patients have any questions relating to heparin, they can direct their questions to Dr. Engelberg in care of Celeste Pepe (see contact information in the Medical Resources section).

Some of the other actions that Dr. Engelberg has discovered suggest that heparin benefits patients suffering from the AIDS virus, stops the metasis of cancer, and helps ALS and Guillain-Barre Syndrome patients. It is also important to note that Dr. Engelberg has found no reported cases of Alzheimer's in patients who have been taking heparin for their TIA or for previous heart attacks in all the years he has been conducting his research.

How to Learn More—Research and Resources

This section contains valuable resources you can utilize in following the treatments I have found successful. Where possible, I have included the Internet web site address of each practice, corporation, organization, or other entity. Each of the resources listed in this section is included to benefit the reader by offering viable points at which additional research can be conducted, or products, vitamins and supplements can be obtained. The resources mentioned here are not the only sources for these materials, assuredly. They are simply institutions, organizations, or companies with whom I have had personal or professional experience and have found to be viable options.

No resource, organization, practitioner, individual, or supplier, including Natural Organics, has tendered any promotional consideration for their inclusion, nor have they received compensation from myself, my writer, agent, or publisher. For convenience and general availability to most readers, I have listed a selection of national vitamin, mineral, and nutritional supplement suppliers only. This should not be construed as an endorsement or judgment as to the quality of products offered in preference to other suppliers or retailers not listed. All resources in any given section are listed in alphabetical order for the reader's convenience. Resources are listed by topic, determined by area of practice, medication, supplement, or treatment-supply applicable to the subject. Although every effort has been made to ensure that the contact information is accurate, some may change over time. Should you find that the information is out of date, I invite you to contact

I hope that you will undertake your own journey to wellness, your personal life quest that will bring you out from the ranks of the MS-afflicted. I truly feel that if you diligently apply these things that I have learned, you will no longer be known as an "MS victim."

me personally, and I will make every effort to give you the latest information I have available on any given resource.

Medical Resources

Physicians, Doctors:
Medical Offices, Centers, and Facilities
Celestial Cybernetics, Inc.
7351 Happy Canyon Rd.
Santa Ynez, CA 93460
(805) 686-4119 ext. 171
Celeste Pepe, D.C., N.D.

The Crawford Center
1 Office Park #404A
Mobile, AL 36609
(334) 461-0660
William Crawford, N.D.

D'Adamo Naturopathic Clinic
56 Lafayette Place
Suite C
Greenwich, CT 06830
(203) 661-7375
Peter J. D'Adamo, N.D.

Matrix, Inc.
5080 List Drive
Colorado Springs, CO 80919
(719) 593-9616
Hal A. Huggins, D.D.S., M.S.
(719) 548-1600
Thomas E. Levy, M.D., J.D.
Dr. Huggins: hahuggins@hugnet.com
Dr. Levy: televy@medmail.com
Internet Address: http://www.hugnet.com

Neiper Clinic (Paracelsus-Klinik)
Oertzeweg 24
30853 Langenhagen
Germany
e-mail: contact@Dr-Ledwoch.de
fax: 011-49-511-318417

The Weeks Clinic
6456 Central Avenue
Clinton, WA 98236
(360) 341-2303
Bradford S. Weeks, M.D.
Internet Address: http://www.weeksmd.com

Scientists, Researchers, Clinical Nutritionists: Centers and Facilities

BioCybernetics, Inc. (BCI)
12 Nearwater
Massapequa, NY 11758
(516) 795-6751
Robert Santoro, C.N.
Alfred Weyhreter, C.N.

Emerson Ecologics, Inc.
18 Lomar Park
Pepperell, MA 01463
(800) 654-4432
William Emerson, Ph.D.
Joseph Emerson, M.A.
Internet Address:
http://www.emersonecologics.com/homepage.htm
Internet e-mail: info@emersonecologics.com

Great Smokies Laboratories, Inc.
63 Zillicoa Street
Asheville, NC 28801
(888) 891-3061

M & M Van Benshoten & Associates
19231 Victory Blvd.
Suite 151
Reseda, CA 91335
(818) 344-9973
Matthew Van Benshoten, C.A.
Joseph McSweyne, C.A.

Surfactant Technologies, Inc.
21 Tioga Way
Marblehead, MA 01945
(800) 346-2703
Barry Sears, Ph.D.

Trace Elements, Inc.
4901 Keller Springs Road
Suite 6
Addison, TX 75001
(972) 250-6410
(800) 824-2314
David L. Watts, D.C., Ph.D.

Apitherapy and BVT Resources
American Apitherapy Society (AAS)
5390 Grand Road
Hillsboro, OH 45133
(937) 364-1108
Internet e-mail: aasoffice@in-touch.net
Internet Address: http://www.apitherapy.org/aas/
Theodore Cherbuliez, M.D., President
(914) 723-0920
Internet Email: tcherbuliez@cyburban.com

The Bee Lady of Waldorf
5431 Lucy Drive
Waldorf, MD 20601-3217
(301) 843-8350
Pat Wagner, Certified Apitherapist
Internet e-mail: beelady@olg.com
Internet Address: http://www.olg.com/beelady/

Ferris Apiaries
P.O. Box 143
Marbury, MD 20658
(800) 787-4669
Michelle Ferris
Internet e-mail: ferris@radix.net
Internet Address: http://www.radix.net/~honeybs/

Vitamin and Nutritional Supplement Resources
Vitamins 4 Less, Inc.
1830 Oakland Avenue
Suite D
Indiana, PA 15701
Phone Orders: 1-888-782-8482
Internet Address: http://www.4lessvitamins.com/

Vitanet
5327 Westpointe Plaza Dr.
Columbus, OH 43228
(614) 274-2722
(800) 807-8080
Internet Address: http://www.healthstyle.com/

Natural Organics
548 Broadhollow Road
Melville, NY 11747
(516) 293-0030

National MS Societies, Nonprofit Organizations, and Support Groups
The National Multiple Sclerosis Society
Main Offices
733 Third Avenue
New York, NY 10017
1-800-Fight-MS (1-800-344-4867)
Internet Address: http://www.nmss.org/

Multiple Sclerosis Association of America
National Headquarters
706 Haddonfield Road
Cherry Hill, NJ 08002
(609) 661-9797
Internet Address: http://www.msaa.com/

Miscellaneous Resources

Amazon.com Online Bookseller
Internet Address: http://www.amazon.com/

Barnes & Noble Online Booksellers
Internet Address: http://www.barnesandnoble.com/

Bibliography

Allison, 1950. Survival in Disseminated Sclerosis: A Clinical Study of a Series of Cases First Seen Twenty Years Ago. *Brain* 73:103-120.

American Apitherapy Society (AAS), 1999. *www.apither apy.org/aas*

American Whole Health, Inc., 1999. Lactase Deficiency in Irritable Bowel Syndrome, *Whole Health Librar.* *www.american whole health.com/library/ibs/ibs038.htm*

Ames, Ellis, Gunn, Copeland, and Abrams, 1999. Vitamin D Receptor (VDR) Gene Fok1 Polymorphism predicts Calcium Absorption and Bone Mineral Density in Children. *Journal of Bone Miner Res* 14: 740–746.

Apitherapy Societies and Associations, 1999. *Apimondia.* *www.sci-fi/~apither/assoc.html*

Bishop, 1999. Rickets Today—Children Still Need Milk and Sunshine. *New England Journal of Medicine* 341: 602-604. *www.nejm.orgcontent/1999/0341/0008/0602.asp*

Bonjour, Carrie, Ferrari, Clavien, Soisman, Theintz, and Rizzoli, 1997. Calcium Enriched Foods and Bone Mass Growth in Prepubertal Girls: A Randomized, Double-blind, Placebo Controlled Trial. *Journal of Clinical Investigations* 99:1287-1294.

Cherbuliez, 1997. Bee Venom Therapy and Safety, *Bee Informed Magazine. www.apitherapy.org/aas*

D'Adamo, James, 1980. *One Man's Food.* Out of Print.

D'Adamo, Peter J, and Whitney, Catherine, 1996. *Eat Right 4 Your Type: The Individualized Diet Solution to Staying Healthy.* New York: G.P. Putnam's Sons.

Dahl-Jorgensen, Joner, and Hanssen, 1991. Relationship between Cow's Milk Consumption and Incidence of IDDM in Childhood *Diabetes Care* 14: 1081–3.

Dawson-Hughes, United States Department of Agriculture Human Nutrition Research Center on Aging, 1996. Calcium and Vitamin D Nutritional Needs of Elderly Women. *Journal of Nutrition* 4(suppl):1165S-1167S.

de Vrese, Sieber, and Stransky, 1998. Lactose in Human Nutrition. *Schweiz Med Wochenschr* 128: 1393-1400.

Diabetes.com Health Library, 1999. *What is Diabetes? www.diabetes.com/health_library/articles/l3t100117.html*

Fava, Leslie, and Pozilli, 1994. Relationship between Dairy Product Consumption and Incidence of IDDM in Childhood in Italy. *Diabetes Care* 17: 1488-1490.

Gallo, 1996. Building Strong Bones in Childhood and Adolescence: Reducing the Risk of Fractures Later in Life. *Pediatric Nursing* 22:369-374,422.

Gilman, et al., Harvard Medical School and Harvard Pilgrim Health Care, Framingham Heart Study, 1997. Some Types of Fat Associated with Reduced Stroke Risk in Men.*The Journal of the American Medical Association* 278:2145-2150.

——, Some Types of Fat Associated with Reduced Stroke Risk in Men, 1997. *Science News Update* (24-31 December).

Hauser, American Apitherapy Society, 1999. Regarding NSAIDs and Anaphylaxis. *www.apitherapy.org/aas/ hauser.html*

Herrmann, Dannemann, Gruters, Radisch, Dudenhausen, Bergmann, Coumbos, Weitzel, and Wahn, 1996. Prospective Study on the Atopy Preventative Effect of Maternal Avoidance of Milk and Eggs during Pregnancy and Lactation. *European Journal of Pediatrics* 155: 770-777.

Hippocrates, 1981. *On Sacred Disease.* From *Works.* Translated by Francis Adams. New York: Loeb. 2:139-183.

Huggins, Hal A., 1993. *It's All in Your Head: The Link Between Mercury Amalgams and Illness.* New York: Avery Publishing Group.

Huggins, Hal A., and Levy, Thomas, E., 1999. *Uninformed Consent: The Hidden Dangers in Dental Care.* Charlottesville, VA: Hampton Roads Publishing Company, Inc.

International Federation of Beekeepers Associations, 1999. *Apimondia. www.apimondia99.ca/index.en.html*

Keller, Burgin-Wolff, Lippold, Wirht, and Lentze, 1996. The Diagnostic Significance of IgG Cow's Milk Protein Antibodies Re-Evaluated. *European Journal of Pediatrics* 155: 331-337.

Knekt, Jarvinen, Seppanen, Pukkala, and Aromaa, National Public Health Intitute, Helsinki, Finland, 1996. Intake of Dairy Products and the Risk of Breast Cancer. *British Journal of Cancer* 73:687-691.

Linus Pauling Institute, Oregon State University, 1999. *Welcome to The Linus Pauling Institute. www.orst.edu/dept/ lpi/*

MacLean and Beckson, 1951. Mortality and Disability in Multiple Sclerosis. *Journal of the American Medical Association* 146: 1367-1369.

Madsen and Henderson, Division of Orthopaedics, University of North Carolina, 1997. Calcium Intake in Children with Positive IgG RAST to Cow's Milk. *Journal of Paediatric Child Health* 33: 209-212.

Miller, 1949. Studies of Disseminated Multiple Sclerosis. *Acta Medica Scandinavia* 222: 1-214.

Mishkin, 1997. Dairy Sensitivity, Lactose Malabsorption, and Elimination Diets in Inflammatory Bowel Disease. *American Journal of Clinical Nutrition* 65:564-567.

Montes, Bayless, Saavedra, and Perman, Department of Pediatrics, David Grant US Air Force Medical Center, 1995. Effect of Milks Inoculated with Lactobacillus Acidophilus or a Yogurt Starter Culture in Lactose Maldigesting Children. *Journal of Dairy Science* 78: 1657-1664.

Muhe, Lulseged, Mason, and Simoes, 1997. Case Control Study of the Role of Nutritional Rickets in the Risk of Developing Pneumonia in Ethiopian Children. *The Lancet* 349: 1801-1804. *www.ncbi.nim.nih.gov*

Netzer, Corrine T., 1997a. *The Complete Book of Food Counts*. New York: Dell Publishing.

——, 1997b. *The Complete Book of Vitamin and Mineral Counts*. New York: Dell Publishing.

Newcomer and McGill, 1983. Irritable Bowel Syndrome. Role of Lactase Deficiency. *Mayo Clinic Procedural* 58:339-341.

New Testament, Matt. 3:4, Mark 1:6.

Nieper, Hans, A., 1999. Reprint. The Treatment of Multiple Sclerosis. *Explore!* Publications. Original publication, *The Townsend Letter for Doctors*, 1990.
URL: http://www.explorepub.com/articles/neiper2.html

——, The Treatment of Multiple Sclerosis 1990. *The Townsend Letter for Doctors*. N A. Keith Brewer Science Library, Admiral Ruge Archives, Richland Center, Wsconsin.
www.mwt.net/~drbrewer/ niep_art.htm

O'Brien, Johns Hopkins University School of Hygiene and Public Health. Combined Calcium and Vitamin D Supplementation Reduces Bone Loss and Fracture Incidence in Older Men and Women. *Nutrition Review* 56:148-150.

Oregon State University, 1999. Linus Carl Pauling: A Biographical Timeline. *www.orst.edu/dept/lpi/resagenda/timeline.html*

Oski, Frank, A., 1992. *Don't Drink Your Milk*. Teach Services.

Reuters Health News, 1999. Low Calcium Intake Raises Kids' Lead Poisoning Risk. (15 June). American Medical Association Health Insight Web Site. *www.ama-assn.org/insight/h_focus/ nemours/news/tmp-news/0615-3f.htm*

Rothfeld, 1999. Bee Venom Therapy. *Spectrum Medical Arts* (June). *www2.shore.net/~spectrum/apitherapy.html*

Santoro and Weyhreter, 1993. Support of Human Gland/Organ Function w/ Raw Protein Concentrate as Measured by Improvement in Serum Chemical Values. *Journal of Applied Nutrition* 45:48-60.

Sawyer, Zenz, Dickerson, and Horvath, 1994. Chromium and Its Compounds. *Occupational Medicine.* Mosby Year-Book, Inc.

Sears, Barry, and Lawren, Bill, 1995. *The Zone: A Dietary Road Map.* New York: Harper Collins.

Smith, 1996. Understanding Prescription Drugs. *Alberta Bee Journal* (November).

Suarez, Adshead, Furne, and Levitt, 1998. Lactose Maldigestion is Not an Impediment to the Intake of 1500mg. Calcium Daily as Dairy Products. *American Journal of Clinical Nutrition* 68: 1118-1122.

Swank, Roy, L., and Brewer Dugan, Barbara, 1987. *The Multiple Sclerosis Diet Book: A Low Fat Diet for the Treatment of MS.* New York: Doubleday.

Teagarden, Lyle, Proulx, Johnston, and Weaver, 1999. Previous Milk Consumption Is Associated with Greater Bone Density in Young Women. *American Journal of Clinical Nutrition* 69:1014-1017.

Texas A&M University, 1999. Africanized Honey Bees. *AgNews* (July). URL: *http://agnews.tamu.edu/bees/*

Thatcher, Fischer, Pettifor, Lawson, Isichei, Reading, and Chan, 1999. A Comparison of Calcium, Vitamin D or Both for Nutritional Rickets in Nigerian Children. *New England Journal of Medicine* 341:563-568.

United States Department of Agriculture, Food and Nutrition Service, 1999. *www.fns.usda.gov/fncs/*

——, USDA Online 1999. *www.usda.gov/*

University of California at Riverside, College of Natural and Agricultural Sciences, 1999. Africanized Honey Bees in USA 1990-1995. URL: *cnas.ucr.edu/~ento/CAAHB/ahb-spread.html*

Vaarala, Knip, Paronen, Hamalainen, Muona, Vaatainen, Ilonen, Simell, and Akerblom, 1999. Cow's Milk Formula Feeding Induces Primary Immunization to Insulin in Infants at Genetic Risk for Type 1 Diabetes, *Diabetes* 48: 1389-94.

Vaarala, Paronen, Otonkosski, and Akerblom, Cow's Milk Feeding Induces Antibodies to Insulin in Children—A Link between Cow Milk and Insulin-Dependent Diabetes Mellitus? *Scandinavian Journal of Immunology* 47:131–135.

Wagner, Pat, 1994. *How Well Are You Willing to Bee?* Waldorf, MD: JBS Publishing.

Woodrow Wilson National Fellowship Foundation, 1999. Linus Pauling: A Biography. *www.woodrow.org/teachers/ci/1992/Pauling.html*

Woods, Weiner, Abramson, Thien, and Walters, 1998. Do Dairy Products Induce Bronchoconstriction in Adults with Asthma? *Journal of Allergy and Clinical Immunology* 101:45-50.

Index

About Celeste Pepe,
D.C., N.D.

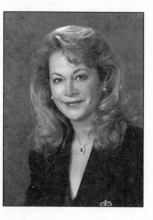

Celeste Pepe, D.C., N.D., brings the unique dual perspective of medical professional and afflicted victim to the writing of this book. Other authors have written of their personal experiences with MS, but none with the particular background of Dr. Pepe. A Doctor of Chiropractic and a Doctor of Naturopathic Medicine prior to the onset of her illness, Dr. Pepe found herself in the singular position of one who not only could choose to accept the challenge of the disease, but also with a real possibility of pursuing and *finding* a cure.

A well-known and highly regarded member of the alternative medical community as well as a practicing chiropractor, nutritionist, and BioCybernetics counselor, Dr. Pepe has been educating audiences on alternative medicine and nutrition through her successful practice, lectures, and other personal appearances.

In addition to being the living picture of health and vitality, Celeste Pepe is an intelligent, articulate, and personable individual. This book is her first endeavor, and she plans to use it as an additional teaching tool in her future lecture commitments.

Founder of The Healing Valley Health & Wellness Center, located in Solvang, California, she has taught guests to apply the nutritional techniques she has learned to their own efforts to bring their health into balance. Mother of college student Sara, Celeste presently enjoys life on the ranch in the beautiful canyon country of California with her longtime companion, Jerry Kessler, a highly successful vitamin and nutritional supplement manufacturer.

Dr. Pepe continues to share her expertise in chiropractic and nutrition with her patients in California. She plans an extensive nationwide teaching and lecture tour to introduce her successful alternative method of healing to fellow medical professionals and MS patients, with the sincere hope of educating them on the alternative healing options available to treat and cure this devastating disease, which currently affects about three hundred thousand people annually in the United States alone.

About Lisa Hammond

Lisa Hammond brings a wealth of talent and writing expertise to this project with her broad base of more than two decades' experience in technical writing for news media, advertising, and commercial clients, and creative writing of full-length fiction and non-fiction works for private clients. A degreed journalist with published works of poetry, short fiction, marketing materials, and technical and informational research publications, Ms. Hammond is an experienced ghostwriter with an excellent industry reputation for quality and readability. A research and statistical expert with a strong educational and corporate background, Ms. Hammond's training in data analysis proved invaluable in the translation of medical data and research into the easily understandable layman's terms so essential to this work.

The owner of URI-Unicorn Research, Inc., a thriving computer science, research, and information technology firm, Lisa resides in her native Southampton, New York, with her two teenagers, son, Thomas and daughter, Casey, and longtime companion, accomplished drummer and author Jim Siegrist. With the publication of this venture, she easily accomplishes the transition from ghost to acknowledged writer. Available for future ghostwritten or coauthored projects, she is presently completing her first solo full-length fiction novel.

Hampton Roads Publishing Company

. . . for the evolving human spirit

Hampton Roads Publishing Company
publishes books on a variety of subjects,
including metaphysics, health, integrative medicine,
visionary fiction, and other related topics.

For a copy of our latest catalog, call toll-free
(800) 766-8009, or send your name and address to:

Hampton Roads Publishing Company, Inc.
1125 Stoney Ridge Road
Charlottesville, VA 22902

e-mail: hrpc@hrpub.com
www.hrpub.com